The RIGHT DOSE_

The RIGHT DOSE

How to Take Vitamins & Minerals Safely

By Patricia Hausman, M.S.
Author of THE CALCIUM BIBLE

Rodale Press, Emmaus, Pennsylvania

Book design: Jane Knutila

Library of Congress Cataloging in Publication Data

Hausman, Patricia.
    The right dose.

    Bibliography: p.
    Includes index.
    1. Nutrition.   2. Vitamins in human nutrition.
3. Minerals in human nutrition.   4. Dietary supplements.
5. Drugs—Dosage.   I. Title.
RA784.H38   1987   615'.328   86–31367
ISBN 0–87857–678–9   hardcover

2   4   6   8   10   9   7   5   3   hardcover

Notice

This book is intended as a reference volume only, not as a medical manual or a guide to self-treatment. If you suspect that you have a medical problem, we urge you to seek competent medical help. Keep in mind that nutritional needs vary from person to person, depending on age, sex, health status, and total diet. Information here is intended to help you make informed decisions about your diet, not to substitute for any treatment that may have been prescribed by your physician.

To Susan, for her dedication

Other Books by Patricia Hausman

The Calcium Bible: How to Have Better Bones All Your Life
(Rawson Associates, 1985; Warner Books, 1986)

At-A-Glance Nutrition Counter
(Ballantine Books, 1984)

Foods That Fight Cancer
(Rawson Associates, 1984; Warner Books, 1985)

Jack Sprat's Legacy: The Science and Politics of Fat and Cholesterol
(Richard Marek Publishers, 1981)

Contents

• Testing for Toxicity • Treating an Overdose: A
Simple Solution • Pregnancy and Other Special
Conditions • Kind Words for Carotene • Call It
Mellow Yellow • When Carotenosis Occurs • A Few
False Alarms • The Case of the Carrot Juice Junkie
• Carotene against Cancer • Converting to Carotene:
Not for Everyone • The Star System Shines on
Carotene • Carotene and Pregnancy

Special Features

Chapter 4: Thiamine (Vitamin B₁)

The Nontoxic Notion • Two Classic Cases • Allergies
and Oddities • One Shot Too Many • The Star
System Shines on Thiamine • How Much Is Too
Much

Special Features

Chapter 5: Riboflavin (Vitamin B₂)

The Slate Is Clean • The Star System Shines on
Riboflavin • Running Up Your Need for Riboflavin
• Special Conditions, Special Needs • A Vitamin for
Vegetarians

Special Features

Chapter 6: Niacin 91

What's in a Name? • The First Outbreak • The Cornmeal Caper • Bagels, Too? • From Food to Supplements—Lessons from the Human Heart • The Liver Protests • Another Liver Complaint • The Diabetic's Experience • The Star System Shines on Nicotinic Acid • Notes for Those with Special Needs • How Much Is Too Much • Safety and Self-Medication • Is Niacinamide Nicer? • Sleuthing a Mysterious Itch • Another Case of Jaundice • Adverse Effects: How Common? • Niacinamide: A Summary

Special Features

Chapter 7: Vitamin B6 120

B_6 Basics • The Bubble Bursts • The Dose Debate • The 500 Mg. Surprise • How Much Is Too Much • The Star System Shines on Vitamin B_6 • A Parting Perspective

Special Features

Chapter 8: Folic Acid 139

The Zinc Link • Tales of Toxicity? • A Healthy Skepticism • Allergies and Epilepsy • Masked Danger • The Star System Shines on Folic Acid • How Much Is Too Much

Chapter 9: Vitamin B₁₂   155

B₁₂ Basics • The Toughest Test • The Allergy
Connection • The Skin Protests • Vegetarianism:
How Risky? • The Star System Shines on Vitamin B₁₂
• A Sigh of Relief

Chapter 10: The Rest of the B's   169

The Roles They Play • From Duties to Deficiencies
• Side Effects? Sometimes • Color Choline Different
• Depressions That Deepened • The Lecithin
Alternative • The Star System Shines on the Rest of
the B's • Turn the Page to Controversy

Chapter 11: Vitamin C   189

Roles to Remember • Generally Recognized as Safe
• The Hidden Hazard • Concern about Kidneys • Has
Anyone Seen a Stone? • The B₁₂ Brouhaha • The
Copper Snatcher? • The Iron Dilemma • More

Cautions for Special Conditions • C Addiction: Real
or Ridiculous? • Why Withdrawal? • The Great
Unknown • The Star System Shines on Vitamin C
• How Much Is Too Much

Special Features

Chapter 12: Vitamin D

What D Does • Distinct Types of D • The Sunshine
Factor • Age and Excesses • Two Classic Cases • High
Calcium Danger • Kidney Complaints • How
Overdoses Are Treated • The Sensitivity Factor
• Caution for Special Conditions • Take Special Care
with Children • Heart Health: The New Issue • Heart
Health: Part Two • D in Your Diet • The Star System
Shines on Vitamin D • How Much Is Too Much
• Checking for Safety

Special Features

Chapter 13: Vitamin E

E's Unique Job • Testimonies of Safety • The Fatigue
Factor • The Controversy Continues • No Fatigue
Here • E and Emotions • Some Serious Charges • To
Clot or Not • Other Special Conditions • E and
Allergy • The Star System Shines on Vitamin E
• How Much Is Too Much

Special Features

Part 3: Minerals

The Old and New • The Magnesium Monitor • More
than the Monitor Could Take • The Underlying
Problem • The Excessive Magnesium Syndrome
• Treatment and Recovery • The Dolomite Debate
• The Star System Shines on Magnesium • How
Much Is Too Much

Special Features

The Care and Feeding of Bones • Better Blood
Pressure • Calcium against Cancer • Which
Supplement Is Best? • The Acid Test • The
Absorption Problem • The Common Carbonates
• The Phosphate Family • Chelates and Chlorides
• Lactate, Gluconate, and Company • Calcium
Powders: Pro and Con • Liquid Calcium, Anyone?
• The "Other" Calciums: Bonemeal and Dolomite
• Better Alternatives? • Decisions, Decisions • Timing
Supplements for Best Effect • Fact versus Fear • How
Calcium Can Hurt • Blood: A Calcium Leach • The
Kidney Connection • Second Opinions • The Experts
Speak • The Milk-Alkali Syndrome • Who Calcium
Can Hurt • The Star System Shines on Calcium
• How Much Is Too Much • A Realistic Safe Dose

Special Features

The Sodium-Potassium Partnership • The Potassium Poor • The Signs of Deficiency • The Blood Pressure Connection • The Salt Assault • Supplement or Drug? • Enter Potassium Chloride • The Expert's Choice • Prescription Status in Perspective • Use versus Abuse • So Far, So Good • The Saga of the Salt Substitute • Generally Recognized as Safe • The Saddest Story in Supplement History • Risky Business • Details on the Drugs • The Best Supplement of All • The Star System Shines on Potassium • How Much Is Too Much

Special Features

Facts and Functions • The Two Faces of Iron • Vitamin C to the Rescue • Heme Isn't Everything • Enter Iron Supplements • Facts and Fallacies • The Road to Anemia • Mistaken Anemia • Risk and Reality • Iron and the Athlete • When Supplementation Is Risky • The Signs of Iron Overload • Heredity versus Environment • Alcohol and Excess Iron • The Lowdown on Overload • Sad News from the Emergency Room • Adults and Acute Ailments • Prevention and Cure • The Star System Shines on Iron • How Much Is Too Much • Sensible Supplementation

Special Features

Supplementation • Manganese and Supplement
Safety • A Flood of Phosphorus • Facts about
Phosphorus Supplements • A Journey's End

Special Features

Acknowledgments

An author's work is never done until she expresses her sincere thanks for the roles others have played in the creation of a book. With *The Right Dose* now complete, I take great satisfaction in introducing the rest of the cast.

The very best round of applause is due to:
• Kalli Tsakos, who cheerfully attended to countless administrative and mathematical details.
• Anita Liss, for the finest in professional library services.
• Debora Tkac, my editor, for her excellent editing skills and pleasant working style.
• Roberta Mulliner, for coordinating editorial and production tasks.
• Judith Hurley and the staff at the Rodale Food Center, for creating and testing each of the recipes.
• Glenn Marcus, who solved many a technical problem and provided a steady dose of emotional support.
• Susan Lee Cohen, my literary agent, who contributed more to the making of this book than any author could ask.

Patricia Hausman
September, 1986

Part 1: It's Time for Supplement Safety

1

Why You Should Know about Supplement Safety

Clint Eastwood does it. Linda Evans does it. Arnold Schwarzenegger, Jane Fonda and Ronald Reagan do it, too.

They take vitamins. Fully 40 percent of Americans take vitamin and mineral supplements. I do, and you probably do, too.

In coming years, more and more Americans are sure to join us. Like us, they will decide to take supplements because of exciting findings such as these:

• Healthy intakes of calcium and vitamin D can help build and keep bones strong.
• At least four nutrients—carotene, vitamins C and E, and selenium—may have the remarkable ability to help guard against cancer, reducing your chances of developing the disease.
• Much to the surprise of its detractors, vitamin E may benefit those with benign breast lumps and premenstrual syndrome.

1

Also, special forms of it are now being studied as treatment for certain eye disorders.
• Certain vitamins may affect important brain chemicals, influencing the quality of your sleep, your mood, and other aspects of feeling good.

And take my word for it, this is just the tip of the iceberg. There are still more ways that nutrients in either food or supplements can help you preserve or regain your precious health.

That's why I expect supplement use to keep climbing. And I also expect the controversy over using them to keep brewing—respected nutritionists and physicians will continue arguing their case against supplements.

Having a master's degree in nutrition, I know firsthand just how strongly my fellow nutritionists frown on supplement use. In fact, I have spent years trying to trace the origins of my profession's prejudice against vitamins and other supplements. I know that this bias is deeply rooted in our history, and there's a good reason for it. Nutritionists, naturally, are deeply concerned about your health. And, frankly, nutritionists like me have seen too many cases of what is best described not as supplement use, but as supplement abuse. That's why I decided to write this book.

This book is about putting supplements to work for you, *safely.* With it, you can have your supplements and your health, too, for in the pages that follow, I am going to tell you *everything* that I have learned about supplement safety. That's a tall order, I will admit, for I have spent several years tracking down the facts on supplement safety. In the process, I have read literally thousands of pages of medical reports. And it is only the beginning of what *The Right Dose* will give you. You'll also find:

• Brand-by-brand comparisons of the common supplements you see on the drugstore shelf.
• Best food sources of each nutrient.
• Fun-to-take quizzes to estimate the amount of certain nutrients in your diet, so you can make the best decision about what dose is right for you.
• Vital information about how nutrients and drugs can interact in your body and affect your health.
• Lots of kitchen-tested recipes that both your taste buds and your body will love.

Are Supplements for You?

Consider this question carefully. If fruits, vegetables, grains, and low-fat animal products are all part of your daily diet, food may be providing for all of your nutritional needs. But if you can answer yes to any one of the following questions, safe use of supplements may give your health a boost that your body will appreciate.

- Do you smoke cigarettes?
- Do you diet frequently?
- Are you pregnant or nursing your baby?
- Do you have high blood pressure?
- Are you petite, thin, and past menopause?
- Do you avoid milk, cheese, and yogurt?
- Do you frequently eat fatty red meat or other high-fat foods?
- Does your doctor say you have benign breast lumps?
- Do you have ulcerative colitis or intestinal polyps?
- Are you fighting a cold?
- Does your work expose you to hazardous chemicals?
- Do you often eat cured or pickled foods (such as bacon, hot dogs, salami, smoked fish)?
- Do you suffer from premenstrual syndrome?
- Do you spend little time outdoors?

WHAT SUPPLEMENTS CAN DO

Supplements can benefit your health in so many ways—far too many to list here. I have already mentioned a few possibilities, such as bone health and resistance to cancer. I will be telling you about the many additional benefits throughout this book.

The point that I want to make now is simply this: that supplements can help make up for shortcomings in your diet. There is no doubt in my mind that an inadequate diet plus a safe supplement program is certainly better than an inadequate diet alone. I don't see how anyone can argue otherwise.

What's more, supplements can make good health simpler for you to achieve. Instead of spending hours planning meals or eating foods that you dislike, you can obtain some of the nutrients you need from supplements. Some decry this route, calling it the easy way out. But what is wrong with the easy way out—as long as it is safe and effective? After all, many respected safety procedures, such as chlorination of public water supplies, are favored over more time-consuming approaches, such as boiling water before each use.

Obviously, I believe that supplements can contribute to the good health of those who learn which supplements to choose and how to take them safely. But there is another side. Supplements can cause harm if abused.

USE OR ABUSE?

Supplement abuse is a real and growing problem. Its victims are often health-conscious people who meant well, but carried a good thing too far. I am not talking about imaginary cases, but of people who arrived in hospital emergency rooms or their doctors' offices complaining of an array of symptoms from head to toe. In upcoming chapters, I will be telling you their stories in detail, but for now, let me briefly describe a few of the recent victims:

• A young woman lost so much feeling in her limbs that one night, while dining out, a waiter ran over her foot with a dessert cart and she felt nothing.
• A 16-year-old boy was admitted to the hospital after weeks of headaches that wouldn't go away. He also suffered from cracked lips and a stiff neck.
• A woman, only 30 years old, had lost so much of her tooth enamel that she needed full crowns on at least 12 of her teeth!

These people had no exotic diseases. They had simply overdosed on vitamins! And in perhaps the saddest known case of supplement abuse, a two-month-old baby died after his mother, acting on extremely dangerous advice in a popular book, administered high doses of a potassium chloride supplement.

You might say that supplements are like fire. Use fire well and it will work for you, keeping you warm and allowing you to cook the foods that keep you healthy and well. But abuse it and it can work against you, harming your precious possessions, your loved ones, or your health.

WHAT SUPPLEMENTS CANNOT DO

Ah, if only a little pill could banish all the ill effects of our bad habits. We could then smoke, drink, or eat whatever we like with abandon.

But you know better than to believe that any supplement, pill, or other approach can eliminate all of the hazards posed by health-threatening habits. I think everyone does.

Nonetheless, those who oppose supplements use the argument that people who take supplements think it gives them license to eat poorly. My own experience is quite the opposite; most of the supplement users I have encountered are more health conscious than nonusers. And a recent survey backs up my personal experience.

Polls taken by the Food and Drug Administration and the Gallup Organization have found that about 40 percent of Americans use supplements. Yet, a recent poll of dieticians found that 60 percent take supplements. In other words, dieticians—who surely are interested in choosing a healthy diet—are much more likely to use supplements than the general public. These findings suggest that people who take vitamins or mineral supplements see healthy food and supplementation as a partnership.

In fact, during the seven years that I served as staff nutritionist for the Center for Science in the Public Interest in Washington, D.C., I never encountered even once an individual who believed that supplements alone could ensure good health. When you consider that my job put me in contact with thousands of health-minded members, dozens of staffers in Congress and in federal agencies, and hundreds of newspaper, radio, and TV reporters, I think my experience shows that most people do understand the importance of sound food habits.

An important survey found much the same. Taken a few years back by the Response Analysis Corporation, it asked people to agree or disagree with the statement that "it is okay to skip meals as long as you take a vitamin supplement." Fully 97 percent of those questioned disagreed with the statement. Enough, I think, to refute the notion that people who take supplements think that doing so can counteract all of the problems posed by unhealthy behavior.

This survey also shows that most people understand another limitation of supplements. No supplement or combination of supplements available today can compensate for a diet containing too few calories. Supplements can supply vitamins and minerals (known to nutritionists as micronutrients). But, from any practical standpoint, supplements cannot meet our needs for calories (which nutritionists refer to as macronutrients). That means that a pregnant woman, for instance, who needs to take in extra calories to ensure the health of her baby, cannot do so by swallowing a few pills. It is vital that she get enough calories to support her pregnancy, and no pill will give her that.

In short, then, just as a balanced diet alone is not the only part of a healthy lifestyle, so supplements alone cannot completely ensure good nutrition.

WHY I CHANGED MY MIND ABOUT SUPPLEMENTS

I never thought I would write a book about vitamin and mineral supplements. But here I am devoting several years' work to one. It reminds me just how much my mind has changed about supplements during the past decade.

Like all university-educated nutritionists, I was taught to scorn supplements. It would have been impossible, I think, to complete my graduate degree in nutrition without having felt a constant pressure to decry their use. Rare was the nutrition textbook that didn't assail supplement use and equate it with "food faddism," an expression that I abhor. And the pressure to deplore supplement use continued after graduation, throughout my seven years at the Center for Science in the Public Interest, and while writing my first two books.

Yet, despite my education and the attitudes of many of my fellow nutritionists, I eventually changed my mind. I did so for many reasons, but I'd like to mention only a few. The nutrition scene has changed dramatically in recent years. Our knowledge has taken off like a rocket, lifting our profession to center stage in health and medicine. (We were waiting in the wings for recognition for longer than I care to remember.)

The great leaps forward in our knowledge have been exciting for nutritionists, but more than a few readers have complained to me that, with more and more nutrients to consider, meal planning has become too complicated. I have to grant that this complaint is valid. I also see how supplements can help simplify meal planning by assuring adequate intake of important vitamins and minerals.

Add to this more and more research finding that some people, such as pregnant women, dieters, and senior citizens, simply cannot obtain the recommended allowances for certain nutrients through food alone. Aren't supplements a sensible solution for them? I think so.

And here is the point that probably won me over: Sometimes supplements are a safer source of nutrients than certain foods. The nutrient that brought me to this conclusion is calcium.

I'm the author of The Calcium Bible: How to Have Better Bones All Your Life. In my research on bone health, I became convinced that millions of women were eating diets shockingly deficient in calcium. Yet, on my bookshelf were two earlier books—Foods That Fight Cancer and Jack Sprat's Legacy: The Science and Politics of Fat and Cholesterol—in which I wrote of the compelling health benefits to be had from reducing your fat intake. This posed a dilemma for me, as some of the foods richest in calcium are also high in fat.

As I wrote and researched The Calcium Bible, no bigger conflict was on my mind. But I resolved it, with no regrets, by concluding that calcium supplements are generally preferable to high-fat calcium-rich foods. Simply stated, the supplement is safer. (You can, of course, rely on low-fat calcium-rich foods; it's just that not everyone likes them.)

Finally, while compiling another of my books—the At-a-Glance Nutrition Counter—I was faced with another troubling truth about the food-only approach to nutrition and health. The nutrition counter was my crusade to simplify nutrition by using symbols to show whether a food's level of important nutrients was good, okay, or poor. To do so, I constructed my own computer database containing nutrition information on 1,500 foods. In the process, I learned just how much nutrition can be lost on the way from the farm to the table.

The chart that follows tells the tale; up to 100 percent of the vitamin C in food, for instance, can be lost through cooking,

The Vanishing Vitamins

Somewhere between the farm (or factory) and the dinner table, vitamin levels in food often decline. Sometimes the changes are small; in other cases dramatic. Here are some estimates from the Vitamin Nutrition Information Service on what causes loss during the cooking process, and the percentage of loss.

Vitamin	Causes of Loss	Estimate of Percent Lost in Food Preparation
Vitamin A	oxygen heat light	0–60
Thiamine (B_1)	water alkaline pH heat	30–70 in vegetables 0–80 in meat 0–50 in baking
Riboflavin (B_2)	water alkaline pH	9–39 in animal foods 10–30 in plant foods
Niacin	water	3–27
Vitamin B_6	water	30–82
Biotin	oxygen alkaline pH	0–50
Pantothenic acid	heat water alkaline pH acid pH	7–56
Vitamin C	oxygen heat alkaline pH water	0–100
Vitamin D	oxygen light	0–40
Vitamin E	oxygen	0–60

Source: *Nutristat*, December 1984, Vitamin Nutrition Information Service, Hoffman-LaRoche, Nutley, NJ 07110.

cutting, storing, and other inevitable practices. And how silly, I realized, to insist that people prepare their food only in the ways that preserve vitamin C. If you would rather take a reasonable dose of supplemental vitamin C than be limited in how you eat your oranges or cook your broccoli, I certainly can understand.

I have decided that playing nutritional dictator isn't the job for me. The rigid attitude of many of my colleagues about how you should meet your nutritional needs (that is, only through food) bothers me. My outlook today is quite the opposite; I consider it part of my job to give you choices. Supplements are one such choice, a way of exercising your options. That's the way it should be, for in my mind, it is your right to choose how to meet your nutritional needs. And if supplements are among your choices, I think that's fine, as long as you take them *safely*.

2

Your Guide to Supplement Safety

B efore we get down to the business of supplement safety, I want to tell you a bit about how I compiled this book, and how you can use it to your best advantage. I'll start by telling you exactly how I define the term "supplement safety."

In my mind, safe use of food supplements is use that has not been reported in the medical journals as hazardous to a healthy adult. In other words, the term "safety," as I use it, refers to current knowledge.

I tell you this for several reasons. First, much as I would like one, I don't have a crystal ball. I would love to be a soothsayer who can predict what tomorrow's research will show, but I don't have the credentials to call myself a prophet. Rather, I make my judgments based on what we know today. Every scientist and doctor that I know does so, too.

You probably noticed that I mentioned adults in my definition of supplement safety. I have tried throughout this book to give you information about supplement safety for children whenever possible. I have been hindered, though, because in some cases there is little information to go on. Most information about supplement safety comes from adults rather than from children. But levels that are safe for adults are not necessarily safe for children, who are smaller in size and have different physiology. So unless I tell you otherwise, keep in mind that my comments apply only to adults.

My search for the facts about supplement safety has been hampered by one other problem: that overdosages of vitamins, minerals, or other supplements are not "reported illnesses." When doctors diagnose a patient's problem as supplement overdose, they do not have to report the case to any health department or government clearinghouse. Other health experts will learn of the case only if the doctors inform medical journals or government agencies of their findings.

So, much as I would like to, I cannot tell you that I have considered every known case of supplement overdose and come up with standards that are guaranteed safe. I can tell you that I have considered those cases reported in leading American medical journals during the past 20 years.

I hope that this notion—that no one can absolutely guarantee supplement safety—does not bother you. If you think about it, I feel you will agree with me that truly nothing in life can be guaranteed harmless. Getting out of bed in the morning can be harmful, for you could fall and break a bone. Staying in bed can be even more harmful, for bedridden people have less resistance to infection and often develop painful bedsores. Every day, you and I make choices, often based on degrees of risk. I know, as do you, that I could fall getting out of bed and hurt myself, but I accept the risk as so small that I take it without a second thought.

I take the same approach to supplement safety—and I had the same attitude when writing my previous books. In fact, I have stopped looking for no-risk situations, not simply because I know they don't exist, but because I believe that where there are no risks, there are no benefits.

So if you want the potential benefits that supplements can offer, I have to ask you to be willing to take the chance, however small, that an unknown or unreported risk may exist. To me, this is a healthy attitude not only toward your supplement program, but toward everything that you do in the interest of your health. Let me explain.

I have known people who demanded guarantees that everything they did for better health would make them healthier. Often they expected benefits almost immediately, too. And do you know what? They had found a good way to drive themselves crazy. By expecting guarantees, they set themselves up for disappointment; as soon as an effort toward better health failed to give them everything they had hoped for, they felt like abandoning everything—diet, exercise, and supplements—and leaving their health to chance.

I have spent enough years in the business of health to know that leaving your health to chance is a lot riskier than taking low-risk efforts to maintain good health. Just think of the impact on our nation's health if all of us who exercise stopped doing so because of the occasional person who suffers a heart attack during physical activity!

What I have done here, then, is my very best job of getting you information to make your supplement program as risk-free as possible. To me, that's what supplement safety is really about.

USE THE STARS TO GUIDE YOU

You know now what I mean by the term "supplement safety." Next, I would like to tell you how I evaluated the safety of each supplement.

In my research, I found five key issues in supplement safety. Since I found five points, the same number of points as a star, I dubbed my evaluation "the star system of supplement safety." Whenever I evaluated a supplement, I looked for any evidence of trouble in these five basic areas. They are:

Side effects—This term, of course, refers to symptoms such as discomfort and drowsiness that often occur when you take a drug. Supplements can cause side effects, too, but are less likely to do so than drugs. As you probably know, side effects are not always grounds to discontinue treatment. Such a decision is usually made on a case-by-case basis, taking into account the degree of discomfort caused by the drug or supplement versus its potential benefits.

Acute ailments—This type of problem is usually more serious than side effects. Often it develops quickly, shortly after a new regimen is begun, and the symptoms can be severe. Doctors frequently use the term "acute toxicity" to describe such ailments. Much more often than not, such a problem calls for the substance in question to be discontinued at once.

Long-term problems—The opposite, so to speak, of acute problems. These can develop slowly, over prolonged use of a supplement. In some cases, a dosage that causes no acute ailments can cause a long-term problem. Chronic toxicity is the medical term commonly used to describe these problems.

Conflicting combinations—These are what I call the troublesome twosomes—health problems that arise not from a supplement alone, but from it combining in the body with some other substance in a way that produces unwanted effects. The other substance is often a drug or another nutrient. This bad marriage is what the medical community commonly terms "drug-nutrient interactions" and "nutrient-nutrient interactions."

Hidden consequences—Occasionally, supplements may cause trouble by interfering with medical detective work. A few nutrients, usually only if taken at high doses, can mask signs of medical conditions. Supplements may also cause false readings in laboratory tests, preventing a correct diagnosis. I am sure you will want to know all about that possibility.

Needless to say, not every supplement can cause all five types of problems if taken unwisely. In fact, most supplements have not been linked to all five—even at high doses. But, information permitting, I will be telling you how each one fares on these five points. I find that following the star system makes it easy to get a clear picture of each supplement's potential to produce unwanted effects.

Of course, I will be telling you about the potential benefits of supplements, too. After you consider both the benefits and the risks, I think you will agree with me that the intelligent approach is to use supplements sensibly—not ban them altogether.

HOW THIS BOOK WAS COMPILED

I truly believe that you have in your hands the most thorough study of supplement safety ever designed for supplement users. That's a big claim, so let me tell you why I feel confident enough to make it.

Ever since I arrived in Washington 12 years ago, I have been a devoted user of the National Library of Medicine, part of the federal government's National Institutes of Health. The library boasts one of the finest collections of medical literature in the world. Today, that means not only books and medical journals, but also computer-based information banks that can identify all articles on a particular subject with mind-boggling speed and accuracy.

Caution—How's Your Health?

It's not unusual to come across a warning that reads: "At moderate doses, this nutrient is essentially nontoxic."

When you read this warning, ask yourself, "Nontoxic to *whom?*"

Supplements that are harmless to healthy people can nonetheless cause trouble for those with special medical conditions. Throughout this book, I will be telling you about certain medical conditions and supplements that do not mix—at least not without planning and medical expertise. Here's a *partial* list of conditions that call for cautious use of certain vitamins, minerals, or other supplements.

- Aplastic anemia
- Cheilosis, if a result of pellagra
- Diabetes
- Gout
- G-6PD deficiency
- Hemochromatosis (an iron metabolism disorder)
- Hemorrhage
- Hepatic (liver) dysfunction

The library's Medline database is a giant index to thousands of medical journals. I had used it to help me find information for each of my four previous books.

But when I began this book, I decided that I wanted to be not just a Medline user, but an expert. So I enrolled in a special course to learn how to get the most out of the Medline. I bought special equipment that allows me to tap into its vast brain from my office. And so, in compiling this book, I have not just consulted the Medline for information on supplement safely; I have *scoured* it. I searched for facts about possible problems related to supplement use and cases of overdosages. In each chapter that follows, I relate these cases to you.

For some supplements, I had not only my own Medline and library research, but also the help of special scientific committees.

- Hypotension (low blood pressure), if active and severe
- Kidney stones, or family history of stones
- Malabsorption syndrome
- Normocytic anemia
- Peptic ulcer
- Polyneuritis
- Refractory anemia
- Sickle cell anemia

If you have a medical condition of any severity, you should discuss your supplement program with your doctor. Drugs and medical conditions can and do interact with nutrients. And while safe levels can often be set for an *isolated* condition or medication, doing so is much more difficult if you have a *combination* of conditions and/or drugs.

This is such an important point that I'm simply going to repeat it: Since it would be impossible to consider every conceivable combination of drugs and/or medical conditions here, discuss supplementation with your doctor, who can prescribe a program personalized just for you.

From time to time, panels of doctors and nutritionists have issued formal statements on safety levels for certain nutrients. And, because nutrients are often added to foods—breakfast cereals, for instance—I had another source of information: an exhaustive study ordered by the Food and Drug Administration during the 1970s.

The study was commissioned by the FDA to review the safety of all substances that were considered Generally Recognized As Safe (GRAS). A panel of university scientists convened by the Federation of American Scientists for Experimental Biology (FASEB) was entrusted with the enormous job of evaluating each GRAS substance. Most vitamins and minerals had the GRAS seal of approval and therefore were included in the review.

For every supplement that was covered by the GRAS review, I have considered carefully the scientists' reports. I always feel better about relying on a committee of experts rather than an individual opinion, as my experience has taught me that the best judgments usually come from a meeting of minds. That's why I have placed special emphasis on these reports in compiling the chapters that follow.

No book on supplement safety would be complete without a careful study of special textbooks and handbooks. I have used far too many to name. Some classic pharmacy handbooks, in particular, were invaluable in educating myself about conflicting combinations, the pesky matter of drug-nutrient and nutrient-nutrient interactions.

What an eye-opening experience this has been for me! I have learned more than I ever expected about supplements. I have concluded that you have much to gain, and little or nothing to lose by taking certain supplements safely. And as you probably have guessed, I have used this information to design my own supplement program. I do hope that you will do the same. Just turn the page and join me as I share the results of my quest for the facts. With them, you can start using supplements safely today.

Part 2: Vitamins

3

Vitamin A and Carotene

Y ou've come a long way, vitamin A. From the turn-of-the-century laboratories where you were known only as an essential growth factor to the proud day years later when you were recognized as the first vitamin. From the universities and research laboratories into the public health clinics where you have saved millions from blindness. And from the days when you could be obtained only from a handful of foods to today when you can be had in many forms, some having their own unique properties.

Since the term "vitamin A" can refer to a number of substances, I would like first to tell you about its various forms. There are two basic types of vitamin A. The first is *preformed* vitamin A, which is basically ready for your body to use. The second is the *precursor* form. Unlike preformed vitamin A, the precursor form must be converted by your body to active vitamin A.

Now for just a few more essential facts.

- *Retinol* is the vitamin A in animal foods. It is preformed—ready for your body to use.
- *Carotene* (or beta-carotene) is a substance in foods that your body can convert to vitamin A—a precursor of the vitamin. (Some

"A" Vitamin of Many Talents

As nutritionists have come to know vitamin A better, we have learned more and more about its powers. At first, we knew only that vitamin A was essential to the growth of young animals. But soon it became clear that this was just the beginning, and vitamin A added other important feathers to its cap. It is now credited with giving you:

- HEALTHY EYES. Vitamin A helps you see in dim light and also prevents the disease xerophthalmia, which can lead to blindness.
- HEALTHY ORGANS. Vitamin A is essential to the health of the tissues lining your lungs, digestive organs, and genito-urinary tract.
- HEALTHY BONES. Without proper intakes of vitamin A, your bones cannot grow normally.
- HEALTHY MEMBRANES. At the microscopic level, vitamin A is busy keeping the membranes of your body cells intact.

Vitamin A deficiency is not very common in the United

nutritionists use the term "provitamin" to describe the precursor form.) Carotene is found almost exclusively in plant foods.

- *Carotenoids*, like carotene, can also be converted to vitamin A. However, these plant-based compounds are not as potent nor as plentiful as carotene. From a practical standpoint, their importance is minor, and like carotene, these are provitamins.
- *Vitamin A palmitate* and *vitamin A acetate* are synthetic forms of vitamin A found in supplements and in foods that have been fortified with added vitamin A. Like retinol, these forms of vitamin A are preformed.
- *Tretinoin and isotretinoin* are special forms of vitamin A used to treat acne. Both can be obtained only by prescription and do not meet your body's needs for vitamin A.
- *Miscellaneous retinoids* are special forms of vitamin A that have been developed for specific uses, such as cancer prevention. Many

States. When it does develop, however, difficulty seeing at night—"night blindness"—is often a first sign. (Of course, vitamin A deficiency is not the only cause of night blindness.) If deficiency of vitamin A continues, skin changes occur. Lumps of hard skin—similar to the texture of nails—appear on the arms, legs, and hands. Finally, severe eye damage may occur as the cornea dries and ulcerates, leading to blindness if vitamin A is not brought to the rescue.

Of course, we all need our fair share of vitamin A. But if you have certain conditions, you are more susceptible to vitamin A deficiency than people not having the disorders. There are several types of conditions that raise concern. First, prolonged diarrhea can prevent you from absorbing sufficient vitamin A. Likewise, the malabsorption syndromes, such as celiac disease, steatorrhea, and sprue, can put you at risk of vitamin A deficiency. So can obstruction of the bile, liver, or gallbladder ducts.

If you have any of these conditions, discuss your vitamin A nutrition with your doctor.

retinoids are used only in research; you cannot buy them in a drugstore, nor can your doctor prescribe them. You may also hear the term "vitamin A analogs" used to describe these compounds.

Only some of these forms of vitamin A are actually available to you as supplements. Two of the preformed types—retinol and vitamin A palmitate (or its rarer cousin, vitamin A acetate)—are commonly found in supplements. And in recent years, the most potent of the precursor forms—carotene—has also become available in supplement form.

The safety of these three basic forms varies dramatically. We'll evaluate each using the star system, then do some figuring about just how much vitamin A, and in what form, is best for you. Then we'll cook up some great-tasting recipes rich in this ever-important vitamin.

RETINOL: THE SAFETY STORY

If retinol is the vitamin A in animal foods, how does it fit into a discussion of supplement safety? Because one favorite vitamin A supplement—cod liver oil—is actually a concentrated source of retinol. So, when we talk about safe use of retinol supplements, we basically are talking about safe use of fish liver oils. Though not as popular today as they were decades ago, these supplements remain in use. And because retinol is a potent form of vitamin A, so is its potential to cause trouble if taken unwisely.

BABY NICK: THE FIRST "OFFICIAL" OVERDOSE

No doubt about it, the first documented case of retinol overdose couldn't be blamed on the victim. He was only 18 months old, and it probably wasn't his idea to start taking halibut liver oil.

Curious? Here is what happened on a history-making occasion back in 1938:

Nicholas had seemed quite healthy, but as he reached the year-and-a-half mark, he began to lose his appetite and interest in playing. Eight months later, while having his tonsils removed, doctors found him to be quite anemic. On further examination, they found both his liver and spleen to be abnormally enlarged. It was obvious to anyone that he had lost a great deal of his hair, and the hair that did grow back no longer appeared healthy. On the contrary, it was dry and rough and grew sparsely—not at all common at so young an age. Also uncommon was the absence of eyebrows and fine hair over other parts of his body and the slight clubbing of his fingers.

For eight more months, Nick's condition failed to change. Because of his anemia and enlarged liver, he was admitted to a hospital. At that time, he was three years old, and both fingers and toes were clubbed somewhat in appearance.

Tests at the hospital showed that Nicholas had an "enormously high content of vitamin A" in his blood. Suddenly, the bewildered doctors had a clue. They talked to his mother, who confirmed that she had given her son a teaspoon of halibut liver oil—containing 240,000 International Units (I.U.) of vitamin A—

daily since he was two or three months old. Occasionally, she said, he took greater amounts.

The doctors sent Nicholas home immediately, with orders that his mother stop giving him any supplemental vitamin A. "Improvement was immediate," reported the doctors.

Two months later, Nicholas's appetite was better, he was gaining weight, and his healthy, normal hair was starting to replace the coarse, sparse hair he had during his illness. With the passing of four more months, the vitamin A level of his blood returned to normal and his appearance was that of a healthy child.

Two and a half years after he was sent home from the hospital, he was "to all external appearances normal and of average height and development." The only remaining signs of his ordeal were a slight clubbing of his fingers and some notable changes in his liver and spleen. It appeared that, for the most part, he had recovered. And doctors had recorded the first diagnosed case of hypervitaminosis A, the official term for vitamin A overdose. Because Nicholas's case developed slowly over more than a year, his was a case of chronic toxicity, or as I call it, a long-term problem.

Was Nicholas's case a fluke, never to be seen by doctors again? Hardly. In the years that followed, many children with similar symptoms were seen in doctors' offices and hospitals, diagnosed, as Nicholas was, as cases of vitamin A overdosages. And as happened with Nicholas, some of these children were first believed to have other, more serious diseases. But once the possibility of vitamin A overdose was considered and the high dosages stopped, steady recovery usually followed.

THE BEAR FACT— ADULTS ARE NOT IMMUNE

Nicholas's case was like the apprehension of a notorious criminal. It reopened the books on cases that had occurred long ago and caused medical detectives to wonder if previously unsolved cases of illness might also have been due to vitamin A overdose. There is every reason to believe that some were.

Of these decades-old cases eventually attributed to overdosages of vitamin A, the most fascinating are tales from voyages to the Arctic or areas inhabited by Eskimos. In his authoritative book, *Vitamin A*, Dr. T. Moore describes several expeditions where the explorers became ill after eating bear liver. Unbeknownst to them, the astronomical vitamin A content of the bear liver probably was responsible.

Here are some engrossing highlights from Dr. Moore's book:

• "The members of an expedition led to Novaya Zembla by Barentzoon as early as 1596 all became ill when they ate bear liver. In three cases the illness was severe, with loss of skin from head to foot."

• On another expedition, this one reported in 1913, Moore relates that "the 19 men who partook of the stew [containing bear liver] on this occasion all became sick." And they were stricken quickly, some within 2 to 4 hours after the meal. Their symptoms? Tiredness and a strong desire to sleep, irritability, violent headaches, and vomiting. Some of the victims also suffered peeling skin.

• In three additional cases, "the skin peeled from head to foot after bear liver had been eaten."

These reactions, of course, were acute ailments, as the victims became ill shortly after taking in extraordinarily high doses of vitamin A. And while supermarkets don't sell polar bear liver, it is possible to take in very high doses of retinol—the vitamin A in bear liver—if you overdo fish oil supplements.

SYNTHETIC VITAMIN A: A MEDICAL MILESTONE

Fish oils may be brimming with vitamin A, but nutritionists recognized long ago that synthetic forms of vitamin A could serve you just as well. And history has proved them right.

Synthetic forms of vitamin A are generally water-soluble supplements, allowing your body to absorb them more quickly than the fat-soluble form of vitamin A in fish liver oils. Just as important, synthetic forms are usually less expensive. And while a dollar here and there may seem insignificant to you, consider the enormous savings when an entire population needs vitamin A supplementation to fight the rampant vitamin A deficiency that has blinded hundreds of thousands in less-developed nations.

In fact, synthetic vitamin A is used routinely in industrialized nations, too—primarily for skin disorders. A diverse range of skin problems—from acne to psoriasis—seem to respond, at least sometimes, to treatment with vitamin A. That's progress, and we love it.

But progress can have its costs. Sure enough, vitamin A toxicity has occurred during medical treatment of skin disorders with high doses. The doctors who prescribe these high doses do monitor their patients for signs of adverse effects. And the patients understand that, as with drugs, there is always some risk. These valiant risk-takers have contributed much to medical knowledge.

In fairness to the doctors, though, some of the patients brought on problems by exceeding the prescribed doses. Taking more than the doctor prescribes can cause as much trouble as not taking the medicine at all. And many people have self-administered high doses of synthetic vitamin A—and paid the price.

Overdoses of synthetic vitamin A know no bounds: infants, children, and adults alike have been affected. The overdosages can develop suddenly (acute ailment) or slowly, over months or years (long-term problem). Let's look first at two cases of acute ailments in infants, since the case of Nicholas described above was a long-term problem.

High as Nicholas's intake of vitamin A might have seemed, some young infants have been given still higher dosages. And as you probably have guessed, they became sick more quickly than did Nicholas. Here are just two of these classic cases (there have been many):

• Richard, a three-and-a-half-month-old infant, was given 350,000 I.U. of vitamin A with his morning feeding. That evening he first vomited, then fell asleep and slept through his usual night feeding. The next day, his mother, alarmed by a bulge in the top of his head, took him to a hospital. That bulge atop the head was established as a hallmark of vitamin A overdose in infants. It is located on the fontanel, the "soft spot" on top of an infant's head where bones have yet to fuse together.
• Two-month-old Jerome had been suffering from a cold for which he received nose drops rich in vitamin A for about a week. The vitamin A in the drops totaled 300,000 I.U. over a six-day period. Within days, he too had the same kind of bulge on his head that affected Richard. But four days after he stopped taking the vitamin A drops, he appeared fine.

(continued on page 28)

The Diet Detective Searches for Preformed Vitamin A

Do you want to know how much preformed vitamin A you are taking in at mealtimes? All you need is a few minutes to take this easy quiz.

Have a pencil and notepad handy. Next, jot down the number of points for any of the following entries that you included in your diet today. After you have added up your total points for the day, see the scoring information at the end of the food listings.

For the best estimate, take the quiz on three separate days. Add up your three-day total, then divide by 3 to get your daily average.

1 point
1 cup milk (skim, low-fat, or whole)

2 points
⅔ cup any of the following cereals:
Crispy Wheats 'n Raisins, Golden Grahams, Grape-nuts flakes, Honey Bran, Raisins, Rice & Rye, Special K, Team, Wheaties
1 cup Cheerios or King Vitaman cereal
1 packet Quaker instant oats
1 cup eggnog

3 points
⅓ cup Bran Buds, granola, or Grape-nuts

⅔ cup Cracklin' Oat Bran, 40% Bran cereal, or Fruit 'n Fibre
1 cup most children's cereals
4 Frosted Mini-Wheats
1 packet Mix 'n Eat cream of wheat
1 cup milk with Pillsbury Instant Breakfast

4 points
⅔ cup Buc Wheats cereal
1 cup milk with Carnation Instant Breakfast
1 cup Tang
1 Carnation Breakfast Bar

7 points
⅔ cup Total or Corn Total cereal
1 cup crabmeat

10 points
¾ cup Product 19 cereal

15 points
⅔ cup Most cereal

24 points
4 ounces chicken liver,
    simmered

75 points
4 ounces calf liver, fried

120 points
4 ounces beef liver, fried

Scoring

Add up your points. Next, add a zero to the total for an estimate of how your preformed vitamin A intake compares to the U.S. RDA for vitamin A.

If your points total 6, for example, add a zero, for a score of 60. That means your diet on the day surveyed contains 60 percent of the U.S. RDA of 5,000 I.U. Since 60 percent of 5,000 I.U. is 3,000, your diet had about 3,000 I.U. of vitamin A. This score is only an estimate, of course, as it would be impractical to list every food containing preformed vitamin A.

If you want to take a vitamin A supplement, subtract this estimate of your dietary intake from the total dosage you want. This is important to help insure that your supplement does not put you beyond the recommended limit. Remember also that your carotene intake qualifies as vitamin A, but the carotene will not push your preformed vitamin A intake beyond the recommended limit. I will tell you why later in this chapter when I discuss carotene.

Do you eat fortified foods such as cereals and snack foods that are not listed in this quiz? If so, you can include them in your tally. Simply divide the percentage of the U.S. RDA listed on the nutrition label by 10 to get the number of points to assign to these foods. If the item contains 30 percent of the U.S. RDA for vitamin A, for instance, it qualifies for 3 points for the purposes of this quiz.

Jerome taught his parents and doctors an important lesson: that the active ingredient in nose drops may be absorbed into the body. Of course, it is also possible that Jerome managed to swallow some of the drops directly.

Regardless, the cure was simple for both Richard and Jerome. Staying away from that bottle of high-potency vitamin A was the answer.

VITAMIN A AND ADOLESCENCE

Since A is for acne (more correctly, for selected acne patients), you probably have guessed that teenagers should be alert for symptoms of too much vitamin A. How right you are!

I would like to tell you about just one case, though. It is a case that illustrates not only the need to be alert during acne treatment but also how a handful of individuals can be far more sensitive to vitamin therapy than most people are.

Eighteen-year-old James, like many teenagers, suffered from acne. He arrived in a neurologist's office one day complaining that, for about six months, he had felt as if some unknown force was pushing him forward. He reported some trouble in keeping his balance, and the doctor did notice that he tended to lean toward one side or the other at times. It was clear to the doctor that the sensations he spoke of were real.

The neurologist worried that James might have a brain tumor and admitted him to the hospital. Fortunately, tests there revealed that he was in fine health—except for a slightly elevated level of vitamin A in his blood. James told the doctor that, because of his acne, he had been taking a modest 10,000 to 20,000 I.U. of vitamin A daily for more than two years.

The case was almost solved. Tests confirmed that James was suffering from benign intracranial hypertension—doctor talk for too much pressure inside his brain. Typically this disorder causes headaches and a range of visual problems including double vision, an enlarged "blind spot," and blurring. Because these can be symptoms of a brain tumor, this disorder is often called pseudotumor cerebri—Latin for false brain tumor. You can imagine the relief for both doctor and patient to learn that it's an impostor, not the real thing!

The ABCs of the RDAs

Like any other profession, nutrition needs standards. Among the standards useful to nutritionists are the Recommended Dietary Allowances, commonly referred to simply as the RDA, set by the National Research Council's Food and Nutrition Board. No doubt, you are familiar with this ever-present standard.

You probably also have heard of the U.S. Recommended Daily Allowances, known as the U.S. RDA. Is the RDA different from the U.S. RDA? Yes! Let me explain.

The RDA varies based on age and sex, and your RDA may differ from that of your children, spouse, or friends of the opposite sex.

The U.S. RDA, however, is a single number that does not vary with age and sex. It is set by the Food and Drug Administration and is intended for use by food manufacturers when giving nutrition information about their products. Since the food label is too small to fit the percent of the RDA for each age and sex group, it simplifies things dramatically to have just one standard—the U.S. RDA—to measure a product's nutrient values.

In setting the U.S. RDA, the FDA usually picks the highest level needed by any age or sex group (excluding pregnant or nursing women). Let's take vitamin A as a case in point. The highest RDA for any age or sex group is 5,000 I.U. Therefore, the FDA has chosen 5,000 as the simple U.S. RDA.

In short, then, both the U.S. RDA and the RDA serve important purposes. The U.S. RDA offers simplicity. The RDA, however, offers you a more precise estimate of your nutrient needs because it considers your age and sex.

The neurologist who treated James asked him to stop taking the vitamin A. He also prescribed some cortisone medication to relieve James's symptoms. Two months later, James was free of symptoms.

James's case illustrates two very important points: First, that vitamin A overdose can be present with only a few of its typical symptoms—in James's case, those of excessive pressure in the brain. He had none of the other classic symptoms, such as skin changes, fatigue, or nausea.

The other important point bears repeating: A few individuals may succumb to vitamin A overdose at levels far below those needed to cause symptoms in most people. James was taking 10,000 to 20,000 I.U. per day—the lowest dose I have found to be associated with signs of overdose in people age 18 or older. The vast majority of cases on record involve larger doses—often many times larger. Perhaps James's diet provided an unusual level of vitamin A, so that the additional 10,000 to 20,000 I.U. from his supplement brought his total intake into the danger zone. But if not, James was simply highly sensitive to vitamin A. The possibility that a few will overdose on amounts that will not harm most always will exist.

Let's look now at more typical cases of vitamin A overdose in adults.

Recommended Dietary Allowances for Vitamin A

Group/Age	I.U.	R.E.*
Infants 0–6 mon.	1,400	420
Infants 6–12 mon.	2,000	400
Children 1–3 yr.	2,000	400
Children 4–6 yr.	2,500	500
Children 7–10 yr.	3,300	700
Males 11–51+ yr.	5,000	1,000
Females 11–51+ yr.	4,000	800
Pregnant and nursing women	5,000	1,000

Note: The U.S. RDA for vitamin A is 5,000 I.U.

*Retinol Equivalents, another way of measuring vitamin A.

ADULTS AND EXCESSIVE A

The cases you have just read about cover most of the symptoms of vitamin A overdose. So rather than tell you about more cases of vitamin A overdose in adults—which involve the same kinds of symptoms as cases already described—I would like simply to give you an idea of the kinds of dosages that have proven troublesome in some adults.

Because hundreds of vitamin A overdosages have been reported in the medical literature, I cannot list the levels associated with each one. Instead, I would like to offer a sampling that will give you a feel for that gray area that I think of as the trouble zone.

Here are some numbers to ponder:

- A 44-year-old woman developed signs of vitamin A overdose one year after taking 600,000 I.U. daily.
- A woman of similar age, 48, showed signs of trouble one year after taking a smaller dose of 150,000 I.U. daily.
- A 52-year-old man found himself in trouble after taking 50,000 I.U. daily for three years.
- Another man, 25, came down with signs of overdose after two months on 200,000 to 275,000 I.U. daily.

Considering still other cases has led me to conclude that, more often than not, vitamin A toxicity in adults involves dosages in the six-figure range. But I have seen a handful of reports of problems in adults who were taking 25,000 I.U. daily and eating large amounts of foods rich in vitamin A, as well as a case that developed after eight years on a supplement of 41,000 I.U. daily.

Needless to say, cases of vitamin A overdose in adults usually fall under the category of long-term problems. Acute ailments are much less common and probably require doses of 250,000 to 300,000 I.U., if not more.

THE STAR SYSTEM SHINES ON RETINOL AND SYNTHETIC VITAMIN A

There you have it—some of the many stories of both infants and adults who took too much vitamin A. Let's now enter these facts into the star system to draw a picture of safety for both synthetic vitamin A and the retinol in fish liver oils.

You will recall that both retinol and synthetic vitamin A are preformed—ready for the body to use. As a result, the medical literature often makes no distinction between retinol or synthetic forms. Because of this, I have had to consider these forms interchangeable for the purposes of the star system. In other words, I have presumed that any symptom known to have been caused by retinol can also be caused by synthetic vitamin A—or vice versa.

The most significant difference between fish oil sources of vitamin A and the synthetic sources is probably the time period before symptoms of overdose appear. Because the synthetic forms are absorbed more readily, toxic reactions are likely to set in sooner than with the same dosage of vitamin A in the form of fish liver oil.

Now, let's put it all together for each of the five points of the star system.

Side effects—In general, side effects from preformed vitamin A are rare in the absence of a toxic reaction. You might consider some of the symptoms mentioned in these cases—such as loss of hair or mild peeling of the skin—as side effects that are not serious. However, when these symptoms occur, changes in the liver, spleen, and/or bones, indicating a toxic reaction, almost always accompany them.

Acute ailments—No doubt about it, very high doses of vitamin A can cause trouble fast—within a few hours to a few weeks of taking high doses. Symptoms of an acute reaction include: severe headache; nausea and vomiting; sluggishness, fatigue, or the desire to sleep; dizziness; and peeling of the skin. In infants, there is another telltale sign: bulging of the fontanel.

Long-term problems—These are more common than acute ailments, especially in teens and adults. Some of the symptoms are the same as for acute ailments, though the violent headaches and vomiting of an acute ailment would probably be replaced by less intense headaches and nausea.

At Minnesota's Mayo Clinic, Manfred Muenter, M.D., and his coworkers analyzed 17 cases of long-term problems with vitamin A. They found some symptoms occurred in most or all of the patients, while other symptoms affected only a handful. Let's break them down into three groups, based on the number of patients affected.

A majority of the 17 patients had these symptoms:

- Bone and joint pain
- Hair loss
- Skin changes: dryness, itching, and flaking
- Tenderness of bones when palpated
- Weakness and fatigue

Six to 9 patients had at one or more of these symptoms:

- Accumulation of fluid in the lower extremities
- Decrease in or loss of menstruation
- Double vision
- Enlarged liver
- Enlarged spleen
- Excessive or frequent urination
- Headache
- Loss of appetite
- Muscle stiffness
- Papilledema (excessive fluid of the eye disk)
- Psychiatric symptoms
- Weight loss

Fewer than one-third of the victims had the following symptoms:

- Bleeding from the nose and lips
- Brittle nails
- Enlargement of the lymph nodes
- Gingivitis (inflammation of the gums)
- Insomnia
- Other nervous system symptoms
- Protruding eyeballs
- Sleepiness
- Yellowing of the skin

Perhaps no other vitamin produces as wide a range of symptoms if taken in excessive doses. Still other problems that have been associated with vitamin A overdoses include: gastrointestinal discomfort; night sweating; slow growth; inflammation of the tongue and lips; visual impairment; growth of sparse and coarse hair; excessive levels of blood fats or calcium in the blood; and both overgrowth of bone and bone fractures.

As the cases I have told you about illustrate, most of the damage from vitamin A overdoses appears to be reversible. But there is one type of damage that sadly is not—harm to the fetus whose mother took high doses in pregnancy. I will be giving you some details shortly, but for now, please note that effective measures to prevent pregnancy are an absolute must for any woman taking high doses of vitamin A.

Conflicting combinations—Ah, the great unknown! I have the feeling that much of what we don't know about vitamin A may fall into this category. Much is known about how vitamin A alone can become toxic. What is not known is whether there is a desirable balance between vitamin A intake and one or more other nutrients.

Preliminary evidence does hint, however, that such a desirable balance may exist between zinc and vitamin A. This research has focused on deficiencies of these nutrients, and the results suggest that a deficiency of one can adversely affect the work of the other. Whether excessive intakes of vitamin A can upset zinc nutrition has not been determined. But, in light of this possibility, I think it wise not to take extreme doses of vitamin A from fish liver oil or synthetic forms without good reason.

An alternative to using these forms of vitamin A, which we will talk about shortly, is to substitute carotene for some of the supplemental vitamin A from fish liver oil or synthetics. From what I have read, I think it less likely that the carotene form of vitamin A might need to be balanced with zinc.

As for prescription drugs, take note of three known interactions with these forms of vitamin A. First, *do not take a vitamin A supplement if you take Accutane, the new anti-acne drug.* The manufacturer warns against use of vitamin A supplements during therapy with this drug.

Second, discuss vitamin A supplementation with your doctor if you take cholestyramine, also known by the brand name Questran. This drug lowers blood cholesterol levels effectively, but can also interfere with the absorption of fat-soluble forms of vitamin A, such as those in animal foods and supplements that contain fish liver oil. Your doctor may want you to take a synthetic, water-soluble vitamin A supplement if you will be taking this drug long-term. Ask for medical advice.

Users of birth control pills should also take vitamin A supplements under a physician's supervision. The Pill can increase the amount of vitamin A in the blood. As a result, Pill users may be more susceptible to overdose.

One over-the-counter drug, mineral oil, can prevent absorption of vitamin A. Four teaspoons of it taken twice daily, for instance, has been shown to interfere with absorption of the vitamin.

Hidden consequences—Vitamin A has been reported to affect laboratory analysis for bilirubin (a component of bile) and one method of determining blood cholesterol.

Remember, too, that vitamin A overdose may be disguised and mistaken for a more serious condition, such as a brain tumor.

HOW MUCH IS TOO MUCH

When it comes to supplement safety, I have learned, one man's safeguard is another man's overdose. A level that confers therapeutic benefits to one person may spell overdose for another. I know of no better example than the case of two 15-year-old brothers, believed to be identical twins, who had both been taking 300,000 I.U. of vitamin A daily for psoriasis. One of the boys developed a severe case of vitamin A overdose, while the other had hardly any symptoms of toxicity at all!

The story of these two brothers illustrates well the concept of nutritional individuality. As the cases I described earlier also made clear, both the dose level required to produce adverse effects as well as the symptoms of the reaction are highly individual. That does not mean, however, that nutritionists cannot offer some basic guidelines. It means only that the guidelines cannot be considered guarantees.

In fact, estimates of potentially troublesome levels have already been offered by various panels of health experts. Let's take a look at their estimates. According to *The Merck Manual*, a popular handbook used by doctors, toxicity in infants can be produced in only a few weeks at dosages of 20,000 to 60,000 I.U. per day of water-soluble vitamin A. Higher doses, of course, can cause acute ailments within hours of ingestion.

As for adults, the American Academy of Pediatrics, echoing sentiments common among nutritionists, advises that doses greater than 25,000 I.U. not be used unless medically indicated. As a rough guide for doctors treating patients with supplemental vitamin A, two researchers designed a formula; they recommend that the daily dose per kilogram of body weight (a kilogram is 2.2 pounds) times the number of days of treatment should not be greater than 1 million I.U.

Perhaps the most precise estimate of your tolerance to vitamin A would be one based on your weight. Nutritionists believe that body weight is a major factor in your ability to tolerate vitamin A. A panel of the Federation of American Societies for Experimental Biology (FASEB) cites a survey showing a level of about 300 I.U. of vitamin A per pound of body weight as the lowest dose associated with adverse effects. That would amount to a maximum dose of 30,000 I.U. for a 100-pound woman. Admittedly, say the scientists, most overdoses involve far higher dosages, often in the six-figure range—100,000 I.U. or more daily.

The 25,000 I.U. limit cited by the American Academy of Pediatrics is the simplest of these guidelines. Most nutritionists, I believe, would endorse it as sound. Of course, teenaged James, mentioned earlier, could not tolerate even this dose. He was an exception rather than the rule, and experience does show that many adults can tolerate substantially more than the 25,000 I.U. limit that nutritionists offer as a rough rule of thumb.

In determining your dosage, remember that the average diet contains 5,440 I.U. of vitamin A. Better yet, calculate your total dietary intake with the two quizzes in this chapter. Deduct this amount from the total dosage you want so that your supplement plus dietary intake doesn't put you above an advisable level.

These guidelines are for healthy, nonpregnant adults. If you are pregnant, have a medical condition, or take any of the drugs I've already mentioned, let your doctor advise you about vitamin A supplements.

TESTING FOR TOXICITY

If you suspect you are suffering from too much vitamin A, a trip to the doctor and a simple blood test called "serum vitamin A" can give you the answer. Because the level of vitamin A in the blood is elevated when toxicity sets in, this test is a simple yet valuable tool for diagnosing overdoses.

What is not as simple, though, is interpreting the results. Standards for normal values do vary. *The Merck Manual* gives 50 to 150 micrograms (mcg.) per 100 milliliters (ml.) of blood as the normal range for vitamin A in the blood. (Unlike the vitamin A in foods, the level in the blood is commonly measured in micrograms rather than international units.)

I have seen other ranges for "normal" vitamin A, however. If your blood vitamin A is above this range but you have no symptoms of vitamin A toxicity, your doctor may feel that there is no cause for concern. I might add that in cases of clear vitamin A toxicity, values for blood vitamin A are often in the range of 100 to 2,000 mcg.

TREATING AN OVERDOSE: A SIMPLE SOLUTION

You'll be happy to know that, for most victims, treating a vitamin A overdose is easy—just take away that bottle!

In the words of Thomas Oliver, M.D., of Ohio State University, "No therapeutic measures are indicated in chronic vitamin A intoxication. Withdrawal of the agent [vitamin A] invariably results in prompt disappearance of symptoms." Says *The Merck Manual*, "Prognosis is excellent. Symptoms and signs usually disappear within one to four weeks after stopping vitamin A ingestion."

Of course, there can be exceptions. In children, for instance, I am not convinced that all damage is reversed quickly. I have read of cases in children and adolescents where all signs of damage took a year or more to subside. So, rather than take high doses with the attitude that any damage can be reversed quickly, I think it far better to prevent vitamin A overdose from occurring by taking or giving it sensibly, within current guidelines.

Drugs have been given occasionally for vitamin A overdose. James, for instance, who suffered from the false brain tumor syndrome, was given cortisone to ease his symptoms quickly. And in patients who have persistent high levels of calcium in their blood as a result of excessive vitamin A, cortisone again may be used along with other measures to reduce the blood calcium level.

PREGNANCY AND OTHER SPECIAL CONDITIONS

Pregnancy deserves a very special place in any discussion of vitamin A. This is a time when you must be cautious about vitamin A supplements, for good intentions have been known to go haywire, inflicting damage instead.

Many studies in test animals show that high doses of vitamin A can cause miscarriages and birth defects. In their report on the safety of vitamin A, the FASEB scientists cited three children whose birth defects were believed to result from their mothers' high intakes of vitamin A during pregnancy. The victims included:

• A baby girl with malformations of the urinary tract, attributed to her mother's daily consumption of a 25,000 I.U. fish oil supplement during the first three months of the pregnancy and a still higher daily dose of 50,000 I.U. during the final six months of her pregnancy.

• A second infant with urinary tract abnormalities, believed to have resulted from the mother's use of 40,000 I.U. of supplemental vitamin A during the sixth through tenth week of the pregnancy.

• An infant with abnormalities of the central nervous system, which were linked to 150,000 I.U. of supplemental vitamin A taken by the mother as an acne treatment for about three weeks during her pregnancy.

In short, the 25,000 I.U. level considered safe for most adults does not apply during pregnancy. I would urge any pregnant woman to discuss her vitamin A intake with her obstetrician, who might prescribe a prenatal supplement with vitamin A. Rest assured that most prenatal vitamins contain only moderate levels—far less than the amounts associated with the birth defects just discussed. Depending on your diet, your doctor may feel that no supplement is needed. Some doctors may prefer to use carotene, which I will discuss shortly, rather than supplements relying on fish liver oils or synthetic forms, which have been associated with birth defects when taken in high doses.

A joint statement of the drug and nutrition committees of the American Academy of Pediatrics dictates that dosages of vitamin

A should not exceed 6,000 I.U. for pregnant women.

One final word to those with another special condition: malabsorption syndrome. Vitamin A supplements are generally unacceptable for those afflicted with these disorders. If you are taking vitamin A and have such a condition, seek your doctor's advice.

KIND WORDS FOR CAROTENE

To know carotene is to love it. Once you understand how your body uses it, you are sure to join its fan club.

As I mentioned at the beginning of this chapter, carotene is a precursor of vitamin A. Your body converts carotene to vitamin A as needed to perform its important functions of contributing to healthy bones, organs, eyes, and membranes. These roles are the nutrient functions of vitamin A. There is no reason to believe that your body will convert carotene to vitamin A for pharmacologic (drug) functions, such as treating acne or psoriasis. When such roles are desired, synthetic vitamin A is the answer.

Medicinal purposes aside, carotene can handle your vitamin A needs as long as you don't have one of the conditions that impairs your body from converting carotene to an active form of vitamin A. And here lies its beauty. Your body changes carotene to vitamin A if you need it, but not if you don't. It's somewhat like a self-regulating pump. When you need vitamin A, the pump turns on, converting carotene to vitamin A. But when you have enough vitamin A, the pump either slows down or shuts off.

In short, this clever pump prevents you from developing toxic levels of vitamin A from carotene. Your body just doesn't let it happen.

CALL IT MELLOW YELLOW

If your body doesn't convert excess carotene to vitamin A, what does it do with it? You may know the answer. Your body deposits at least some of the extra carotene in various places—most notably in your skin, and possibly in other tissues of your body. And since carotene is a pigment, yellow to orange in color, high levels of carotene rarely go undetected. The skin turns color, usually most noticeably on the palms of the hands and soles of the feet. The yellow to orange cast that you see as a result of taking excessive carotene can be alarming, but you can rest assured that nutritionists know of no harm from this condition, which goes by several names:

• Carotenemia or hypercarotenemia, terms referring to the high levels of carotene in the blood that accompany the yellow skin syndrome.
• Carotenosis or hypercarotenosis, technical terms meaning nothing more than abnormal levels of carotene in the body.
• *Xanthis cutis* or *Cutaneous xanthosis*, which translated from Latin mean "yellow skin."

You may be wondering how doctors distinguish carotenosis from that serious symptom—jaundice—that also causes a yellowing of the skin. And the answer is simple. Doctors don't distinguish between the two until they see the whites of the eyes. In carotenosis, the whites of the eyes are unchanged; no carotene pigment is deposited there. In jaundice, however, the reverse is true; a yellow tint in the whites of the eyes is the giveaway.

WHEN CAROTENOSIS OCCURS

Of course, most people don't want to walk around with yellow or orange hands and faces. So, if this happens to you, relax. When signs of carotenosis appear, cutting back on your intake of foods and/or supplements rich in carotene will reverse the process, usually within a few weeks. In severe cases, a few months might be needed before your natural color is fully restored.

Because carotenosis is considered harmless, little research has been done to determine the level at which the condition develops. For adults, however, a consistently high intake is probably needed before signs of carotenosis appear. A half-cup serving of carrots a day, for instance, is unlikely to cause your skin to change color. On the other hand, eating several pounds of carrots a week might. Carrot consumption was encouraged by the British government during World War II, and carotenosis developed in citizens who characteristically ate 4 or more pounds weekly of the officially endorsed vegetable. Four pounds a week translates into more than a cup and a half of sliced carrots daily.

Based on my own experience with a few cases of carotenosis, I would guess that 20,000 I.U. daily over a period of months might cause mild symptoms in some people; much lower intakes from foods rich in carotene have caused the condition in infants. I also have seen a few truly marked cases that probably resulted from daily intakes in the range of 50,000 I.U. or more. But whether mild or severe, and whether in infants or adults, prevailing medical opinion holds that the condition is harmless.

A FEW FALSE ALARMS

Carotene research has been hampered by more than the attitude that the substance is harmless. Until recently, carotene capsules were not widely available. The carotene supplements that did exist were used mainly by doctors in the treatment of a rare condition that is marked by adverse reactions to sunlight. Thanks to carotene supplements, the severity of this problem has been eased in many of the affected patients.

But since few people have this condition, studies of the general effects of carotene supplements have been all but non-existent. The research that is available invariably has involved diets containing carotene-rich foods. And that's not the same thing as a carotene supplement. Carotene is but one of many substances in carrots and other rich sources of the nutrient. So if and when untoward effects occur on carotene-rich diets, no one can be sure whether the carotene alone, or some other substance in the foods, caused the problem.

I have read reports of two hypercarotenemic patients who also had abnormally low levels of white blood cells, a condition that lowers resistance to infection. Both patients were eating enormous quantities of carrots. One of the patients, Jennifer, had been drinking the juice from two pounds of carrots every day for years. The report of her low white blood cell count in a medical journal prompted researchers treating sun-sensitive people with carotene supplements to examine the white blood cell counts of their patients. They found nothing abnormal.

It seems that the two cases of low white cell counts in these carrot-lovers probably resulted from some substance other than carotene in the carrots. Alternatively, these two cases might represent atypical reactions. But the evidence that carotene itself is responsible simply isn't convincing in light of the research showing that purified carotene supplements did not adversely affect the blood count.

Likewise, another doctor linked diets containing enormous amounts of high-carotene foods to menstrual irregularities. His subjects were five women who were eating huge quantities of squash, pumpkins, and carrots. One of his patients, Elizabeth, was eating six pounds of carrots and up to seven pounds of pumpkin per week, for a daily carotene intake of 30,000 I.U. from these foods alone. Another patient, Jane, was eating almost nothing but carrots and pumpkins.

Was it the carotene in the diets of Jane and Elizabeth that caused their problems, or the overall diet? When you consider how unbalanced these diets were—low or deficient in protein and other vital nutrients—you probably will have a hard time blaming carotene. I do. If their problems were in fact nutritional, I doubt that it was the carotene, but rather the overall inadequacy of their diets that was responsible.

So, these alarms were probably false ones, and the evidence still supports the widely held belief that carotene is nontoxic.

THE CASE OF THE CARROT JUICE JUNKIE

I would like to tell you about the most famous false alarm ever attributed to carotene. Here, word-for-word, is a news item that appeared in a respected European medical journal in 1974.

Briton, 48, Killed by Carrot Juice

Croydon, England, Feb. 15 (Reuters). Health food enthusiast Basil Brown became addicted to carrot juice and was bright yellow when he died of cirrhosis of the liver.

The 48-year-old scientific advisor was drinking up to a gallon of carrot juice a day, an inquest was told here yesterday. He was also consuming vitamins by the handfull [sic] and was found to have taken 70 million units of vitamin A in 10 days.

A doctor warned Mr. Brown about the vitamin pills because his liver was already enlarged—but he had a low opinion of doctors. The doctor was not told about the carrot juice.

I found this story so unbelievable that I donned my detective cap and set out to get to the bottom of this case. And when I did, I found quite a different story.

I found the true story about Mr. Brown in another medical journal, which carried the scientific report of his case. Yes, Mr. Brown had been consuming enormous amounts of carrot juice. But he died of liver cirrhosis, which has never been linked to carotene. The vitamin A supplements, on the other hand, might have contributed to the liver damage. Brown also had suffered from pneumonia and other health problems, such as fluid buildup in his organs, in the year or two before his death.

The scientists who reported his story to the medical journal were slow to blame the carrot juice. "How far the carrots should be incriminated," they said, "seems uncertain. Possibly carrot addiction may have lowered the patient's condition through a reduced intake of more nourishing food." That I can agree with. But to call carrot juice the killer? The basis for that escapes me.

I am not the only one who can't buy this story. In a recent paper, four vitamin A experts commented that "there is no evidence that one man reputed to have died of carrot juice actually did."

There certainly isn't.

CAROTENE AGAINST CANCER

A little extra carotene might do our health a world of good.

As I noted earlier, your body converts carotene to vitamin A only as needed; beyond that, the carotene remains in its original state. This unconverted carotene may serve you well by helping to guard against the cancer process.

Carotene, like vitamins C and E and the mineral selenium, is an antioxidant. Cancer researchers believe that antioxidants may help ward off cancer, preventing the development of cancer-causing chemicals in the body. And dozens of studies support this possibility. When scientists have compared the diets of cancer victims to that of nonvictims, they frequently have found that the nonvictims reported diets richer in carotene.

Only certain types of cancer have been linked to diets low in carotene. Research on the protective effect of carotene is most convincing for cancers of the lung, stomach, and esophagus. Some

The Diet Detective Searches for Carotene

Is your curiosity about your carotene intake mounting? If so, then grab a pencil and take my carotene quiz. To use it, simply check off any of the following entries that you included in your diet today. Add up your total points, then see the tips for interpreting your score at the end of the food listings.

1 point
1 cup orange juice
10 pods okra
½ grapefruit
1 cup zucchini
1 avocado
1 cup green beans

2 points
1 cup yellow corn
1 cup brussels sprouts
1 cup summer squash
1 cup peas
1 cup romaine lettuce
1 medium tomato
½ cup tomato sauce (or entrée with tomato sauce)
⅙ peach pie (9-inch size)

3 points
1 cup asparagus

4 points
¾ cup vegetable juice cocktail (V-8, 6-ounce can)
1 cup tomato juice

5 points
1 nectarine
1 cup apricot nectar
1 cup papaya
1/16 watermelon
3 apricots, fresh
1 cup minestrone or vegetable soup
⅛ pumpkin pie (9-inch size)

10 points
1 cup spinach, raw
1 cup apricots, canned with syrup
1 cup broccoli

research suggests promising effects against the chances of developing cancer of the mouth, bladder, colon, and prostate. If you have any characteristic, such as smoking, that puts you at high risk for any of these forms of cancer, you'll want to make sure you get your fair share of carotene. Actually, almost everyone should.

There are, however, a few conditions that interfere with carotene metabolism. Please read on so you can learn about them.

1 cup bok choy
1 cup dried peaches
1 cup "chunky" soup with
   vegetables

15 points
1 cup beet greens
1 large carrot
1 cup mustard greens
1 cup turnip greens
1 cup winter squash

20 points
1 cup mixed vegetables
1 cup kale
½ cantaloupe
1 sweet potato, baked

25 points
1 cup spinach
1 cup collard greens
1 cup carrots

Scoring

Add up your points. Then add a zero to the total for an estimate of how your carotene intake compares to the U.S. RDA for vitamin A.

For example, if your points total 9, add a zero, for a score of 90. That means your diet on the day surveyed contains enough carotene to give you 90 percent of the U.S. RDA of 5,000 I.U. Add to this your score from the preformed vitamin A quiz on page 26 and you'll have a rough estimate of your total vitamin A intake from food. (I would hazard a guess that you might take in another 1,000 I.U. of vitamin A from foods not mentioned in the quizzes.) Unless your doctor directs otherwise, this total vitamin A intake, including from carotene, should be considered whenever making a decision about a vitamin A supplement.

CONVERTING TO CAROTENE: NOT FOR EVERYONE

By now, it is clear that most people can be assured of getting enough vitamin A without the risk of overdose by using carotene instead of synthetic vitamin A or fish liver oil. But there are exceptions. Are you one of them?

The ability to convert carotene to vitamin A is impaired in three types of disorders:

- Diabetes
- Hypothyroidism
- Severe liver malfunctioning

If you have any of these conditions, it is best not to rely solely on carotene to meet your vitamin A needs. If your doctor does want you to take some vitamin A in the form of carotene, an increase in dosage is recommended to compensate for the reduced ability to convert carotene to vitamin A.

These conditions, of course, make you more susceptible to the yellowing of skin that is the hallmark of carotenosis. But the excess carotene is nonetheless not known to be harmful to you.

THE STAR SYSTEM SHINES ON CAROTENE

Let the star system shine on carotene and carotene shines back! Just compare these facts to those of the star system for synthetic vitamin A and retinol. What a difference!

Side effects—The only known side effect of excess carotene is the yellowing of skin.

Acute ailments—There are no acute ailments associated with high intakes of carotene. I found one very minor exception— a report of a patient whose skin reacted to an externally applied sunscreen containing carotene. His doctor attributed the reaction to the carotene, but there is no proof that this was the guilty ingredient, and no other cases have been reported. At most this was a highly atypical reaction to carotene; at worst it was another false alarm, with some other substance actually causing the skin reaction.

Long-term problems—I have found no long-term health problems that can be reasonably blamed on carotene itself.

Conflicting combinations—A few prescription drugs do interact with carotene. Clofibrate, a drug used to treat high blood triglyceride levels (and also known by the brand name Atromid-S), can decrease your body's ability to absorb carotene. So can colchicine, a drug useful in the treatment of gout. In addition to plain colchicine pills, multi-ingredient drugs such as ColBenemid and ProBenecid with colchicine also contain it.

Unlike these drugs, birth control pills increase the rate at which the body converts carotene to vitamin A. It's best to discuss use of carotene with your doctor if you take any of these drugs.

Mineral oil, on the other hand, decreases the absorption of carotene. Four teaspoons of it twice daily can produce malabsorption of carotene, so be careful not to overdo it.

Hidden consequences—As I mentioned earlier, carotenosis will not prevent your doctor from diagnosing jaundice. Because of its color, it can affect laboratory tests of bilirubin, blood vitamin A, and the icteric index, a liver function test that many doctors no longer use.

The only hidden consequence of excessive carotene that I can foresee would relate to any condition that is diagnosed on the basis of actual skin color. One condition comes to my mind, and it is one that I will be telling you more about in the chapter on iron.

This condition is hemochromatosis, a disorder that causes the body to store harmful amounts of iron. One sign of hemochromatosis is a bronze coloring of the skin. It's conceivable that carotenosis might mask it, though I have not read of any cases where this actually occurred.

CAROTENE AND PREGNANCY

Since nutritionists consider carotene to be basically innocuous, its effect on pregnancy has not been a high priority for researchers. I have but two facts to relate:

• A very high intake of carrots during pregnancy has been reported to cause yellowing of the skin in both the mother and the newborn baby. That is not to say that the mother or baby are actually harmed.
• A study in rats did show that "large doses" of carotene adversely affected bone development and ability to maintain the pregnancy. I'm not ready to draw any conclusions from this, however.

What do I advise pregnant women? As always, to take supplements under their doctor's supervision. I might add that I belong to the school of thought favoring cautious use of all pills during pregnancy. So take at most modest amounts of any supplement during this time and seek regular medical supervision.

C O O K I N G
for Vitamin A

LIVER WITH ONIONS AND ROSEMARY

(Makes 2 servings)

Vitamin A: 25,602 I.U. per serving
Calories: 336 per serving

½ pound calf's liver, cut into ¾-inch slices
1 tablespoon minced fresh rosemary or 1 teaspoon dried rosemary
3 cloves garlic, minced
¼ teaspoon mustard seed, crushed

2 tablespoons olive oil
¼ cup malt vinegar
1 medium-size onion, sliced into thin rings
2 leeks, white part only, sliced into julienne pieces

Place liver in a 9-inch glass baking dish. Mix the rosemary, garlic, mustard seed, oil, and vinegar in a small bowl and pour over the liver. Let marinate at room temperature for 1 hour.

Spray a no-stick sauté pan with no-stick spray and heat to medium. Add the onions and leeks and sauté for about 3 minutes, adding a bit of marinade, if needed. Add the liver and remaining marinade and sauté for about 10 minutes, or until liver is cooked to your taste.

C O O K I N G
for Vitamin A—*continued*

SWEET POTATO PANCAKES
WITH CARROTS AND RAISINS

(Makes 8 pancakes or 4 waffles)

Vitamin A: 3,298 I.U. per pancake
            6,596 I.U. per waffle
Calories: 189 per pancake (without topping)
           278 per waffle (without topping)

2	tablespoons wheat germ	¼	cup raisins
1¼	cups flour	⅔	cup shredded raw sweet potatoes
1	teaspoon baking powder	2	tablespoons maple syrup
	pinch of cinnamon	¼	teaspoon vanilla extract
	pinch of nutmeg		
¼	teaspoon ground ginger	1	egg, beaten
¼	cup shredded raw carrots	1	cup skim milk

In a large bowl, combine the wheat germ, flour, baking powder, cinnamon, nutmeg, ginger, carrots, raisins, and sweet potatoes. In a separate bowl, combine the maple syrup, vanilla, egg, and milk. Stir the wet ingredients into the dry until ingredients are just moistened.

Spray a no-stick pan or griddle with no-stick spray and spoon 2 tablespoons of the batter onto the heated pan. Cook the pancakes on both sides until puffy and brown. Repeat with the remaining batter.

If making waffles, use 4 tablespoons (¼ cup) of batter for each waffle and bake in a waffle iron, according to the manufacturer's instructions.

(continued)

C   O   O   K   I   N   G
for Vitamin A—*continued*

SALMON-STUFFED TOMATOES

(Makes 2 servings)

Vitamin A: 3,889 I.U. per serving
Calories: 234 per serving

2 large, ripe, firm tomatoes	2 tablespoons plain yogurt
2 scallions, minced	2 tablespoons mayonnaise
⅓ cup minced fresh spinach	½ teaspoon prepared coarse mustard
½ cup canned pink salmon, drained	1 tablespoon minced fresh parsley
1 hard-cooked egg, chopped	½ teaspoon dried dillweed

With a sharp knife, slice away the top of each tomato. Carefully scoop out the pulp, leaving enough so that tomatoes retain their shape.

Drain the pulp and chop coarsely. In a medium bowl, mix the pulp, scallions, spinach, salmon, and egg.

In a small bowl, combine the yogurt, mayonnaise, mustard, parsley, and dillweed. Gently toss with salmon mixture. Spoon into the shells.

Vitamin A Content
of Selected Supplements

Dosage is one tablet or capsule unless otherwise indicated.

Supplement	Manufacturer	I.U.
Abdec Baby Drops (per 0.6 ml.)	Parke-Davis	5,000
Abdec Kapseal	Parke-Davis	10,000
Abdol with Minerals	Parke-Davis	5,000
Abron	O'Neal, Jones & Feldman	8,000
Aqua-A	Anabolic	25,000
AVP Natal	A.V.P.	5,000
Bugs Bunny	Miles	2,500
Bugs Bunny Plus Iron	Miles	2,500
Bugs Bunny with Extra C	Miles	2,500
Cal-Prenal	North American	4,000
Centrum	Lederle	5,000
Chew-Vite	North American	5,000
Cluvisol 130	Ayerst	10,000
Cluvisol Syrup (per tsp.)	Ayerst	2,500
Cod Liver Oil Concentrate Capsules	Schering	10,000
Cod Liver Oil Concentrate Tablets	Schering	4,000
Cod Liver Oil Tablets with Vitamin A	Schering	4,000
Dayalets	Abbott	5,000
Dayalets plus Iron	Abbott	5,000
Engram-HP	Squibb	8,000
Feminins	Mead Johnson	5,000
Femiron with Vitamins	J.B. Williams	5,000
Filibon Tablets	Lederle	5,000
Flintstones	Miles	2,500
Flintstones Plus Iron	Miles	2,500
Flintstones with Extra C	Miles	2,500
Ganatrex (per 0.6 ml.)	Merrell Dow	5,000
Gerilets	Abbott	5,000
Geriplex	Parke-Davis	5,000
Geriplex-FS Kapseals	Parke-Davis	5,000
Geritinic	Geriatric Pharm.	5,000
Geritol Junior Liquid (per tsp.)	J.B. Williams	8,000

(continued)

Supplements—*continued*

Supplement	Manufacturer	I.U.
Geritol Junior Tablets	J.B. Williams	5,000
Gest	O'Neal, Jones & Feldman	4,000
Gevral	Lederle	5,000
Gevral Protein	Lederle	2,167
Gevral T Capsules	Lederle	5,000
Gevrite	Lederle	5,000
Multicebrin	Lilly	10,000
Multiple Vitamins	North American	5,000
Multiple Vitamins with Iron	North American	5,000
Multivitamins	Rowell	5,000
Myadec	Parke-Davis	10,000
Natabec	Parke-Davis	4,000
Natalins Tablets	Mead Johnson	8,000
Norlac	Rowell	8,000
Nutra-Cal	Anabolic	1,250
Obron-6	Pfipharmecs	5,000
One-A-Day	Miles	5,000
One-A-Day Core C 500	Miles	5,000
One-A-Day Plus Iron	Miles	5,000
One-A-Day Vitamins Plus Minerals	Miles	5,000
Optilets-500	Abbott	10,000
Optilets-M-500	Abbott	10,000
Os-Cal Forte	Marion	1,668
Os-Cal Plus	Marion	1,666
Paladec (per tsp.)	Parke-Davis	5,000
Paladec with Minerals	Parke-Davis	4,000
Panuitex	O'Neal, Jones & Feldman	6,000
Poly-Vi-Sol Chewable	Mead Johnson	2,500
Poly-Vi-Sol Drops (per 0.6 ml.)	Mead Johnson	1,500
Poly-Vi-Sol with Iron Chewable	Mead Johnson	2,500
Poly-Vi-Sol with Iron Drops (per 0.6 ml.)	Mead Johnson	1,500
Selenace	Anabolic	10,000
Stuart Formula	Stuart	5,000
Stuart Prenatal	Stuart	8,000
Super D Cod Liver Oil (per tsp.)	Upjohn	4,000
Super D Perles (per tsp.)	Upjohn	10,000

Supplements—*continued*

Supplement	Manufacturer	I.U.
Super Plenamins	Rexall	8,000
Theragran	Squibb	10,000
Theragran Liquid (per tsp.)	Squibb	10,000
Theragran-M	Squibb	10,000
Theragran-Z	Squibb	10,000
Therapeutic Vitamins	North American	1,000
Thera-Spancap	North American	10,000
Tri-Vi-Sol Chewable	Mead Johnson	2,500
Tri-Vi-Sol Drops (per 1 ml.)	Mead Johnson	1,500
Tri-Vi-Sol with Iron Drops (per 1 ml.)	Mead Johnson	1,500
Unicap	Upjohn	5,000
Unicap Chewable	Upjohn	5,000
Unicap T	Upjohn	5,000
Vi-Aqua	USV	5,000
Vicon Plus	Glaxo	4,000
Vigran	Squibb	5,000
Vigran Chewable	Squibb	2,500
Vigran plus Iron	Squibb	5,000
Vio-Geric	Rowell	5,000
Vi-Penta Infant Drops (per 0.6 ml.)	Roche	5,000
Vi-Penta Multivitamin Drops (per 0.6 ml.)	Roche	5,000
Vitagett	North American	5,000
Vita-Kaps-M Tablets	Abbott	5,000
Vita-Kaps Tablets	Abbott	5,000
Vitamin-Mineral Capsules	North American	5,000
Viterra	Pfipharmecs	5,000
Viterra High Potency	Pfipharmecs	10,000
Vi-Zac	Glaxo	5,000
Zymacap Capsules	Upjohn	5,000
Zymasyrup (per tsp.)	Upjohn	5,000

Source: Adapted from the American Pharmaceutical Association, *Handbook of Nonprescription Drugs*, 7th ed. (1982), 240–57.

Note: This chart is intended only as a guide. Vitamin formulations change periodically; always read product labels for accurate and up-to-date information on their nutrient levels.

4

Thiamine (Vitamin B₁)

T hiamine. It's the vitamin that almost rhymes with diamond. And whether you judge it by its benefits to your health or by its record for safety, this one really is a gem.

It's thiamine that helps your body release energy from food—specifically from the carbohydrates that nutritionists are now cheering for so wildly. Because of its energy-releasing role, thiamine is credited with helping you to keep three things healthy: your appetite, your digestive tract, and your nervous system.

And many nutritionists consider thiamine to be one of the leader nutrients. That means that it's often a marker for other important nutrients—a sort of divining rod that alerts you to a nutrient-rich food.

Supplements often are no different from food on this count. Most supplements that contain thiamine have other B vitamins, too; many contain still other vitamins and minerals as well. But in this chapter, we'll look at the safety story for just thiamine. That way it will get a fair hearing—untarnished by problems that might result not from it alone, but from the company it often keeps.

THE NONTOXIC NOTION

Too little thiamine spells trouble. But too much—well, it happens, but rarely.

As you probably know, thiamine is a water-soluble vitamin. Vitamin A, on the other hand, is fat-soluble. Nutritionists long believed that this characteristic was the key factor in nutrient toxicity. It was believed that fat-soluble vitamins could collect in the body and become toxic, while water-soluble ones could not.

But the nutritionists have proven themselves wrong. Some people have reacted to high doses of the water-soluble B vitamins, making it clear that these vitamins can be toxic. However, while water-soluble vitamins can become toxic, they are much less likely to do so than the fat-soluble ones. Just as importantly, the toxicity of water-soluble vitamins varies from one to another, with some being all but harmless and others having a significant potential for harm at high doses.

As nutritionists have become better acquainted with thiamine, some time-honored basics have emerged. From the standpoint of supplement safety, it is important to remember these basics about B_1:

• Your body can absorb only so much thiamine at a time. That is, just as a car can go only so many miles per hour, your body can absorb only so much thiamine from a single dose.

• Your body has a limit to how much thiamine it can retain. Once that limit is reached, your body rapidly excretes thiamine that it does not absorb, much of it within a day or two after it's consumed.

TWO CLASSIC CASES

It was the summer of 1940 when Clarence Mills, M.D., professor at the University of Cincinnati College of Medicine, reported a classic case of thiamine overdose. The patient was Annamarie, age 47.

For two and a half weeks, Annamarie had been taking 10,000 milligrams (mg.) of thiamine daily. There was no Recommended Dietary Allowance (RDA) at the time. But by today's standards, she was taking in 5,000 times the U.S. Recommended Daily Allowance (U.S. RDA). Little wonder that her body protested!

(continued on page 58)

The Diet Detective Searches for Thiamine

If you have a few minutes, you can estimate the thiamine content of your diet. Just read down the list of foods that follows, jotting down the point values for any of the items that you included in your diet yesterday or today. Then see the scoring information at the end of the food listings.

1 point
1 ounce crackers (for example, 26 Cheese Nips, 10 Rich and Crisp, 14 Sociables, 9 Wheatsworth)
⅔ cup instant cream of wheat
1 cup hot wheat cereal (for example, Wheatena)
1 waffle
3 pancakes (4 inches in diameter)
Any of the following: 1 bagel, 2 biscuits, 1 sandwich, 2 small rolls
½ cup bread stuffing
½ cup rice
½ cup chopped almonds
4 ounces chicken liver
4 ounces duck meat
4 ounces tuna
1 cup lobster meat
4 ounces fish fillets
4 ounces oysters
4 ounces salmon
2 slices pork luncheon meat
4 ounces roast lamb or lamb chops
1 veal chop

4 slices bacon
1 slice Canadian bacon
½ cup pumpkin seeds
1 cup spaghetti or macaroni

2 points
2 slices bread
1 piece corn bread
1 English muffin
1 cup egg noodles
1 packet Quaker instant oats
⅔ cup any of the following cereals: Corn Bran, Crispy Wheats 'n Raisins, Golden Grahams, Grape-nuts flakes, Honey Bran, Raisins, Rice & Rye, Special K, Wheaties
1 cup Cheerios or Quisp cereal
1 ounce Brazil nuts
½ cup cashews
½ cup filberts
½ cup peanuts
2 ounces luncheon ham
1 cup lima or Great Northern beans
1 cup split peas

4 ounces beef or calf liver
⅕ recipe Hamburger
    Helper
⅕ recipe Tuna Helper
1 cup crabmeat

3 points
⅓ cup granola, Grape-nuts,
    or 100% bran cereal
⅔ cup any of the following
    cereals:
    Bran Buds, Bran Chex,
    Cracklin' Oat Bran, 40%
    Bran cereal, Fruit 'n
    Fibre, Life, Wheat Chex
1 cup Corn Chex or most
    children's cereals
1 packet Mix 'n Eat cream
    of wheat
1 cup soybeans
1 cup black-eyed peas
½ cup chopped pecans
1 "Grillers" soy-based
    imitation breakfast meat
2 slices "Luncheon slices"
    soy-based imitation
    lunch meat

2 slices ham
4 ounces veal roast

4 points
⅔ cup Buc Wheats cereal
1 Italian sandwich roll
¼ cup sunflower seeds
4 ounces ham roast

5 points
1 cup Kaboom cereal
3 soy-based imitation
    sausage links

7 points
⅔ cup Total or Corn Total
    cereal
4 ounces pork chop or
    roast

9 points
2 soy-based imitation
    sausage patties
⅔ cup Product 19 cereal

13 points
⅔ cup Most cereal

Scoring
    Add up your points. To that number, attach a zero. The result is an estimate of the percentage of the U.S. RDA for thiamine in your diet. For instance, if your points total 7, add a zero for a level of 70 percent of the U.S. RDA.
    Of course, the quiz provides only an estimate. Your total intake of thiamine is probably above the level estimated by the quiz, for it was impossible to include all foods that supply any amount of thiamine. Such a list would be very, very long.

(continued)

The Diet Detective—
Thiamine (continued)

If you want to take a thiamine supplement, do consider the level in your diet before determining your dosage.

If your diet includes foods not listed here that you know to be good sources of thiamine, you can account for them. After you have your final score and have converted it to a percent of the U.S. RDA, add the percent of U.S. RDA for thiamine listed on the food's nutrition label. For example, if you scored 70, but ate a food not listed that contains 30 percent of the U.S. RDA, add 70 and 30 for a score of 100 percent of the U.S. RDA.

Congratulations!

Dr. Mills found that Annamarie's symptoms were similar to those produced by overdosing on thyroid medication:

- Headache
- Insomnia
- Irritability
- Rapid pulse
- Trembling
- Weakness

Dr. Mills had Annamarie do the obvious; stop taking the thiamine supplement. In two days the troubling symptoms were gone. Annamarie was more or less recovered.

But then she invited trouble to return. A week later, she started taking thiamine again, this time at a level of 5 mg. daily. That was quite a drop from the 10,000 mg. level she had been taking when her overdose developed. But four and a half weeks later, the same symptoms recurred.

Annamarie stopped the thiamine once more. And like clockwork, her symptoms vanished promptly.

Annamarie was cured, but Dr. Mills remained concerned. He continued his study of thiamine overdose. While traveling in Panama, he learned that doctors there often prescribed daily thiamine supplements in the range of 20 to 40 mg. (10 to 20 times the current U.S. RDA). He found another woman, Johanna, who like Annamarie had symptoms suggestive of too much thyroid hormone: irritability, rapid pulse, and muscle tremors.

Laboratory tests revealed that Johanna was excreting at least 12 mg. of thiamine a day. She had been taking about 17 mg. per day. And obviously that was too much.

ALLERGIES AND ODDITIES

The cases of thiamine toxicity mentioned above were caused by taking too much thiamine. Annamarie and Johanna simply took in too much of a substance that otherwise would not have harmed them. Their bodies responded with signs similar to that of thyroid malfunctioning.

Around the same time that Dr. Mills reported the cases of Annamarie and Johanna, other doctors found that some patients could not tolerate thiamine injections or regimens of injections and oral supplements. These reactions, however, are believed to be allergic reactions rather than the type of toxic reactions that affected Annamarie and Johanna. That is, just as some people are allergic to dust, pollen, animal hair, and other substances that are harmless to most people, so some people are allergic, or hypersensitive, to thiamine injections.

Since these allergic reactions resulted from thiamine injections or injections plus supplements, the results are not easily applied to the issue of supplement safety. There is no assurance, I feel, that an injection of 25 mg. of thiamine affects the body in exactly the same way as an oral supplement containing the same amount. But I'd nonetheless like to tell you about a classic case so you can appreciate the possible difference between various types of thiamine supplementation.

ONE SHOT TOO MANY

Ellen, age 59, had been taking an oral thiamine supplement on and off for about two years. At that point, her doctor began giving her thiamine shots "fairly regularly and usually twice weekly in doses ranging from 8 to 90 mg." He had her continue the oral supplement also.

One day about six months later, her doctor gave her the usual shot. This time, however, she had an unusual reaction: She felt weak and about to faint. These sensations of weakness and faintness occurred on and off soon after the shot.

The Seldom-Seen Signs
of Thiamine Deficiency

Amidst all the commentary about what is wrong with our diet, we sometimes lose sight of what is right with it. And one such right thing is our thiamine intake. Except for those afflicted with alcoholism, genetic diseases, or metabolic disorders, thiamine intake is generally adequate in the United States.

But take in too little thiamine and before long deficiency may pay you a visit. When deficiency occurs, it comes in stages, each one marked by its own set of symptoms.

As thiamine deficiency first sets in, you would be apt to feel tired and lacking energy. Emotions might run amok, with irritability, depression, anger, and fear dominating your mood. You might find your appetite lessening, and as a result, lose some weight.

Should the deficiency continue uncorrected, physical discomfort might heighten. You might experience headaches, indigestion, and constipation. Your heartbeat might speed up at levels of exertion that normally would not cause it to do so. Finally, you might experience the signs of nerve damage in the legs that nutritionists know to be a hallmark of thiamine deficiency. The condition is called peripheral neuritis, and those afflicted experience heavy, weak feelings in

---

Four days later, her doctor again gave her the shot. This time she complained of an unusual amount of nervousness. Her pulse rose from 70 to 120, and the skin of her face and hands was flushed. It was obvious to the doctor that something was wrong.

Two weeks later, after still another shot, the same symptoms occurred with greater intensity. From that point on, Ellen also developed flushing and rapid heartbeat if she took her usual multivitamin containing thiamine. Even a fairly small dose of thiamine—3 mg.—could no longer be injected without symptoms, which lasted about a half hour.

To confirm his belief that Ellen was hypersensitive to thia-

their legs. Leg cramps, burning sensations, and a feeling of numbness in the feet may happen as well. These are strong clues that peripheral neuritis is developing.

If these symptoms remain unchecked, the final stage of thiamine deficiency eventually arrives. It's called beri-beri, and though highly unusual in the United States, it is no stranger in some parts of the world.

Beri-beri occurs in two forms, which doctors refer to as "wet" and "dry," depending on the symptoms. Signs of the body retaining too much fluid and abnormal heart functioning predominate in the wet form, while nerve and muscle problems in the muscles and nerve problems in the limbs stand out in the dry form. Severe pain often accompanies the disorder, which can lead to death if left untreated.

Happily, the heart and digestive malfunctioning that accompanies beri-beri can be reversed with therapeutic doses of thiamine. Symptoms of nerve malfunctioning, however, are more difficult to correct.

How long does it take for thiamine deficiency to develop? That depends, but inadequate intakes have been shown to cause signs of deficiency within two to three weeks of a grossly inadequate intake.

mine, the doctor prepared a skin test similar to the kind allergists use to test for common allergies. When the test was given to Ellen, she developed the raised red bump indicative of an allergic reaction. Five others, however, voluntarily took the skin test and had no reaction. It seemed clear that Ellen was allergic to the thiamine regimen she had been receiving.

Needless to say, the shots were stopped. Some months later, Ellen's doctor began prescribing very small amounts of an oral thiamine supplement for her. Slowly, he increased the amount to 0.3 mg. which she was able to tolerate without any ill effects.

There have been others, who, like Ellen, were allergic to

thiamine injections, and there have also been cases of "drug rash" from these injections. Sadly, even death has been reported from a thiamine injection in an allergic individual.

As I mentioned earlier, all of these cases of hypersensitivity involved either thiamine injections alone or a combination of injections and oral supplements. Might the oral supplements have been safe had it not been for the injections? Quite possibly. But it's my policy to be careful.

What, then, should you do about an oral thiamine supplement if you are allergic to thiamine injections? That's simple; you should take no supplements containing thiamine without your doctor's expressed approval. Keep in mind that some of the people who proved allergic to thiamine injections also developed intolerance to oral supplements. Through trial and error, it became apparent that these people could tolerate small amounts of oral

Recommended Dietary Allowances for Thiamine

Group/Age	Mg.
Infants 0–6 mon.	0.3
Infants 6–12 mon.	0.5
Children 1–3 yr.	0.7
Children 4–6 yr.	0.9
Children 7–10 yr.	1.2
Males 11–18 yr.	1.4
Males 19–22 yr.	1.5
Males 23–50 yr.	1.4
Males 51+ yr.	1.2
Females 11–22 yr.	1.1
Females 23–50 yr.	1.0
Females 51+ yr.	1.0
Pregnant women	1.4–1.5
Nursing women	1.5–1.6

Note: The U.S. RDA for thiamine is 1.5 mg.

thiamine, but not large doses.

Some experts recommend that doctors give a skin test before administering thiamine by injection. This allows screening for allergy before giving thiamine shots.

THE STAR SYSTEM SHINES ON THIAMINE

Now let's sort these facts about thiamine safety into each of the five categories of the star system. First, though, I would like to say that no matter how diverse these reactions, and no matter how severe, it serves us well to remember that these reactions apparently are rare.

Side effects—As is the case for some of the other vitamins, side effects from thiamine don't seem to occur in the absence of an actual toxic reaction. So I feel that these signs are better classified under acute ailments or long-term problems.

Acute ailments—I have found no reports of acute ailments occurring within a few hours or days of taking an oral thiamine supplement. For thiamine injections, the reverse is true; within minutes or hours there are reports of itching, weakness, pain, sweating (sometimes intense), nausea, sensations of tingling or feeling about to faint, and tightness of the throat. Serious symptoms of heart and lung distress, as well as death, have occurred from these injections also. Sometimes these reactions to the injections develop over a short period of taking them; in other cases, the reactions occur only after many injections have been given.

Long-term problems—For oral thiamine supplements, long-term toxicity can produce signs of too much thyroid hormone: headache, irritability, trembling, rapid pulse, and insomnia. Intolerance to thiamine injections can develop over long-term use, producing the same symptoms listed under acute ailments.

Conflicting combinations—These fall into several categories. First, common antacids can inactivate thiamine. The reason is simple; thiamine has trouble surviving in their acid-neutralizing presence. This should be of concern, however, only among people who use antacids routinely. If you do, consult your doctor.

One type of diuretic, or "water pill," is known to increase excretion of thiamine. This type is known as the "mercurial" class. Common diuretics, such as Diuril, Hydrodiuril, Dyazide, and Renese, do not fall into this category.

Barbiturates, notorious for their potential to be abused, can also decrease absorption of thiamine. Seconal, Amytal, Butisol, Nembutal, and phenobarbital, as well as some lesser-known drugs, belong to this class of drugs. Though these interactions have been recorded, I found no evidence that their use is causing widespread problems with thiamine nutrition.

Finally, high doses of thiamine may enhance the effects of drugs known as neuromuscular blocking agents. These are sometimes used along with anesthesia to relax certain types of muscle during surgery. The possibility of this affecting you is small, but if you ever are a candidate for surgery, you should be sure to discuss your supplement habits with your doctor, surgeon, and the anesthesiologist.

Hidden consequences—Thiamine has been linked to false positive results in two laboratory tests: for uric acid (of importance in gout) and for urobilinogen. It may also interfere with a correct reading in a test for the level of theophylline in the blood. Theophylline is not a substance that occurs naturally in the body; it is a drug used to treat bronchial asthma and to dilate blood vessels.

HOW MUCH IS TOO MUCH

For thiamine, it's not easy to say how much is too much, simply because there are so few reports of toxicity from oral supplements.

Of course, the absence of reports sends a very strong message that few of us are likely to get too much. When you consider that preparations containing many times the RDA of 2 mg. have been marketed for decades, with only a handful of adverse effects reported, you tend to agree with the American Society of Hospital

Pharmacists, which advises, "Thiamine is usually nontoxic even following administration of large doses." The pharmacists note, however, that serious reactions and even death have been associated with thiamine injections. But it is not accurate to equate these with oral thiamine supplements.

Of course, there are exceptions, such as Annamarie and Johanna. Based on their stories, I would have to say that 5 mg. daily is the lowest oral dose known to have caused ill effects. But Annamarie, the victim here, may have sensitized herself to even this modest level of thiamine by taking enormous amounts (10,000 mg. daily) not long before. I would estimate, then, that doses lower than 5 mg. are unlikely to harm a healthy adult. At the same time, I feel that with so few other reports of toxic reactions, it is likely, but not guaranteed, that many healthy adults could tolerate substantially more.

Said pharmacologists Joseph DiPalma and David Ritchie in a recent review of the subject, "Aside from hypersensitivity reactions, few instances of toxicity of thiamine have been reported in the recent literature." That is pretty convincing evidence that the chance of overdosing is low.

These comments, of course, assume that you are not allergic or taking any drugs that interact with thiamine. If you are allergic to thiamine injections you should not take any supplement containing thiamine unless recommended by your doctor. Moreover, these findings should not be applied to infants or children, whose ability to handle high doses of thiamine is not established. Especially for infants, only supplementation prescribed by a doctor should be given.

These ifs, ands, and buts aside, thiamine seems like a nutrient that's not likely to cause problems. And what a relief that is.

C O O K I N G
for Thiamine

UNFORGETTABLE FOUR WHEAT BREAD
(Makes 1 loaf, 18 slices)

Thiamine: 0.31 mg. per slice
Calories: 157 per slice

This bread freezes well and makes excellent toast.

½ cup cracked wheat
1½ cups hot water
¼ cup safflower oil
½ teaspoon salt
1   package active dry
      yeast
2   tablespoons molasses
1   tablespoon malt
      extract (syrup)

2   tablespoons brewer's
      yeast
2   cups whole wheat
      flour
2   cups unbleached flour
¼ cup toasted wheat
      germ

In a large bowl, combine the cracked wheat, water, oil, and salt. Let stand for 10 minutes. Add active dry yeast, stirring to dissolve. Add molasses and malt and stir to combine. Add brewer's yeast, flours, and wheat germ, mixing to form a stiff dough. Turn out onto a floured surface and knead for about 7 minutes, kneading in additional flour if necessary.

Turn dough into an oiled bowl, turning to grease the top. Cover with plastic wrap and let rise in a warm place for 1 hour or until doubled in bulk.

Punch dough down and form into a loaf. Turn into a well-oiled 9 × 5-inch loaf pan and let rise again for about 30 minutes.

Mist the top with water and bake in a preheated 350°F oven for about 45 to 50 minutes, misting the top with water 15 and 30 minutes into baking. Remove from pan and let cool on wire rack.

C   O   O   K   I   N   G
for Thiamine—*continued*

MOO SHIU PORK

(Makes 4 servings)

Thiamine: 1.08 mg. per serving
Calories: 165 per serving

¾ pound lean pork, such
    as center cut chops
2 cloves garlic, minced
½ teaspoon minced fresh
    ginger
½ teaspoon cornstarch
½ teaspoon soy sauce
2 tablespoons beef stock

⅔ cup bamboo shoots,
    sliced
3 scallions, sliced into
    thin 1-inch pieces
2 tablespoons hoi sin
    sauce*
8 romaine lettuce leaves

Slice pork against the grain into 2½ × ½-inch slices and place in a small bowl. In a cup, mix together garlic, ginger, cornstarch, and soy sauce and pour over pork.

Spray a wok or sauté pan with no-stick spray and heat on medium-high for about 2 minutes. Add the stock, swirl around and quickly add the pork. Stir-fry for about 3 minutes, or until pork is cooked through. Quickly add the bamboo shoots, scallions, and hoi sin sauce and toss until combined. Remove from heat and serve the pork with romaine by wrapping a leaf around a portion of pork and eating by hand.

*Available at Oriental markets.

(continued)

C   O   O   K   I   N   G

for Thiamine—*continued*

CREAMY BEANY BROCCOLI SAUCE

(Makes about 2 cups)

Thiamine: 0.17 mg. per ¼ cup
Calories: 141 per ¼ cup

Toss this sauce with pasta (cook ½ pound for each cup of sauce), or serve over chicken, steamed vegetables, or fish. Or use as a topping for baked potatoes. It's also delicious as a sandwich spread or dip for raw vegetables.

1½ cups broccoli florets	½ cup ricotta cheese
2 cups cooked navy beans	½ cup milk
1 clove garlic	½ teaspoon dried oregano
¼ cup sunflower seeds	⅛ teaspoon ground nutmeg
1½ tablespoons olive oil	

Steam the broccoli until tender, about 8 to 10 minutes. When cool enough, puree broccoli with the beans, garlic, sunflower seeds, and oil in a food processor or blender until smooth. Add the ricotta, milk, oregano, and nutmeg and puree until smooth. The sauce will keep, covered and refrigerated, for about a week, or frozen for up to three months. Bring to room temperature before serving.

Thiamine Content
of Selected Supplements

Dosage is one tablet or capsule unless otherwise indicated.

Supplement	Manufacturer	Mg.
Abdec Baby Drops (per 0.6 ml.)	Parke-Davis	1.00
Abdec Kapseal	Parke-Davis	5.00
Abdol with Minerals	Parke-Davis	2.50
Abron	O'Neal, Jones & Feldman	3.00
Allbee C-800	Robins	15.00
Allbee C-800 plus Iron	Robins	15.00
Allbee-T	Robins	15.50
Allbee with C	Robins	15.00
B6-Plus	Anabolic	10.00
B-C-Bid Capsules	Geriatric Pharm.	15.00
B-Complex Capsules	North American	1.50
B Complex Tablets	Squibb	0.70
Becomco	O'Neal, Jones & Feldman	2.25
Belfer	O'Neal, Jones & Feldman	2.00
Beminal 500	Ayerst	25.00
Beminal Forte with Vitamin C	Ayerst	25.00
Beta-Vite Liquid (per tsp.)	North American	10.00
Beta-Vite with Iron Liquid (per tsp.)	North American	10.00
Bewon Elixir (per tsp.)	Wyeth	0.25
Brewers Yeast	North American	0.06
Bugs Bunny	Miles	1.05
Bugs Bunny Plus Iron	Miles	1.05
Bugs Bunny with Extra C	Miles	1.05
Cal-M	Anabolic	45.00
Cal-Prenal	North American	2.00
C-B Bone Capsules	USV	25.00
Cebefortis	Upjohn	5.00
Cebetinic	Upjohn	2.00
Centrum	Lederle	2.25
Cherri-B Liquid (per 0.6 ml.)	North American	1.50
Chew-Vite	North American	3.00
Cluvisol 130	Ayerst	10.00
Cluvisol Syrup (per tsp.)	Ayerst	1.00

(continued)

Supplements—*continued*

Supplement	Manufacturer	Mg.
Dayalets	Abbott	1.50
Dayalets plus Iron	Abbott	1.50
Engram-HP	Squibb	1.70
Feminins	Mead Johnson	1.50
Femiron with Vitamins	J.B. Williams	1.50
Feostim	O'Neal, Jones & Feldman	3.00
Ferritrinsic	Upjohn	2.00
Filibon Tablets	Lederle	1.50
Flintstones	Miles	1.05
Flintstones Plus Iron	Miles	1.05
Flintstones with Extra C	Miles	1.05
Folbesyn	Lederle	10.00
Ganatrex (per 0.6 ml.)	Merrell Dow	1.50
Geralix Liquid (per tbsp.)	North American	3.30
Geriamic	North American	15.00
Gerilets	Abbott	**2.25**
Geriplex	Parke-Davis	5.00
Geriplex-FS Kapseals	Parke-Davis	5.00
Geriplex-FS Liquid (per 2 tbsp.)	Parke-Davis	1.20
Geritinic	Geriatric Pharm.	3.00
Geritol Junior Liquid (per tsp.)	J.B. Williams	5.00
Geritol Junior Tablets	J.B. Williams	2.50
Geritol Liquid (per tsp.)	J.B. Williams	5.00
Geritol Tablets	J.B. Williams	5.00
Gerix Elixir (per 2 tbsp.)	Abbott	6.00
Gerizyme (per tbsp.)	Upjohn	3.30
Gest	O'Neal, Jones & Feldman	1.70
Gevrabon (per 2 tbsp.)	Lederle	5.00
Gevral	Lederle	1.50
Gevral Protein	Lederle	2.20
Gevral T Capsules	Lederle	2.25
Gevrite	Lederle	1.50
Golden Bounty B Complex with Vitamin C	Squibb	4.00
Hi-Bee Plus	North American	20.00
Hi-Bee W/C Capsules	North American	15.00
Iberet	Abbott	6.00
Iberet-500	Abbott	6.00

Supplements—*continued*

Supplement	Manufacturer	Mg.
Iberet-500 Oral Solution (per tsp.)	Abbott	1.50
Iberet Oral Solution (per 0.6 ml.)	Abbott	1.50
Iberol	Abbott	3.00
Incremin with Iron Syrup (per tsp.)	Lederle	10.00
Lederplex Capsules	Lederle	2.00
Lederplex Liquid (per tsp.)	Lederle	2.50
Lederplex Tablets	Lederle	2.00
Lipoflavonoid Capsules	Cooper Vision Pharm.	0.33
Lipotriad Capsules	Cooper Vision Pharm.	0.33
Lipotriad Liquid (per tsp.)	Cooper Vision Pharm.	1.00
Livitamin Capsules	Beecham Labs	3.00
Livitamin Chewable	Beecham Labs	3.00
Livitamin Liquid (per tbsp.)	Beecham Labs	3.00
Lufa Capsules	USV	2.00
Methischol Capsules	USV	3.00
Multicebrin	Lilly	3.00
Multiple Vitamins	North American	3.00
Multiple Vitamins with Iron	North American	2.00
Multivitamins	Rowell	2.50
Myadec	Parke-Davis	10.00
Natabec	Parke-Davis	3.00
Natalins Tablets	Mead Johnson	1.70
Norlac	Rowell	2.00
Obron-6	Pfipharmecs	3.00
One-A-Day	Miles	1.50
One-A-Day Core C 500	Miles	1.50
One-A-Day Plus Iron	Miles	1.50
One-A-Day Vitamins Plus Minerals	Miles	1.50
Optilets-500	Abbott	15.00
Optilets-M-500	Abbott	15.00
Orexin Softabs	Stuart	10.00
Os-Cal Forte	Marion	1.70
Os-Cal Plus	Marion	0.50
Paladec (per tsp.)	Parke-Davis	3.00
Paladec with Minerals	Parke-Davis	3.00

(continued)

Supplements—continued

Supplement	Manufacturer	Mg.
Panuitex	O'Neal, Jones & Feldman	1.50
Peritinic	Lederle	7.50
Poly-Vi-Sol Chewable	Mead Johnson	1.05
Poly-Vi-Sol Drops (per 0.6 ml.)	Mead Johnson	0.50
Poly-Vi-Sol with Iron Chewable	Mead Johnson	1.05
Poly-Vi-Sol with Iron Drops (per 0.6 ml.)	Mead Johnson	0.50
Probec-T	Stuart	15.00
Roeribec	Pfipharmecs	10.00
S.S.S. Tablets	S.S.S.	5.00
S.S.S. Tonic (per tbsp.)	S.S.S.	1.70
Stresscaps Capsules	Lederle	10.00
Stresstabs 600	Lederle	15.00
Stresstabs 600 with Iron	Lederle	15.00
Stresstabs 600 with Zinc	Lederle	20.00
Stuart Formula	Stuart	1.50
Stuart Hematinic Liquid (per tsp.)	Stuart	1.70
Stuartinic	Stuart	6.00
Stuart Prenatal	Stuart	1.70
Super Plenamins	Rexall	2.30
Surbex	Abbott	6.00
Surbex 750 with Iron	Abbott	15.00
Surbex 750 with Zinc	Abbott	15.00
Surbex-T	Abbott	15.00
Surbex with C	Abbott	6.00
Thera-Combex H-P Kapseals	Parke-Davis	25.00
Theragran	Squibb	10.30
Theragran Liquid (per tsp.)	Squibb	10.00
Theragran-M	Squibb	10.00
Theragran-Z	Squibb	10.30
Therapeutic Vitamins	North American	10.00
Thera-Spancap	North American	6.00
Thex Forte	Medtech	25.00
Tonebec	A.V.P.	15.00
Tri-B-Plex	Anabolic	50.00
Unicap	Upjohn	1.50
Unicap Chewable	Upjohn	1.50
Unicap T	Upjohn	10.00

Supplements—*continued*

Supplement	Manufacturer	Mg.
Vi-Aqua	USV	5.00
Vicon-C	Glaxo	20.00
Vicon Iron	Glaxo	2.00
Vicon Plus	Glaxo	10.00
Vigran	Squibb	1.50
Vigran Chewable	Squibb	0.70
Vigran plus Iron	Squibb	1.50
Vio-Bec	Rowell	25.00
Vio-Geric	Rowell	5.00
Vi-Penta Multivitamin Drops (per 0.6 ml.)	Roche	1.00
Vitagett	North American	3.00
Vita-Kaps-M Tablets	Abbott	3.00
Vita-Kaps Tablets	Abbott	3.00
Vitamin-Mineral Capsules	North American	3.00
Viterra	Pfipharmecs	3.00
Viterra High Potency	Pfipharmecs	10.00
VM Preparation (per 2 tbsp.)	Roberts	3.00
Z-Bec	Robins	15.00
Zymacap Capsules	Upjohn	2.25
Zymalixir Syrup (per tsp.)	Upjohn	1.00
Zymasyrup (per tsp.)	Upjohn	1.00

Source: Adapted from the American Pharmaceutical Association, *Handbook of Nonprescription Drugs*, 7th ed. (1982), 240–57.

Note: This chart is intended only as a guide. Vitamin formulations change periodically; always read product labels for accurate and up-to-date information on their nutrient levels.

5

Riboflavin
(Vitamin B$_2$)

Considering thiamine's safety record, it deserves a reputation as one hard act to follow. But I wouldn't hesitate to put riboflavin to the test. In fact, I'm going to give you a sneak preview right here. Riboflavin's safety record is even better than thiamine's.

Like thiamine, riboflavin is often considered a "leader nutrient"—a marker for other healthful nutrients in food. Riboflavin works at the most basic level in your body—helping you to metabolize proteins, fats, and carbohydrates.

Deficiency of riboflavin, when it occurs, often does not do so alone. Rather, it is often only a part of a multiple deficiency of B vitamins. Naturally, treatment in such cases emphasizes the B complex, not just riboflavin alone.

But riboflavin intake in the United States is generally good, so it's a rare day when American nutritionists see riboflavin deficiency. Such is not the case in some parts of the world, however, where mild symptoms of riboflavin deficiency are not uncommon.

Symptoms of riboflavin deficiency can affect various parts of the body. Often the eyes are the first to react, becoming sensitive to light and quick to tire. Itching, watering, and soreness of the eyes are still other signs. Later, cracks in the skin around the corners of the mouth may occur. This is perhaps the best-known symptom of riboflavin deficiency, and you might have heard nutritionists refer to it by its official name: cheilosis.

THE SLATE IS CLEAN

But what about the chances of overdosing on riboflavin?

Such chances are very slim indeed. In fact, I hardly can believe the safety record that riboflavin boasts.

My trusty computer searched through 4.5 million journal articles, seeking out cases of riboflavin overdoses. And it didn't find a single one!

The results of my research match those of others who have studied the issue of riboflavin overdose. My favorite nutrition textbook, *Human Nutrition and Dietetics*, comments, "Thus far, no one seems to have been adversely affected by treatment with synthetic riboflavin." And the nutritionist's bible, the ninth edition of *Recommended Dietary Allowances*, says simply, "No cases of toxicity have been reported."

In my quest for information, however, I did find some things that you should know about riboflavin. It can interact with certain drugs. It can interfere with laboratory tests, too.

Let's turn, then, to the star system and take a look at the facts.

THE STAR SYSTEM SHINES ON RIBOFLAVIN

This is going to be a breeze, so here goes.

Side effects—High doses of riboflavin are known to make the urine very yellow. This is not surprising to the laboratory scientist, for in its pure form, riboflavin is yellow to orange-yellow in color.

Acute ailments—No such reactions to riboflavin are known.

Long-term problems—No toxic reactions to long-time use of riboflavin have been reported.

Conflicting combinations—Certain prescription drugs seem to be fond of interacting with riboflavin, and I'll be telling you about them right here. First, though, I want to comment that although these interactions exist, their effects don't fall under the now nonexistent category of riboflavin overdose. More often than not, the drugs in question decrease your body's absorption of riboflavin. That is much different than causing a toxic reaction. There are other types of interactions, however, so let's look at the complete picture.

GOUT DRUGS. The antigout drug, probenecid, decreases the body's absorption of riboflavin. This drug is also known by the brand names Benemid and ColBenemid. Combination pills containing both probenecid and antibiotics are also available (by prescription only, of course).

ANTIBIOTICS. Riboflavin doesn't fare well in the company of three antibiotics—tetracycline, erythromycin, and streptomycin. It's not that the combinations will make you sick, but rather that riboflavin is unstable in the presence of these drugs and may not survive. So if you're taking any of them, try to remember not to take a supplement containing riboflavin at the same time. That way, you're better assured that usable riboflavin from the supplement will be available to your body. A different and infrequently used antibiotic, chloramphenicol, may actually increase the need for riboflavin.

CENTRAL NERVOUS SYSTEM DRUGS. Three drugs that affect the central nervous system also may interact with riboflavin. These include:

• Amitriptyline, an antidepressant better known by the brand name Elavil
• Chlorpromazine, an antipsychotic drug commonly called by its best-known brand name, Thorazine
• Imipramine, an antidepressant related to Elavil, that you may also know by the brand name, Tofranil

Just how important these interactions may be remains to be determined, but if you have any concerns, ask your doctor.

DIURETICS. Diuretics ("water pills") that belong to the thiazide class of drugs can cause an increase in the amount of riboflavin that your body excretes. Again, this is a matter to take up with your doctor if you take these drugs. The list of drugs that fall under this category is very long, but a partial list including the most common brand names follows:

- Aldactizide
- Aldoril
- Apresazide
- Apresoline
- Corzide
- Diuril
- Dyazide
- Hydrodiuril
- Hydropres
- Naturetin
- Rauzide
- Ser-Ap-Es

ORAL CONTRACEPTIVES. Rounding out the list of drugs that interact with riboflavin is the birth control pill. Studies have found that the Pill may change the way that the body uses vitamins such as riboflavin. Whether these changes in fact increase the riboflavin needs of Pill users remains to be determined.

A SPECIAL NOTE TO CANCER PATIENTS. Riboflavin appears to affect the way that cancer cells respond to one of the anticancer drugs, methotrexate. Other research has shown that riboflavin deficiency inhibits growth of cancerous tumors. So, even though I have already stated my opposition to cancer patients' self-administering a supplement program, I want to underscore that cancer patients should not take riboflavin supplements without the approval of their cancer specialists.

Hidden consequences—There are no reports of riboflavin supplements masking the symptoms of disease. However, because of its yellow-orange color, excess riboflavin can interfere with medical tests where color is the basis for a correct reading. Some of the tests that may be affected are uncommon ones. Blood tests for the enzyme acetoacetate decarboxylase or for catecholamines (substances that transmit impulses in the brain) may be affected. Excess riboflavin may also prevent accurate readings of urine tests for catecholamines and for urobilin. Of course, you may never have tests for any of these.

As for common tests that might be affected by high intakes of riboflavin, the one to note is a simple urinalysis. If the color of the

(continued on page 80)

The Diet Detective Searches for Riboflavin

Ready to find out how much riboflavin your diet contains? All you need is a pencil and pad to check off any of the following foods that you ate today or yesterday and record the point values for each.

1 point
½ avocado
1 cup brussels sprouts
1 cup kale
1 cup mustard or beet greens
1 cup summer squash
10 okra pods
1 cup cocoa from mix
1 cup dry curd cottage cheese
1 wedge Camembert cheese
½ chicken breast, fried
4 ounces chicken
⅕ recipe Tuna Helper
4 ounces salmon
4 ounces oysters
1 tin sardines
2 ounces chipped, dried beef
1 cup corned beef hash
4 ounces ground beef
2 slices bread
3 pancakes (4 inches in diameter)
1 waffle
1 packet Quaker instant oats
⅓ cup 100% Natural cereal

2 points
1 cup asparagus
1 cup broccoli
1 cup mushrooms
1 cup spinach
1 cup turnip or collard greens
1 cup winter squash
⅓ cup chopped almonds
1 Italian sandwich roll
2 slices Hollywood dark bread
1 English muffin
⅔ cup any of the following cereals: Corn Bran, Crispy Wheats 'n Raisins, Golden Grahams, Grape-nuts flakes, Honey Bran, Raisins, Rice & Rye, Special K, Team, Wheaties
1 cup Cheerios or Quisp cereal
1 packet instant cream of wheat
1 chicken thigh
4 ounces dark meat chicken
4 ounces duck or goose, with skin

4 ounces turkey
4 ounces beef round or
  sirloin
⅕ recipe Hamburger
  Helper
4 ounces veal
4 ounces lamb
4 ounces pork loin or roast
4 ounces baked shad
4 ounces mackerel, canned
  or fresh
1 cup whole milk yogurt
1 cup flavored low-fat
  yogurt
1 cup creamed cottage
  cheese, 4 percent fat
1 cup ice cream
1 Fudgsicle
½ cup pudding or custard

3 points
1 cup low-fat cottage
  cheese
1 cup milk, plain or
  flavored
1 cup plain low-fat yogurt
1 cup ricotta cheese
1 fast-food milk shake
1 cup soft-serve ice milk
1 cup most children's
  cereals
⅔ cup any of the following
  cereals: Cracklin' Oat
  Bran, 40% Bran cereal,
  Fruit 'n Fibre, Life
⅓ cup any of the following

cereals: Bran Buds,
  granola, Grape-nuts,
  100% bran cereal
1 cup Cheerios or King
  Vitaman cereal
¼ frozen medium pizza
4 ounces duck or goose
1 meat or chicken pie

4 points
¼ cup Scramblers egg
  substitute
4 ounces Cornish hen
⅔ cup Buc Wheats cereal

5 points
½ cup chicken liver
2 slices braunschweiger
1 cup Kaboom cereal

7 points
⅔ cup Total or Corn Total
  cereal

9 points
⅔ cup Product 19 cereal

10 points
2 slices liver cheese

13 points
⅔ cup Most cereal

28 points
4 ounces beef liver, fried
4 ounces calf liver, fried

(continued)

The Diet Detective—
Riboflavin (continued)

Scoring

Add up your points. To that number, attach a zero. The result is an estimate of the percentage of the U.S. RDA for riboflavin in your diet. For instance, if your points total 8, add a zero for a level of 80 percent of the U.S. RDA.

Of course, the quiz provides only an estimate. Your total intake of riboflavin probably exceeds the level estimated by the quiz, for it was impossible to include all foods that supply any amount of riboflavin. Such a list would be extremely long.

If you want to take a riboflavin supplement, do consider the level in your diet before determining your dosage.

If you ate foods not listed here that you know to be good sources of riboflavin, you nonetheless can account for them. After you have your final score and have converted it to a percent of the U.S. RDA, add the percent of the U.S. RDA for riboflavin listed on the food's nutrition label. For example, if you scored 80, but ate a food not listed that contains 30 percent of the U.S. RDA, add 80 and 30 for a score of 110 percent of the U.S. RDA. You obviously make the grade!

---

urine is to be used as a basis for diagnosis, be sure to let the laboratory know if you are taking a high-dose riboflavin supplement. You might want to skip the supplement for a few days to a week preceding your test.

RUNNING UP YOUR NEED FOR RIBOFLAVIN

The idea that athletes have unique nutrient needs has been around for decades. What there hadn't been was first-rate research to support the idea, so nutritionists tended to dismiss the notion as undocumented. But the times they are a-changing.

Daphne Roe, M.D., professor of nutrition at Cornell University, has pioneered one important aspect of the athlete's kitchen: how activity affects the need for riboflavin. And her findings in one study deserve our attention.

Dr. Roe found that women aged 21 to 32 who jogged 30 to 50 minutes a day for six weeks needed almost twice the Recommended Dietary Allowance (RDA) for riboflavin. Those who lost weight while on the jogging program needed still more riboflavin.

These results came as a surprise to all, but it's not hard to make sense out of them. Riboflavin is intimately involved in the process of burning calories for energy, something that you do more of when you are active.

Recommended Dietary Allowances for Riboflavin

Group/Age	Mg.
Infants 0–6 mon.	0.4
Infants 6–12 mon.	0.6
Children 1–3 yr.	0.8
Children 4–6 yr.	1.0
Children 7–10 yr.	1.4
Males 11–14 yr.	1.6
Males 15–22 yr.	1.7
Males 23–50 yr.	1.6
Males 51+ yr.	1.4
Females 11–22 yr.	1.3
Females 23–51+ yr.	1.2
Pregnant women	1.5–1.6
Nursing women	1.7–1.8

Note: The U.S. RDA for riboflavin is 1.7 mg.

SPECIAL CONDITIONS, SPECIAL NEEDS

Dr. Roe's findings join a time-honored list of life stages and conditions known to increase riboflavin needs. Chief among these are growth, pregnancy, and breast-feeding. Note the differences in the RDA allowances for various ages and conditions in the table on page 81.

Hepatitis, cirrhosis, and biliary obstruction decrease your body's ability to absorb riboflavin. Illnesses involving fevers, diarrhea, vomiting, or other physical stress can also increase the need for riboflavin.

It's important, though, to make a distinction between minor physical stress—a short-lived fever or stomach upset—and major physical stress. Major surgery, serious burns, and broken bones are good examples of the latter. In 1952, the National Academy of Sciences published a book, *Therapeutic Nutrition*, recommending a riboflavin intake of almost six times the RDA during severe physical trauma.

The average American daily diet contains almost 2.5 milligrams (mg.) of riboflavin. That's almost more than twice the RDA for adult women and a good bit more than the recommended level for men, too.

A VITAMIN FOR VEGETARIANS

But the ill and the stressed aren't the only ones who have a special need for riboflavin. There is concern that vegans—vegetarians in the strictest sense, who eat no animal products whatsoever—may not get enough of the vitamin in their diets. Strict vegetarians need to eat large amounts of green vegetables, legumes, grains or wheat germ, and seeds just to meet their RDA allowance for riboflavin. And many of them don't. In one study, for instance, about a fourth of strict vegetarians consumed less than 60 percent of the dietary standard for riboflavin.

However, their riboflavin needs may be smaller than those of other adults because strict vegetarians usually consume fewer calories than those who eat animal products. And your body's need for riboflavin directly corresponds to the number of calories consumed.

Nevertheless, if you're a strict vegetarian and also from the better-safe-than-sorry school, you will probably want to take a riboflavin supplement. At best it will enhance your health, and at worst should do no harm.

C O O K I N G
for Riboflavin

LEMON CHICKEN WITH BROCCOLI AND ALMONDS

(Makes 4 servings)

Riboflavin: 0.45 mg. per serving
Calories: 421 per serving

1 pound skinless, boneless chicken breast	2 cups broccoli florets boiling water for blanching
2 tablespoons freshly squeezed lemon juice	1½ teaspoons peanut oil
½ teaspoon minced fresh ginger	½ teaspoon cornstarch dash of soy sauce dash of sesame oil
1 clove garlic, minced	¼ cup sliced almonds
2 teaspoons white grape juice	

Cut the chicken into 1-inch chunks and place in a shallow glass baking dish. In a cup, combine the lemon juice, ginger, garlic, and grape juice and pour over chicken. Cover and refrigerate for 1 hour.

Meanwhile, blanch the broccoli for 1 minute in the boiling water. Remove it with a strainer to let it cool.

Heat a wok or large sauté pan for about 30 seconds on high heat. Add the peanut oil and let it heat for about 10 seconds. Use a slotted spoon to add the chicken, leaving the marinade in the dish. Stir-fry the chicken for about 5 minutes, or until cooked through.

(continued)

C O O K I N G
for Riboflavin—continued

While the chicken is cooking, prepare a sauce by adding the cornstarch to the marinade. Combine well. Add the soy sauce and sesame oil.

Add the broccoli to the chicken and let it heat through. Make a well in the center of the wok and add the sauce, stirring constantly, until it thickens. Toss so the sauce coats all the ingredients. Add the almonds, toss again, and serve.

SPINACH AND RICOTTA PIE

(Makes 4 servings)

Riboflavin: 0.33 mg. per serving
Calories: 323 per serving

Crust:

⅓ cup whole wheat pastry flour
⅓ cup unbleached white flour
¼ teaspoon dried thyme
2 tablespoons safflower oil
1 to 2 tablespoons ice water

Filling:

1 cup fresh spinach, tightly packed
2 tablespoons fresh basil
1 clove garlic
15 ounces part-skim ricotta cheese
1 egg
¼ cup grated mozzarella cheese
½ teaspoon dijon-style mustard

Preheat oven to 375°F.

To make the crust, place the flours and thyme into a food processor. With the motor running, gradually add the oil. Then add the ice water, a teaspoon at a time, until the mixture forms a ball of dough. Wrap the ball in wax paper

C   O   O   K   I   N   G
for Riboflavin—*continued*

and refrigerate while you prepare the filling.

To make the filling, add the spinach, basil, and garlic into the food processor and process until finely minced. With the motor running, add the ricotta cheese, egg, mozzarella cheese, and mustard, and process until creamy and well combined.

Lightly oil a 9-inch pie plate. Sprinkle a rolling pin with flour, then roll out the dough on a floured pastry board, making it large enough to fit the pie plate. Set the dough in the pie plate, trim if necessary and crimp the edges. Scoop in the filling and bake for about 35 minutes. Let stand for 5 minutes, then serve.

NOTE: If you don't have a food processor, make the crust by working the oil into the flour with a pastry blender or long-tined fork. Prepare the filling in a blender.

FUZZY PEACH NECTAR

(Makes 2 servings)

Riboflavin: 0.37 mg. per serving
Calories: 130 per serving

2	medium peaches, peeled and pitted	¼	teaspoon vanilla extract
	dash of freshly grated nutmeg	1	tablespoon honey
3	drops almond extract	1½	cups skim milk

Slice peaches into a blender and add the nutmeg, almond extract, vanilla extract, and honey and process until smooth. With the motor running, add the milk and combine well. Serve immediately.

Riboflavin Content
of Selected Supplements

Dosage is one tablet or capsule unless otherwise indicated.

Supplement	Manufacturer	Mg.
Abdec Baby Drops (per 0.6 ml.)	Parke-Davis	1.20
Abdec Kapseal	Parke-Davis	3.00
Abdol with Minerals	Parke-Davis	2.50
Abron	O'Neal, Jones & Feldman	3.00
Allbee C-800	Robins	17.00
Allbee C-800 plus Iron	Robins	17.00
Allbee-T	Robins	10.00
Allbee with C	Robins	10.00
B6-Plus	Anabolic	2.40
B-C-Bid Capsules	Geriatric Pharm.	10.00
B-Complex Capsules	North American	2.00
B Complex Tablets	Squibb	0.70
Becomco	O'Neal, Jones & Feldman	2.60
Belfer	O'Neal, Jones & Feldman	2.00
Beminal 500	Ayerst	12.50
Beminal Forte with Vitamin C	Ayerst	12.50
Brewers Yeast	North American	0.02
Bugs Bunny	Miles	1.20
Bugs Bunny Plus Iron	Miles	1.20
Bugs Bunny with Extra C	Miles	1.20
Cal-Prenal	North American	2.00
C-B Bone Capsules	USV	10.00
Cebefortis	Upjohn	5.00
Cebetinic	Upjohn	2.00
Centrum	Lederle	2.60
Cherri-B Liquid (per 0.6 ml.)	North American	0.30
Chew-Vite	North American	2.50
Cluvisol 130	Ayerst	5.00
Cluvisol Syrup (per tsp.)	Ayerst	1.00
Dayalets	Abbott	1.70
Dayalets plus Iron	Abbott	1.70
Engram-HP	Squibb	2.00
Feminins	Mead Johnson	3.00
Femiron with Vitamins	J.B. Williams	1.70

Supplements—*continued*

Supplement	Manufacturer	Mg.
Feostim	O'Neal, Jones & Feldman	1.00
Ferritrinsic	Upjohn	2.00
Filibon Tablets	Lederle	1.70
Flintstones	Miles	1.20
Flintstones Plus Iron	Miles	1.20
Flintstones with Extra C	Miles	1.20
Folbesyn	Lederle	5.00
Ganatrex (per 0.6 ml.)	Merrell Dow	1.70
Geralix Liquid (per tbsp.)	North American	1.70
Geriamic	North American	5.00
Gerilets	Abbott	2.60
Geriplex	Parke-Davis	5.00
Geriplex-FS Kapseals	Parke-Davis	5.00
Geriplex-FS Liquid (per 2 tbsp.)	Parke-Davis	1.70
Geritinic	Geriatric Pharm.	3.00
Geritol Junior Liquid (per tsp.)	J.B. Williams	5.00
Geritol Junior Tablets	J.B. Williams	2.50
Geritol Liquid (per tsp.)	J.B. Williams	5.00
Geritol Tablets	J.B. Williams	5.00
Gerix Elixir (per 2 tbsp.)	Abbott	6.00
Gerizyme (per tbsp.)	Upjohn	3.30
Gest	O'Neal, Jones & Feldman	2.00
Gevrabon (per 2 tbsp.)	Lederle	2.50
Gevral	Lederle	1.70
Gevral Protein	Lederle	2.20
Gevral T Capsules	Lederle	2.60
Gevrite	Lederle	1.70
Golden Bounty B Complex with Vitamin C	Squibb	4.80
Hi-Bee W/C Capsules	North American	10.00
Iberet	Abbott	6.00
Iberet-500	Abbott	6.00
Iberet-500 Oral Solution (per tsp.)	Abbott	1.50
Iberet Oral Solution (per 0.6 ml.)	Abbott	1.50
Iberol	Abbott	3.00
Lederplex Capsules	Lederle	2.00

(continued)

Supplements—continued

Supplement	Manufacturer	Mg.
Lederplex Liquid (per tsp.)	Lederle	2.50
Lederplex Tablets	Lederle	2.00
Lipoflavonoid Capsules	Cooper Vision Pharm.	0.33
Lipotriad Capsules	Cooper Vision Pharm.	0.33
Lipotriad Liquid (per tsp.)	Cooper Vision Pharm.	1.00
Livitamin Capsules	Beecham Labs	3.00
Livitamin Chewable	Beecham Labs	3.00
Livitamin Liquid (per tbsp.)	Beecham Labs	3.00
Lufa Capsules	USV	2.00
Methischol Capsules	USV	3.00
Mucoplex	ICN	1.50
Multicebrin	Lilly	3.00
Multiple Vitamins	North American	2.50
Multiple Vitamins with Iron	North American	2.50
Multivitamins	Rowell	2.50
Myadec	Parke-Davis	10.00
Natabec	Parke-Davis	2.00
Natalins Tablets	Mead Johnson	2.00
Norlac	Rowell	2.00
Obron-6	Pfipharmecs	2.00
One-A-Day	Miles	1.70
One-A-Day Core C 500	Miles	1.70
One-A-Day Plus Iron	Miles	1.70
One-A-Day Vitamins Plus Minerals	Miles	1.70
Optilets-500	Abbott	10.00
Optilets-M-500	Abbott	10.00
Os-Cal Forte	Marion	1.70
Os-Cal Plus	Marion	0.66
Paladec (per tsp.)	Parke-Davis	3.00
Paladec with Minerals	Parke-Davis	3.00
Panuitex	O'Neal, Jones & Feldman	2.50
Peritinic	Lederle	7.50
Poly-Vi-Sol Chewable	Mead Johnson	1.20
Poly-Vi-Sol Drops (per 0.6 ml.)	Mead Johnson	0.60
Poly-Vi-Sol with Iron Chewable	Mead Johnson	1.20
Poly-Vi-Sol with Iron Drops (per 0.6 ml.)	Mead Johnson	0.60
Probec-T	Stuart	10.00

Supplements—*continued*

Supplement	Manufacturer	Mg.
Roeribec	Pfipharmecs	10.00
S.S.S. Tablets	S.S.S.	2.40
S.S.S. Tonic (per tbsp.)	S.S.S.	0.80
Stresscaps Capsules	Lederle	10.00
Stresstabs 600	Lederle	15.00
Stresstabs 600 with Iron	Lederle	15.00
Stresstabs 600 with Zinc	Lederle	10.00
Stuart Formula	Stuart	1.70
Stuart Hematinic Liquid (per tsp.)	Stuart	1.70
Stuartinic	Stuart	6.00
Stuart Prenatal	Stuart	2.00
Super Plenamins	Rexall	2.35
Surbex	Abbott	6.00
Surbex 750 with Iron	Abbott	15.00
Surbex 750 with Zinc	Abbott	15.00
Surbex-T	Abbott	10.00
Surbex with C	Abbott	6.00
Thera-Combex H-P Kapseals	Parke-Davis	15.00
Theragran	Squibb	10.00
Theragran Liquid (per tsp.)	Squibb	10.00
Theragran-M	Squibb	10.00
Theragran-Z	Squibb	10.00
Therapeutic Vitamins	North American	10.00
Thera-Spancap	North American	6.00
Thex Forte	Medtech	15.00
Tonebec	A.V.P.	10.00
Tri-B-Plex	Anabolic	20.00
Unicap	Upjohn	1.70
Unicap Chewable	Upjohn	1.70
Unicap T	Upjohn	10.00
Vi-Aqua	USV	5.00
Vicon-C	Glaxo	10.00
Vicon Iron	Glaxo	2.00
Vicon Plus	Glaxo	5.00
Vigran	Squibb	1.70
Vigran Chewable	Squibb	0.80
Vigran plus Iron	Squibb	1.70
Vio-Bec	Rowell	25.00

(continued)

Supplements—continued

Supplement	Manufacturer	Mg.
Vio-Geric	Rowell	5.00
Vi-Penta Multivitamin Drops (per 0.6 ml.)	Roche	1.00
Vitagett	North American	2.50
Vita-Kaps Tablets	Abbott	2.50
Vita-Kaps-M Tablets	Abbott	2.50
Vitamin-Mineral Capsules	North American	2.50
Viterra	Pfipharmecs	3.00
Viterra High Potency	Pfipharmecs	10.00
VM Preparation (per 2 tbsp.)	Roberts	2.00
Z-Bec	Robins	10.20
Zymacap Capsules	Upjohn	2.60
Zymalixir Syrup (per tsp.)	Upjohn	1.00
Zymasyrup (per tsp.)	Upjohn	1.00

Source: Adapted from the American Pharmaceutical Association, *Handbook of Nonprescription Drugs*, 7th ed. (1982), 240–57.

Note: This chart is intended only as a guide. Vitamin formulations change periodically; always read product labels for accurate and up-to-date information on their nutrient levels.

6

Niacin

It's inevitable. Whenever nutritionists talk of thiamine and riboflavin, niacin joins the conversation too. The three just go together like red, white, and blue.

Yet the safety picture for niacin differs distinctly from that of thiamine and riboflavin, clearly two of the safest vitamins on the shelf. Niacin, by contrast, can cause a laundry list of side effects when taken in high doses. I will be telling you the whole story, but first some basic facts.

Niacin, like riboflavin, works at a very basic level in your body. It teams up with other substances to form compounds that play a key role in the metabolism of fats and proteins. It also helps you use carbohydrates for energy.

These traditional roles of niacin are textbook stuff that nutritionists have known for decades. But niacin has also been on the cutting edge of new and exciting research. Today, it has earned its place in the treatment of certain blood fat disorders that increase the risk of heart disease. And some physicians say that it shows promise as part of new treatments for psoriasis.

In fact, these pioneering new uses of niacin have had an unanticipated benefit. In addition to exploring new treatments for disease, the scientists and doctors involved have collected useful information on the safety of niacin. Time now to tell the story.

WHAT'S IN A NAME?

Just as vitamin A comes in various forms, so does niacin. In fact, niacin is really a generic term referring to several substances. As far as supplements are concerned, only two are important: nicotinic acid and niacinamide. The term "nicotinamide," incidentally, is synonymous with niacinamide. The two terms can be used interchangeably. I prefer the term niacinamide; it more closely resembles the term niacin, which is what we are talking about.

Both nicotinic acid and niacinamide can perform the traditional functions of niacin. But only nicotinic acid combats high blood fats and dilates blood vessels. As a result, however, it possesses some side effects that niacinamide does not.

In light of the differences, it makes sense to examine the safety record of the two individually. That way niacinamide isn't held responsible for toxic reactions that only nicotinic acid can cause.

Incidentally, you may hear of substances called "nicotinic acid analogues" or "niacin analogues." These are actually drugs, not vitamins, and are designed to treat medical conditions. The analogues have no nutrient activity in your body; that is, they cannot be substituted for the niacin in food or supplements. Scientists are experimenting with a number of these analogues. Since they lack any vitamin activity, however, we won't be considering their safety record here.

THE FIRST OUTBREAK

The year was 1957, and the place Omaha, Nebraska. An alarmed physician notified the Omaha-Douglas County Health Department that two families in his care had phoned him reporting a bizarre illness after eating dinner. The two families had one factor in common; both had served hamburger at the evening meal. The first family affected told the following story, which is quoted exactly from the Nebraska State Medical Journal.

Is It Nicotinic Acid or Niacinamide?

Now that you know the difference between nicotinic acid and niacinamide, you may be scratching your head when you read "niacin" on food labels. Which form of niacin? you may be wondering.

Sometimes you have no choice but to wonder, because food manufacturers use both forms in certain classes of food. In certain foods, however, only niacinamide is used. And food companies that prepare bakery goods for infants use only nicotinic acid, not niacinamide in their products.

Here's a list for those curious to know which type is used where. It's based on a survey of food manufacturers conducted by the National Research Council.

Niacinamide Only
Baby cereals
Baby dinners
Baby formulas
Beverages, nonalcoholic
Fillings (e.g. pie)
Gelatins
Imitation dairy products
Poultry products
Puddings

Nicotinic Acid or Niacinamide
Baked goods
Baking mixes
Breakfast cereals
Grain products (pasta, rice)
Meat products
Milk products
Snack foods
Sweet sauces
Toppings and syrups
Vegetable proteins, reconstituted

The J.L. family ate supper at home Saturday night. Mrs. J.L. ate one hamburger with onion, garlic salt, mustard, chili, and dill pickle. She also had black coffee. As she arose from the table, she felt nauseated, but had no vomiting or diarrhea. The blood seemed to rush to the head and caused her ears to pound. The face and chest became fiery red. A slight headache developed. She went to bed and began to feel better in 20 minutes; after napping for 2 hours, she was fully recovered. Mr. J.L. consumed three hamburgers with no ill effect. A son, five years old, who ate less than one-half hamburger, had no trouble. A four-year-old daughter, after eating one hamburger with catsup, turned splotchy red in her face and upper body soon after her mother became ill. Swelling occurred about the eyes. The youngest daughter ate one-half hamburger and became fiery red over her entire body. She complained of severe itching. Neither girl was nauseated, and no one in the family had ever been sick like this before.

The J.L. family was but 1 of 38 affected by these bizarre symptoms. A total of 88 people reported symptoms similar to those

The Plague That Was Pellagra

It's the plague that was, but is no more. Nutritionists knew it as the notorious "plague of corn," but gave it an official name, too—pellagra.

At the turn of the century, pellagra was killing thousands of Americans every year. In fact, no other nutritional deficiency disease claimed nearly as many American lives. But the plague came to an end with the discovery that it was caused not by a germ, as originally believed, but by a diet deficient in niacin.

And why the nickname the "plague of corn"? Nutrition research established that the niacin in some foods is a form that the body does not absorb. Corn proved to be particularly troublesome in this regard, unless combined with an alkaline substance, such as the lime water often used in the making of tortillas. To this day, pellagra occurs most often where corn or grains dominate the diet.

But in the United States, niacin intake is generally good, thanks to widespread availability of foods containing niacin in a form the body can absorb. For decades now, bread has been enriched with usable niacin, and in recent years food manufacturers have been adding niacin to other foods such

of the mother and daughters of the J.L. family. Additional symptoms included sweating and abdominal cramps. According to the medical report, one man "became so warm that he undressed at once in the living room. His wife was frantic, thinking he was having a fatal seizure." The culprit: not the meat itself, but nicotinic acid that had been added to it to preserve the red color. Such an addition, incidentally, had not been approved by the state.

What does this experience have to do with supplement safety? That's simple. Though the problem here was food, not a supplement, this episode offers clues about how much niacin—in the form of nicotinic acid—will cause an acute reaction. And as you can imagine, your body will react the same way to excessive niacin from a supplement as the members of the affected families did.

---

as cereals and snacks. Moreover, Americans often consume ample amounts of tryptophan, a constituent of protein that the body usually can convert to niacin. As a result, deaths from pellagra plummeted from 5,418 in 1927 to 0 in 1977.

Niacin deficiency still does occur on occasion. Most commonly, the victims are alcoholics who have poor diets. Other possible causes of deficiency include chronic diarrhea, malabsorption diseases, cancer, prolonged fever, and deficiency of vitamin B_6. A lack of B_6 impairs the body's ability to turn the amino acid tryptophan into niacin. The first part of the body to show signs of niacin deficiency is usually the skin. Parts of the skin that are exposed to the sun or to heat appear to be sunburned. Later, ulcers and sores may develop on the skin; diarrhea, anxiety, depression, and irritability may follow. In the more advanced stages, niacin deficiency may lead to hallucinations, delirium, and confusion and ultimately to coma and death.

But none of these advanced symptoms have to happen. Accurate diagnosis and proper treatment can intervene successfully and promptly alleviate the disease that is an epidemic no more.

How much niacin had the victims consumed? Plenty! Health department officials obtained six samples of the meat in question. It contained 14 to 56 milligrams (mg.) of niacin per ounce. Some quick arithmetic reveals that a typical hamburger made from this meat would have supplied 42 to 168 mg. of niacin; that's two to nine times the U.S. Recommended Daily Allowance (U.S. RDA).

In the years that followed, five more outbreaks similar to this one were reported to medical journals. One of these outbreaks occurred at a Northwestern University sorority house in Evanston, Illinois. Of the experience, one victim said simply, "[I] felt funny as though I were under an oven lamp."

Another victim gave more detail. "[I] got pain in my stomach five minutes after dinner, chilled immediately after the pain started and then I turned red and my face felt as if sandpaper were being rubbed against my face. My knees were very hot and red, my eyes burned, and my elbows itched."

Health department investigators suspected that it might have been a practical joke, as it was pledge week at the sorority. But that suspicion proved false. The problem once again was meat that had been treated with nicotinic acid by the supplier, again in violation of local law.

Investigation of the other four outbreaks also revealed that the victims had eaten ground meat that had been treated with nicotinic acid to prolong that fresh red color that we associate with freshly ground beef. They had all had an unpleasant and alarming experience, but fortunately, no one seemed permanently harmed.

THE CORNMEAL CAPER

Meat isn't the only food that has caused niacin toxicity. Here's a story from a nursing home in Illinois that likewise tested the detective skills of the local health department.

On December 17, 1980, 42 percent of the patients in the nursing home became sick within 15 to 30 minutes after eating breakfast. More than half had a red rash on the face and arms; four developed redness from head to toe, in varying degrees; three experienced flushing and tingling in the face. The least affected were sick for only 15 minutes; the worst cases lasted almost 2 hours.

All the victims had eaten cornmeal mush for breakfast. The

staff noted, in retrospect, that the cornmeal had seemed unusually green—like "pea soup."

Chemists at the Food and Drug Administration (FDA) went to work, analyzing the cornmeal. According to its label, it contained added thiamine, riboflavin, niacin, and iron. Analysis showed that the cornmeal in question contained more than 100 times the amount of each nutrient declared on the label. Thus, a bowl of the cornmeal might have contained in the range of 100 to 150 mg. of niacin. (This is just a very rough estimate, as the reporting scientists did not calculate the amount per serving.)

At the Illinois Department of Health and the Center for Disease Control, there seemed little doubt that the niacin alone, apparently in the form of nicotinic acid, was responsible for the ill effects. How can we be confident that this was so? Because the symptoms experienced by the victims had never been associated with thiamine, riboflavin, or iron. But the symptoms involved here had been linked to excessive nicotinic acid in food many times before. It only follows that the nicotinic acid form of niacin was the culprit once again.

BAGELS, TOO?

Lest you think that only meat and cornmeal have been tainted with too much niacin, consider this brief report from Rochester, New York. At a 1983 brunch, about 20 percent of the guests became ill with rash, itching, and sensations of warmth.

Health investigators immediately suspected the pumpernickel bagels because they seemed unusually light in color. Sure enough, the bagels had been tainted with excessive niacin—about 190 mg. per bagel (about 10 times the U.S. RDA). Normally, such bagels would contain perhaps only 3 mg. of niacin.

Again, the symptoms were alarming, but no one was reported to have been significantly harmed.

FROM FOOD TO SUPPLEMENTS— LESSONS FROM THE HUMAN HEART

Of course, acute ailments such as these have also occurred from the use of niacin supplements. But the symptoms and effects are the same, so I won't be repeating the litany of complaints that

(continued on page 100)

The Diet Detective Searches for Niacin

Want to figure out how much niacin your diet actually contains? As usual, all you need is a little time and a pencil and pad to check off any of the following foods that you ate yesterday or today. Record the point values for each.

1 point
1 cup asparagus
1 boiled or baked potato
1 cup mashed potatoes
1 cup mixed vegetables
1 cup corn
1 cup peas
1 cup collard greens
2 slices bread
1 English muffin
3 pancakes (4 inches in diameter)
1 waffle
1 cup pasta or macaroni
1 cup barley
¼ cup sunflower seeds
2 ounces corned beef
2 ounces chipped beef
2 slices boiled ham
4 fish sticks
4 ounces bluefish
4 ounces flounder or sole
4 ounces oysters
2 slices turkey bologna
2 slices turkey pastrami
1 chicken wing or drumstick, fried
1 cup coconut milk

2 points
1 cup raw mushrooms
2 tablespoons peanut butter

1 Italian sandwich roll
⅔ cup any of the following cereals:
   Crispy Wheats 'n Raisins, Golden Grahams, Grape-nuts flakes, Honey Bran, Raisins, Rice & Rye, Special K, Team, Wheaties
1 cup Cheerios cereal
1 packet Quaker instant oats, any flavor
4 ounces beef rib roast
4 ounces ham roast
1 cup crabmeat
4 ounces cod
2 slices turkey ham
1 cup chicken liver
1 chicken thigh, fried

3 points
⅓ cup any of the following cereals:
   Bran Buds, granola, Grape-nuts, 100% bran cereal
⅔ cup any of the following cereals:
   Bran Chex, Corn Bran, 40% Bran cereal, Fruit 'n Fibre, Wheat Chex

1 cup Corn Chex or
   Cracklin' Oat Bran
1 cup most children's
   cereals
1 packet Mix 'n Eat cream
   of wheat
4 ounces ground beef or
   ground round
4 ounces beef round roast
⅕ recipe Hamburger
   Helper
4 ounces veal cutlet
1 lamb chop
1 veal chop
⅕ recipe Tuna Helper
1 tin sardines
4 ounces turkey

4 points
⅔ cup Buc Wheats cereal
⅓ cup peanuts
4 ounces lean sirloin steak
4 ounces leg of lamb
4 ounces pork roast
2 slices liver cheese
4 ounces veal rib roast
4 ounces red salmon

5 points
1 cup Kaboom cereal
4 ounces veal scallopini
4 ounces pink salmon
4 ounces mackerel
4 ounces broiled chicken
4 ounces Cornish hen

6 points
½ chicken breast, fried
4 ounces turkey breast

7 points
⅔ cup Total or Corn Total
   cereal
4 ounces oil-packed tuna
4 ounces chicken breast

8 points
4 ounces water-packed
   tuna

9 points
⅔ cup Product 19 cereal
4 ounces beef or calf liver,
   fried

10 points
4 ounces veal rump roast

13 points
⅔ cup Most cereal

Scoring
   Add up your points. To that number, attach a zero. The result is an estimate of the percentage of the U.S. RDA for niacin in your diet. For instance, if your points total 8, add a zero for a level of 80 percent of the U.S. RDA. Consider this level before determining whether to take supplemental niacin, and if so, how much.

(continued)

The Diet Detective—
Niacin (continued)

Of course, the quiz provides only an estimate. Your niacin intake is probably greater than the level estimated by the quiz. In the interest of brevity, only some of the many foods that supply a substantial amount of niacin could be included. This is particularly a problem for the B vitamins, because food manufacturers so often add extra amounts of them to countless foods.

If you ate foods not listed here that you know to be good sources of niacin, you nonetheless can account for them. After you have your final score and have converted it to a percent of the U.S. RDA, add the percent of the U.S. RDA for niacin listed on the food's nutrition label. For example, if you scored 70, but ate a food not listed that contains 30 percent of the U.S. RDA, add 70 and 30 for a score of 100 percent of the U.S. RDA. Right on the money!

---

sometimes accompany use of high-dose niacin supplements.

Instead, I would like to use the medical reports on niacin supplementation to explore the long-term problems that can result from high doses of supplemental niacin. By far the greatest source of these reports is the field of heart health. For almost a quarter century, heart experts have been using the nicotinic acid form of niacin to treat high blood fat levels.

Before I tell you about some of the adverse effects involved, I would like to mention a curious fact about the flushing and tingling that so often accompanies high doses of niacin. Many of the victims who ate tainted food reported this feeling. Those who begin to take high-dose supplements experience it, too, finding that this effect often subsides with regular use. As mentioned earlier, only the nicotinic acid form of niacin, not niacinamide, causes the flushing reaction.

The dose necessary to produce the flushing varies dramatically, but I estimate that a sensitive individual might experience it with as little as 50 to 75 mg. Others, however, will tolerate such a dose easily. In fact, a level of 50 to 75 mg. is high relative to the Recommended Dietary Allowances (RDA), but extremely small when compared to the levels used for treatment of high blood fats and other medical disorders. And many practitioners consider even enormous doses, such as 3,000 to 6,000 mg. daily, to be relatively safe for most patients.

THE LIVER PROTESTS

Not everyone, however, can tolerate thousands of milligrams of nicotinic acid with only some bothersome flushing. The liver, in particular, seems sensitive to excessive niacin and can make its objection known in a variety of ways. One such way is with jaundice, the liver disorder that causes deposits of yellow pigment in the whites of the eye. A number of cases apparently due to high-dose niacin have been reported in medical journals. I have chosen the following one because it involves the lowest dose that I have found linked to jaundice.

Here is the doctor's report, condensed from the *Journal of the American Medical Association.*

> A 69-year-old white man became bored with his inactive retirement and attempted suicide by car exhaust fumes. Five months earlier he had had an apparent stroke and developed a parkinsonian tremor, difficulty in walking, episodic memory difficulties, and increasing depression. He was lethargic but not comatose when admitted to a general hospital for emergency treatment after his suicide attempt, and three days later he was transferred to a psychiatric hospital.

> The patient was treated with supportive psychotherapy as well as thiamine, 500 mg. twice daily; niacin, 250 mg. three times daily; and ascorbic acid, 100 mg. three times daily. After recovery from the depression in five weeks, he was discharged to a nursing home, and while there he continued to receive niacin in the same dosage.

> Because of recurrent episodes of forgetfulness and confusion, he was readmitted to the psychiatric hospital for reevaluation six weeks later. At that time, the patient was jaundiced; results of physical examination were oth-

erwise normal. Niacin therapy was discontinued, and during the next two weeks the jaundice deepened.

The patient was transferred to a general hospital. After another ten days of increasing jaundice, further recovery was uneventful, with gradual disappearance of jaundice during the next several months.

A. Arthur Sugerman, M.D., and Charles G. Clark, M.D., the doctors who treated this man, underscored that his jaundice began to lessen within a month of stopping the niacin. But they conclude, "This case was alarming, however, in that the jaundice became more severe in the three weeks following discontinuation

Recommended Dietary Allowances for Niacin

Group/Age	Mg.*
Infants 0–6 mon.	6
Infants 6–12 mon.	8
Children 1–3 yr.	9
Children 4–6 yr.	11
Children 7–10 yr.	16
Males 11–18 yr.	18
Males 19–22 yr.	19
Males 23–50 yr.	18
Males 51+ yr.	16
Females 11–14 yr.	15
Females 15–22 yr.	14
Females 23–50 yr.	13
Females 51+ yr.	13
Pregnant women	15–16
Nursing women	18–19

Note: The U.S. RDA for niacin is 20 mg.

*60 mg. of the amino acid tryptophan can be substituted for 1 mg. of niacin.

of the drug therapy." Why things got worse before getting better, no one really knows for sure.

As I noted above, this was the lowest dose of niacin that I have found associated with jaundice. The other cases I have found involved much larger doses and may be more typical of the levels that are likely to cause problems. It might be, for instance, that the victim's age, 69, made him more susceptible to toxic effects than younger, relatively healthier people would be.

Other cases I have found involved doses in the 1,500 to 3,000 mg. range. Some of the affected patients were taking timed-release forms of nicotinic acid that doctors consider more likely to cause toxicity than the plain nicotinic acid in vitamin supplements. It also seems that toxicity develops more quickly on these timed-release forms, which require a doctor's prescription.

If jaundice is not apparent during high-dose nicotinic acid therapy, this does not mean all is well with the liver. Perhaps a third of patients on such high-dose therapy show abnormal results in one or more tests of liver function. So high doses call for regular monitoring, though abnormal test results are not a certain sign of actual damage to the liver.

On the positive side, it seems that the chances are quite good for full recovery from jaundice resulting from too much nicotinic acid. Stopping the medication is often the only treatment required.

ANOTHER LIVER COMPLAINT

In addition to cases of jaundice, I found the following case of "niacin hepatitis" believed to have been caused by high doses of nicotinic acid. It was reported in *Southern Medical Journal* by David J. Patterson, M.D., and his colleagues at the Veterans Administration Hospital in Houston and the Baylor College of Medicine. Here is a condensed version of their comments:

> A 41-year-old male schoolteacher was admitted to the Houston Veterans Administration Hospital in May 1980 with a five-day history of nausea, vomiting, anorexia [loss of appetite], weakness and dull abdominal and low back pain. Jaundice and [itching] had started only one day earlier.
>
> In June 1978 he had begun to take steadily increas-

ing daily doses of self-prescribed vitamin B complex for depression. After he had increased the amount of nicotinic acid from 900 mg. to 4,500 mg. per day over a six-month period, nausea, vomiting, and jaundice developed and he was seen as an outpatient. Liver function tests yielded abnormal results, and all medication was discontinued. The symptoms rapidly resolved. Two weeks later, he again started taking the vitamin B complex in small doses, gradually increasing the amount over the next 18 months. At that time he was taking 3,000 mg. [niacinamide], 4,500 mg. nicotinic acid, 1,000 mg. of vitamin B_1, 300 mg. vitamin B_6, and 250 mg. vitamin B_5 per day. He had discontinued all medication the day before admission [to the hospital].

Studies of the man's liver showed that it had sustained severe injury. He was treated with injected vitamin K; after four days in the hospital, the symptoms were gone. Follow-up tests performed one month and one year later yielded normal results.

THE DIABETIC'S EXPERIENCE

The schoolteacher I just told you about had self-prescribed the nicotinic acid. Many cases of vitamin overdose have happened the same way. Still others have resulted when people exceeded the levels prescribed by their doctors.

Other cases, though, begin and end with a doctor's best intentions. In the case I would like to tell you about next, doctors learned something important about nicotinic acid's effects on diabetes.

About two decades ago, a diabetic woman named Mae was admitted to the psychiatric ward of a Midwestern hospital. At the time, her blood sugar level was 108. Two weeks later, doctors began treating her with nicotinic acid, gradually increasing the dose to 3,000 mg. a day. After three weeks of treatment, Mae's blood sugar had skyrocketed to an alarming 372 and her urine contained large amounts of sugar.

The alarmed doctors made various changes in her insulin, to no avail. At the same time, doctors noticed that another diabetic patient being treated with nicotinic acid was showing similar signs of worsening diabetes. The nicotinic acid was stopped for both of them. Within two days, Mae's diabetic signs improved, and she was released shortly from the hospital. At home, she continued to improve.

Other cases like Mae's have been reported, and the lesson is clear: High doses of nicotinic acid should be taken with great caution by diabetics, and only with good reason and close follow-up.

THE STAR SYSTEM SHINES ON NICOTINIC ACID

Not harmless, you must be thinking about nicotinic acid. That's for sure, though most of the trouble has been either transient or the result of extremely high doses. Let's turn now to the star system for a complete wrap-up, including some facts about nicotinic acid safety that I haven't mentioned yet.

Side effects—Almost everyone will experience flushing from substantial doses of nicotinic acid. The amount necessary to produce flushing will vary, from a low of perhaps 50 to 75 mg. to much higher doses. Some people abandon nicotinic acid because of the flushing, but those who continue taking it often find that the flushing subsides in about two weeks.

There is no known harm to the flushing, although one doctor suspected that the anxiety it caused worsened the psychotic experience of a patient who was admitted to the hospital for psychiatric care a few days later. It is reasonable, I think, for anyone who experiences anxiety from this type of physical symptom to substitute niacinamide for nicotinic acid or lower the dosage. Of course, if only high-dose nicotinic acid will do, this isn't an alternative. The flushing, incidentally, doesn't necessarily bother everyone who experiences it.

Other side effects include the following skin afflictions: itching and dryness, rashes, a sensation of warmth, and brown pigmentation. These skin reactions reportedly disappear after use is discontinued. Also reported from large doses are the following: bloating, gas, hunger pains, heartburn, and dizziness.

Acute ailments—Acute reactions to accidental ingestion of nicotinic acid have been frightening because the victims had no idea that they had consumed (quite accidentally) a substance that can cause the rashes, tingling, itching, and flushing that accompanied these outbreaks. Those who know what to expect, of course, are not taken by surprise. Regardless, these symptoms are generally short-lived and leave no lasting harm. Fainting, rapid heartbeat, and low blood pressure have also occurred.

Long-term problems—People who regularly take high doses of nicotinic acid may experience some of the side effects listed above. In addition, the liver, digestive tract, and body metabolism can be affected, and it is these reactions that have the most potential to cause serious health problems.

First, the digestive complaints. Nausea, vomiting, diarrhea, and ulcers may occur. Whether the ulcers affect only those with a history of ulcers or emotional trauma has been a topic of debate. And as noted earlier, cases of jaundice and other signs of liver malfunction have been documented at high-dose levels (750 mg. or more).

Abnormal glucose tolerance has been found in both diabetics and normal subjects taking high doses of nicotinic acid. Blood levels of uric acid often increase dramatically on high doses, and as a result, those with gout may find their condition worsening.

Finally, there are isolated reports of nervousness and panic attributed to high doses of nicotinic acid: one case of hypothyroidism, and also blurring of vision and other eye problems.

Conflicting combinations—I found nothing particularly noteworthy to report in this department. The one exception pertains to a few drugs, known as ganglionic blocking drugs, that are used in severe cases of high blood pressure. Nicotinic acid may enhance the pressure-lowering effects of these medications, which are often used by injection. Also, the tuberculosis drug, isoniazid, may increase the need for niacin.

Hidden consequences—Nicotinic acid can interfere with accurate results in several laboratory tests. Most important, perhaps, is that testing for sugar in the urine with Benedict's reagent can be foiled by high doses.

Large doses of nicotinic acid also can interfere with the laboratory's ability to measure substances called catecholamines in either the blood or urine. These catecholamines play an important role in the functioning of the brain and nervous system and include the substances epinephrine, norepinephrine, and dopamine. Doctors don't routinely measure levels of these substances, but in the event that you do have such a test, be sure to inform your doctor about your supplement habits.

Finally, there is one report of nicotinic acid interfering with a liver scan. The patient was taking 3,000 mg. of nicotinic acid daily for six months. Her doctors found that while she was on this regimen, her liver would not take up the chemical used to make her liver visible to the scanning equipment. The woman stopped taking nicotinic acid for six weeks; the scanning technique then worked successfully.

NOTES FOR THOSE WITH SPECIAL NEEDS

Doctors consider nicotinic acid to be off-limits for people having hypersensitivity to it, abnormal liver function, duodenal ulcers or active peptic ulcers, severe low blood pressure, hemorrhaging, or bleeding of the arteries. As you probably realize from reading the section above, those who have diabetes or gout must take nicotinic acid only with utmost caution.

You also should be cautious with high doses if you have allergies, as nicotinic acid reportedly stimulates the body to release histamine. Histamine is the substance that your body secretes when you have an allergic reaction.

The safety of nicotinic acid for pregnant women has not been established, as most research has involved middle-aged men with high blood fat levels. Because of the lack of information, doses above the standard amounts given during pregnancy should be avoided.

HOW MUCH IS TOO MUCH

It's not easy to set a "safe" level for nicotinic acid, unless I play supercautious and tell you not to take a supplement containing more than the RDA. I don't think that route is fair, though, because many people obviously can tolerate much more. Saying exactly how much more is where I get mixed feelings.

On the one hand, there are thousands of people who have taken 3,000 to 6,000 mg. of nicotinic acid daily for months or years (to control blood fats) with no signs of toxicity. On the other hand are case reports of problems at doses as low as 750 mg. daily for three months. And of course the notorious, but not harmful, flushing can occur at doses under 100 mg.

Looking at the niacin content of common supplements on pages 115 to 119, it's apparent that quite a few products, particularly the "stress" formulas, contain 100 mg. of niacin. Most of these contain niacinamide, not nicotinic acid, but for the sake of argument, let's ask if those that do contain 100 mg. of nicotinic acid are safe. I think so.

How about doses in the 200 to 300 mg. range? I think that most people could tolerate such doses without harm. Five hundred to 750 mg.? More likely than not, but it is hard to give guarantees. The lowest toxic dose I found was 750 mg. taken for three months, but it is impossible to know whether 500 mg. taken for a longer period would be safe for all.

As for doses in the 1,000 mg. or higher range, many people have taken such doses without problems; others have had minor to major ones. I feel that you should have professional follow-up while on such a dose.

Because nicotinic acid is used as a food additive, its safety was recently assessed as part of an FDA review of food additives. The scientists who studied it concluded that "the adverse effects reported in animals and man have been associated with intakes at least a hundredfold greater than those likely to be achieved from fortification of foods." How much would you have to take to consume this trouble level of 100 times the amount added to foods? Conservatively, about 1,000 mg. daily. Obviously, these scientists believe that there is a wide margin of safety for nicotinic acid, and for most of us, I'd bet they are right.

I think you could argue that the most important issue isn't defining a level that is guaranteed not to cause unwanted effects in everyone. After all, the damage caused by too much nicotinic acid has rarely proved permanent in adults. So, for those who want to take the risk of high doses, perhaps the most important thing is to be aware of and alert for any of the signs of toxicity that we've discussed here. Should they occur, stop the supplement and see a doctor. So far, recovery has generally been the rule when medical attention is sought.

SAFETY AND SELF-MEDICATION

As someone who has been battling a high cholesterol level for more than a decade, I can understand the temptation to take high doses of nicotinic acid in an effort to treat high blood fats yourself. But I hope I can convince you that it's not a good idea.

There are five basic types of blood fat problems. Within these five groups, there are several subgroups. Nicotinic acid is recommended only for certain types, not all. A doctor will know whether nicotinic acid is appropriate for your type. The doctor will probably take tests periodically to ensure that your signs of liver function and other important indicators of good health remain normal.

So, if like me, you have a blood fat problem, please treat it right... let a doctor you trust handle it.

IS NIACINAMIDE NICER?

Take a look at the chart on pages 115 to 119 and you'll see that more supplements contain the niacinamide form of niacin than the nicotinic acid form. Does this mean that niacinamide is safer than nicotinic acid?

Actually, though niacinamide is used more often in multiple vitamin products, there is far less research on its safety than is the case for nicotinic acid. Why? Because nicotinic acid has been used therapeutically for blood fat problems, while niacinamide has not. As a result, little research has been published on its safety. Why, then, is niacinamide used so much more by supplement manufacturers? Because, unlike nicotinic acid, niacinamide does not cause flushing. That might lead you to think that it's less toxic. Actually, one animal test has indicated otherwise. As for research in humans, there hasn't been any that compared the two forms side by side to determine if one is safer than the other. Although reports on the safety of niacinamide are few and far between, here are two stories that I think you will want to know about.

SLEUTHING A MYSTERIOUS ITCH

A 71-year-old man, Jerome, visited a dermatologist complaining of itching and burning sensations. At first, the doctor was stumped, finding "nothing revealing" in the man's current health history.

Jerome had neglected to tell the doctor that he had been

taking Stresstabs, a common high-potency supplement, at the recommendation of another doctor. He stopped taking the Stresstabs, and the mysterious itch disappeared at once. A few days later, Jerome started taking Stresstabs again; the itch returned. Apparently a true scientist at heart, he waited another month or two, then repeated the experiment. The itching returned once more.

The next step was to determine which of the ingredients in Stresstabs might be responsible for the itching. The 100 mg. of niacinamide that the Stresstabs contained proved to be the suspect because Jerome experienced the same symptoms when he took another product containing only 50 mg. of niacin.

Jerome, unfortunately, went on to commit suicide for an unrelated reason, but his doctor, Frank Bures, M.D., continued to research his patient's problem. He found itching listed as a potential side effect of niacinamide in the prescribing information for two niacinamide supplements. His report of Jerome's case in a medical journal prompted four doctors experienced in the use of niacinamide to report their experience with its safety. I'll be telling you about their findings shortly.

ANOTHER CASE OF JAUNDICE

Jerome's case, no doubt, represents a highly unusual reaction to niacinamide, especially at the moderate dose contained in Stresstabs. The itching he suffered can hardly be considered a serious, or even toxic, reaction to niacinamide; rather, it is a side effect. But at a much higher dose—30 to 90 times as much—one man did sustain serious injury.

Stephen, age 35, was a graduate student in Chicago. One September day he was admitted to the hospital, complaining of a six-month period of nausea and vomiting that had already resulted in four hospitalizations. On one of these four occasions, doctors determined that he had a case of infectious hepatitis, a liver disease.

He told doctors that for a year and a half, he had been taking 3,000 mg. of niacinamide daily, which was discontinued at the hospital. Tests performed on this, his fifth admission, revealed abnormal liver function and Stephen was diagnosed as having jaundice. A liver biopsy showed that the organ had sustained serious injury. The symptoms improved quickly, however, and in three weeks, lab tests indicated that liver function had been restored to normal levels.

Stephen then revealed to the doctors that before each of his previous episodes of nausea and vomiting, he had increased his daily intake of niacinamide to 9,000 mg. to "feel better."

Wanting to get an idea of how much niacinamide was too much, his doctors asked Stephen if he would be willing to participate in a experiment in which he would be "rechallenged" with large doses of niacinamide. He agreed. Over a four-day period, doctors gave him increasing doses, starting with 3,000 mg. and building to the 9,000 mg. he had been taking before his previous illnesses.

After four days on 9,000 mg. of niacinamide, Stephen developed diarrhea. Two days later, he awoke with nausea, vomiting, loss of appetite, and fatigue. Once again, his liver function tests were abnormal.

The experiment ended, and in about three weeks, Stephen's lab tests were again back to normal. He abstained from niacinamide for the next six months, and during this time did not experience the troubling symptoms even once.

ADVERSE EFFECTS: HOW COMMON?

As you would expect, your chances of experiencing side effects from niacinamide will vary with the amount you take, among other factors. Again we are hampered in our search for facts by the relatively few reports that have been made on niacinamide safety. The few that are available, though, shed some light, so let's take a look.

The first report comes from a group of dermatologists who treated 204 psoriasis patients with 100 to 3,000 mg. of niacinamide daily. Most patients received 300 to 600 mg. daily. Of these 204 subjects, 8 complained of such symptoms as red patches on the face, dull headache, mild nausea, or flushing. (I, as well as the doctors, suspect that those who experienced flushing had inadvertently purchased nicotinic acid instead of niacinamide at the drugstore.)

A similar survey among 262 patients who received 3,000 mg. daily for 3 to 36 months found that only 5 percent of the patients complained of adverse effects. Their symptoms included: headaches, heartburn, nausea and other digestive complaints, sore mouth, hives, fatigue, and lightheadedness. One patient complained of difficulty focusing his eyes, dry hair, and a tight feeling in his face. Skin irritations also have been reported.

At higher doses, usually above 8,000 mg., more serious effects, such as vomiting and other flu-like symptoms, have been reported, as well as the liver problems that we talked about above.

NIACINAMIDE: A SUMMARY

That's everything I have to report on niacinamide. Since I have told you about everything I think you should know in the few preceding pages, I won't repeat myself with the usual star system listings.

Despite the small amount of research that has been done on niacinamide, what is known seems reassuring to me. So far, only a small minority of healthy adults have developed side effects at doses below 1,000 mg. Of course, no one has followed people on such a dose for a lifetime, and whether ill effects might occur after many years of use simply isn't known.

Certainly the 100 mg. of niacinamide found in high-potency supplements can be considered safe, save for Jerome's case of itching. Clearly, many people can tolerate quite a bit more. My advice is to use the same guidelines given earlier for nicotinic acid when determining doses of niacinamide.

C   O   O   K   I   N   G
for Niacin

JUST-FOR-BREAKFAST BARS

(Makes 8 bars)

Niacin: 21 mg. per bar
Calories: 221 per bar

2 tablespoons safflower oil
¼ cup honey

¼ cup maple syrup
2 cups Product 19 cereal
¼ cup chopped peanuts

Preheat oven to 350°F.

In a small skillet, slowly bring the oil, honey, and maple syrup to a boil. In a medium-size bowl, combine the cereal and peanuts and add the syrup mixture, stirring until all pieces are coated.

Line an 8 × 8-inch baking dish with foil and spray with no-stick spray. Press the mixture into the dish and bake for 15 minutes. Refrigerate for 20 to 30 minutes. Lift from baking dish, peel off foil, and cut into eight 2 × 4-inch bars.

TANGY TUNA WITH LIME DRESSING

(Makes 2 servings)

Niacin: 10 mg. per serving
Calories: 153 per serving

1 can (6½ ounces) water-packed tuna, drained
1 teaspoon minced fresh mint
1 teaspoon minced fresh parsley
2 scallions, minced

1 celery stalk, minced
freshly ground black pepper
1 teaspoon freshly squeezed lime juice
2 tablespoons plain yogurt
1 tablespoon mayonnaise

(continued)

C O O K I N G
for Niacin—*continued*

In a medium-size bowl, combine the tuna, mint, parsley, scallions, celery, and pepper.

In a small bowl, combine the lime juice, yogurt, and mayonnaise. Stir into the tuna mixture.

Serve as a salad, in lettuce cups; as a sandwich on whole grain bread; or with crackers as an appetizer.

VEAL SCALLOPINI WITH WILD MUSHROOMS

(Makes 4 servings)

Niacin: 7 mg. per serving
Calories: 204 per serving

¼ cup dried wild mushrooms, such as porcini, cepes, or mountain black
⅔ cup beef stock

¾ pound thinly sliced veal
2 tablespoons flour
2 teaspoons olive oil
juice of 2 limes
¼ teaspoon dried thyme

In a small bowl, soak the mushrooms in the stock for 20 minutes, or until soft.

Sprinkle the veal with the flour. Heat the oil in a 10-inch no-stick skillet and sauté the veal for about 2 minutes on each side. You may need to sauté the veal in batches.

Remove the veal to a heated platter. Add the lime juice, thyme, mushrooms and their stock to the skillet and cook over medium-high heat until sauce is reduced by half. Pour over the veal and serve immediately.

Niacin Content
of Selected Supplements

Dosage is one tablet or capsule unless otherwise indicated.

Supplement	Manufacturer	Mg.
Abdec Baby Drops (per 0.6 ml.)	Parke-Davis	10.0*
Abdec Kapseal	Parke-Davis	25.0*
Abdol with Minerals	Parke-Davis	20.0*
Abron	O'Neal, Jones & Feldman	20.0
Allbee C-800	Robins	100.0*
Allbee C-800 plus Iron	Robins	100.0*
Allbee-T	Robins	100.0*
Allbee with C	Robins	50.0*
B6-Plus	Anabolic	20.0
B-C-Bid Capsules	Geriatric Pharm.	50.0*
B-Complex Capsules	North American	10.0*
B Complex Tablets	Squibb	9.0
Becomco	O'Neal, Jones & Feldman	30.0
Beminal 500	Ayerst	100.0*
Beminal Forte with Vitamin C	Ayerst	50.0*
Bugs Bunny	Miles	13.5
Bugs Bunny Plus Iron	Miles	13.5
Bugs Bunny with Extra C	Miles	13.5
Cal-M	Anabolic	90.0
Cal-Prenal	North American	10.0*
C-B Bone Capsules	USV	74.0*
Cebefortis	Upjohn	50.0*
Cebetinic	Upjohn	10.0*
Centrum	Lederle	20.0*
Cherri-B Liquid (per 0.6 ml.)	North American	6.0*
Chew-Vite	North American	20.0*
Cluvisol 130	Ayerst	50.0*
Cluvisol Syrup (per tsp.)	Ayerst	5.0*
Dayalets	Abbott	20.0*
Dayalets plus Iron	Abbott	20.0*
Engram-HP	Squibb	20.0
Feminins	Mead Johnson	15.0
Femiron with Vitamins	J.B. Williams	20.0*

(continued)

Supplements—*continued*

Supplement	Manufacturer	Mg.
Ferritrinsic	Upjohn	10.0*
Filibon Tablets	Lederle	20.0*
Flintstones	Miles	13.5
Flintstones Plus Iron	Miles	13.5
Flintstones with Extra C	Miles	13.5
Folbesyn	Lederle	50.0*
Ganatrex (per 0.6 ml.)	Merrell Dow	20.0*
Geriamic	North American	30.0*
Gerilets	Abbott	30.0*
Geriplex	Parke-Davis	15.0*
Geriplex-FS Kapseals	Parke-Davis	15.0*
Geriplex-FS Liquid (per 2 tbsp.)	Parke-Davis	15.0*
Geritinic	Geriatric Pharm.	10.0*
Geritol Junior Liquid (per tsp.)	J.B. Williams	100.0*
Geritol Junior Tablets	J.B. Williams	20.0*
Geritol Liquid (per tsp.)	J.B. Williams	100.0*
Geritol Tablets	J.B. Williams	30.0*
Gerix Elixir (per 2 tbsp.)	Abbott	100.0*
Gerizyme (per tbsp.)	Upjohn	33.3*
Gevrabon (per 2 tbsp.)	Lederle	50.0*
Gevral	Lederle	20.0*
Gevral Protein	Lederle	6.5*
Gevral T Capsules	Lederle	30.0*
Gevrite	Lederle	20.0*
Golden Bounty B Complex with Vitamin C	Squibb	4.7
Hi-Bee Plus	North American	100.0*
Hi-Bee W/C Capsules	North American	50.0*
Iberet	Abbott	30.0*
Iberet-500	Abbott	30.0*
Iberet-500 Oral Solution (per tsp.)	Abbott	7.5*
Iberet Oral Solution (per 0.6 ml.)	Abbott	7.5*
Iberol	Abbott	15.0*
Lederplex Capsules	Lederle	10.0*
Lederplex Liquid (per tsp.)	Lederle	12.5*
Lederplex Tablets	Lederle	10.0*
Lipoflavonoid Capsules	Cooper Vision Pharm.	3.3*

Supplements—continued

Supplement	Manufacturer	Mg.
Lipotriad Capsules	Cooper Vision Pharm.	3.3*
Lipotriad Liquid (per tsp.)	Cooper Vision Pharm.	10.0*
Livitamin Capsules	Beecham Labs	10.0*
Livitamin Chewable	Beecham Labs	10.0*
Livitamin Liquid (per tbsp.)	Beecham Labs	10.0*
Lufa Capsules	USV	5.0*
Methischol Capsules	USV	10.0*
Multicebrin	Lilly	25.0
Multiple Vitamins	North American	20.0*
Multiple Vitamins with Iron	North American	20.0*
Multivitamins	Rowell	20.0*
Myadec	Parke-Davis	100.0*
Natabec	Parke-Davis	10.0*
Natalins Tablets	Mead Johnson	20.0
Norlac	Rowell	20.0
Obron-6	Pfipharmecs	20.0
One-A-Day	Miles	20.0
One-A-Day Core C 500	Miles	20.0
One-A-Day Plus Iron	Miles	20.0
One-A-Day Vitamins Plus Minerals	Miles	20.0
Optilets-500	Abbott	100.0*
Optilets-M-500	Abbott	100.0*
Os-Cal Forte	Marion	15.0*
Os-Cal Plus	Marion	3.3*
Paladec (per tsp.)	Parke-Davis	20.0*
Paladec with Minerals	Parke-Davis	20.0*
Panuitex	O'Neal, Jones & Feldman	15.0*
Peritinic	Lederle	30.0*
Poly-Vi-Sol Chewable	Mead Johnson	13.5
Poly-Vi-Sol Drops (per 0.6 ml.)	Mead Johnson	8.0
Poly-Vi-Sol with Iron Chewable	Mead Johnson	13.5
Poly-Vi-Sol with Iron Drops (per 0.6 ml.)	Mead Johnson	8.0
Probec-T	Stuart	100.0*
Roeribec	Pfipharmecs	100.0*
S.S.S. Tablets	S.S.S.	30.0
S.S.S. Tonic (per tbsp.)	S.S.S.	6.6*

(continued)

Supplements—*continued*

Supplement	Manufacturer	Mg.
Stresscaps Capsules	Lederle	100.0*
Stresstabs 600	Lederle	100.0*
Stresstabs 600 with Iron	Lederle	100.0*
Stresstabs 600 with Zinc	Lederle	100.0*
Stuart Formula	Stuart	20.0*
Stuart Hematinic Liquid (per tsp.)	Stuart	10.0*
Stuartinic	Stuart	20.0*
Stuart Prenatal	Stuart	20.0*
Super Plenamins	Rexall	18.0
Surbex	Abbott	30.0*
Surbex 750 with Iron	Abbott	100.0*
Surbex 750 with Zinc	Abbott	100.0*
Surbex-T	Abbott	100.0*
Surbex with C	Abbott	30.0*
Thera-Combex H-P Kapseals	Parke-Davis	100.0*
Theragran	Squibb	100.0*
Theragran Liquid (per tsp.)	Squibb	100.0*
Theragran-M	Squibb	100.0*
Theragran-Z	Squibb	100.0
Therapeutic Vitamins	North American	100.0
Thera-Spancap	North American	60.0*
Thex Forte	Medtech	100.0*
Tonebec	A.V.P.	5.0*
Tri-B-Plex	Anabolic	100.0*
Unicap	Upjohn	20.0
Unicap Chewable	Upjohn	20.0*
Unicap T	Upjohn	100.0*
Vi-Aqua	USV	20.0*
Vicon-C	Glaxo	100.0*
Vicon Iron	Glaxo	20.0*
Vicon Plus	Glaxo	25.0*
Vigran	Squibb	20.0
Vigran Chewable	Squibb	9.0
Vigran plus Iron	Squibb	20.0
Vio-Bec	Rowell	100.0*
Vio-Geric	Rowell	20.0
Vi-Penta Multivitamin Drops (per 0.6 ml.)	Roche	10.0*

Supplements—*continued*

Supplement	Manufacturer	Mg.
Vitagett	North American	20.0*
Vita-Kaps-M Tablets	Abbott	20.0*
Vita-Kaps Tablets	Abbott	20.0*
Vitamin-Mineral Capsules	North American	20.0*
Viterra	Pfipharmecs	25.0
Viterra High Potency	Pfipharmecs	100.0
VM Preparation (per 2 tbsp.)	Roberts	20.0*
Z-Bec	Robins	100.0
Zymacap Capsules	Upjohn	30.0*
Zymalixir Syrup (per tsp.)	Upjohn	8.0*
Zymasyrup (per tsp.)	Upjohn	10.0*

Source: Adapted from the American Pharmaceutical Association, *Handbook of Nonprescription Drugs*, 7th ed. (1982), 240–57.

Note: This chart is intended only as a guide. Vitamin formulations change periodically; always read product labels for accurate and up-to-date information on their nutrient levels.

*Indicates use of niacinamide rather than nicotinic acid as the source of niacin. As the manufacturer may have changed niacin sources since this survey was taken, always check the label of the product for current information about the type of niacin it contains.

7

Vitamin B$_6$

If a waiter ran over your foot with a dessert cart and you felt nothing, would you suspect something was wrong?

It may sound incredible, but it happened to one victim who had taken too much vitamin B$_6$. It was at that moment that she admitted to herself that she was "in trouble." She was. In fact, her story became a textbook case in the annals of supplement safety.

In a moment, I'll tell you even more stories like that one. But first, I think you will want to know some basic information about vitamin B$_6$—the positive side of the B$_6$ story. For while the potential of vitamin B$_6$ to cause toxic reactions has been big news in recent years, its potential to benefit your health in new ways has also been under investigation. And the evidence shows that B$_6$ is an important vitamin, one whose talents are just beginning to unfold.

Today, doctors are experimenting with B$_6$ for a variety of health problems, such as premenstrual syndrome and the nerve disorder known as carpal tunnel syndrome. Its effectiveness as an antidote to the abuse of certain prescription drugs is widely accepted. And the effects of B$_6$ on the brain are also under study, with possible importance to conditions such as depression.

As for what's long been known about vitamin B$_6$ ... here's the story.

B$_6$ BASICS

For years, nutritionists have credited vitamin B$_6$ with the following roles:

• Helping your body convert tryptophan, a constituent of protein, to niacin and to the important brain chemical called serotonin
• Assisting in the metabolism of proteins, carbohydrates, and fats
• Allowing your body to make heme, an important component of your blood

As for deficiencies of vitamin B$_6$, two groups have given nutritionists the most cause for concern: the elderly and women who are pregnant or nursing. Surveys show that many of them don't meet the recommended allowance for B$_6$. Of course, that is not a guarantee of deficiency, which includes these symptoms:

• Digestive problems, such as abdominal distress and vomiting
• Nervous system complaints, such as depression, confusion, irritability
• Skin problems, such as flaking, irritation, cracking
• Weight loss

You may already know that technically, vitamin B$_6$ is not a single substance, but a complex of three different ones that all can meet your body's need for this vitamin. However, supplemental B$_6$ generally contains but one of these—pyridoxine—so that's what we will be talking about from now on.

THE BUBBLE BURSTS

Until recently—1983 to be exact—nutritionists believed B$_6$ to be reasonably nontoxic, with little potential for harm. In 1976, for instance, the National Academy of Sciences published an authoritative book on vitamin B$_6$ which predicted that even overuse of B$_6$ supplements probably would cause no harm. The authors lived to eat their words.

(continued on page 124)

The Diet Detective Searches for Vitamin B₆

Nutritionists were taken by surprise not long ago when the U.S. Department of Agriculture reported an analysis of vitamin B₆ intake among pregnant and nursing women. The study of women (not poor, but upper middle class) found that the average diet during pregnancy supplied only about half of the RDA for pregnancy. B₆ intakes during nursing were not much better, at an average 60 percent of the recommended level.

How does your B₆ intake stack up? Sharpen your pencil and check off any of the following foods that you ate on the day of your choosing. Then follow the scoring directions that follow for the verdict.

1 point
1 cup canned apricots
1 cup canned asparagus
1 cup frozen wax beans
1 cup raw cabbage
1 cup canned sweet potato
1 tomato
1 cup cooked white rice
1 cup milk
1 cup yogurt
1 cup oysters, raw

2 points
1 cup raw carrots
1 cup raw cauliflower
1 cup frozen peas
1 cup raw spinach
1 cup canned tomatoes

10 French fries (4 inches long)
1 12-ounce can or bottle of beer
⅓ cup peanuts
1 3-ounce hamburger patty
½ cup all-bran cereal
1 tablespoon brewer's yeast

3 points
1 cup broccoli, raw or frozen
1 medium baked potato
1 cup frozen brussels sprouts
1 cup frozen cauliflower
1 cup canned corn

1 cup brown rice
1 cup frozen lima beans
1 cup canned Great
   Northern beans
1 cup lentils
1 cup soybeans
4 ounces lean beef
4 ounces lamb
4 ounces tuna
1 cup crabmeat
½ cup raisins

4 points
1 cup pearled barley
4 ounces dark meat
   chicken
4 ounces dark meat turkey
4 ounces canned ham

4 ounces salmon
4 ounces herring
1 cup frozen corn

6 points
⅓ cup sunflower seeds
4 ounces light meat turkey

7 points
4 ounces light meat
   chicken

8 points
1 cup canned kidney beans

9 points
1 medium banana

13 points
1 avocado

Scoring

Add up your total points. Multiply the total by 5. The result is an estimate of the percent of the U.S. RDA for vitamin B₆ that you took in on the day in question. If you scored 13 points, for example, multiply 13 by 5 for a score of 65 percent of the U.S. RDA.

Of course, with facts about the B₆ content of foods so hard to come by, this quiz probably overlooks some of the B₆ in your diet. But if your score is substantially below the U.S. RDA—by a third or more—chances are your diet falls short of the allowance.

In 1983, Herbert Schaumburg, M.D., and his coworkers turned the conventional wisdom on its ear with their now classic report of 7 cases of B_6 overdose. And that was just the tip of the iceberg; within months, Dr. Schaumburg's team had recorded a total of 30 cases. Some of the victims had been seriously hurt. Here is a description of a typical victim, quoted from his original report in the *New England Journal of Medicine*.

> A 27-year-old woman sought medical attention be-cause of increased difficulty in walking. Approximately two years previously she had been told that vitamin B_6 provided a natural way to get rid of body water and she had begun to take 500 mg. per day for premenstrual edema [water retention].
>
> One year before presentation [for medical advice], she had started to increase her intake, until she reached a daily dose of 5 g [5,000 mg.] per day. During this period of increase in dosage, she initially noticed that flexing her neck produced a tingling sensation down the neck and into the legs and soles of her feet. In the four months before neurological evaluation, she became progres-sively unsteady when walking, particularly in the dark, and noticed difficulty in handling small objects. She also noticed some change in the feeling in her lips and tongue ... [and] could walk only with the assistance of a cane.

That last line really caught my attention—a 27-year-old woman with the kind of disability we associate with people many years her senior. And that's not all. The doctors who examined her found that her ability to sense touch, pinpricks, vibration, and the position of her joints was severely impaired.

What was she to do? For starters, stop the B_6. Sure enough, that was the answer. Two months later, she was better able to walk and feel normal sensations. That was a relief, to be sure. But it wasn't for a full *seven months* off the B_6 regimen that she was able to toss away that cane and return to work. Full recovery, however, was still not at hand. Despite the improvements, her sense of touch still remained abnormal in both feet and limbs.

The same held true for other victims. After six months with-out the vitamin B_6, four more patients had improved, but not fully recovered. After two years for one patient and three years for another, however, Dr. Schaumburg reported "almost complete" recovery.

And while we're on the subject, how about a name for this syndrome? It's a strange-sounding but important one—sensory neuropathy. That means nerve disorder that damages the ability to feel normal sensations. And within months of Dr. Schaumburg's report, the condition had become a hot topic of conversation in the nutrition world. Medical journals were alive with commentary, concern, and still more cases brought on by doses of B$_6$ in the 2,000 to 6,000 milligram (mg.) range.

THE DOSE DEBATE

But as I told you earlier, doctors have not only been talking about this nerve damage syndrome from vitamin B$_6$, but also of its potential in treating disease. So it was inevitable that doctors who actively prescribe B$_6$ would speak up, urging a debate of not just the risks, but also the benefits.

And the debate has been lively. No one has denied the seriousness of the syndrome reported by Dr. Schaumburg. But, they argue, his victims were consuming enormous doses—2,000 to 6,000 mg. daily. That's 10 to 30 times more than the 200 mg. that advocates of B$_6$ sometimes prescribe. And so the dose debate continues: Are moderately high doses, in the 200 to 500 mg. range, safe?

Here are some sample comments on this important issue. First from Herman Baker, Ph.D., and Oscar Frank, Ph.D., of New Jersey Medical School: "We have given 75 mg. of vitamin B$_6$ by mouth three times a day (daily total, 225 mg.) to six elderly subjects every day for a year without untoward effects, despite the increases in blood levels of vitamin B$_6$ to five to eight times normal that were maintained for the year."

And from Toronto Western Hospital in Canada, three physicians said "Pyridoxine [vitamin B$_6$] in doses of 250 to 500 mg. [daily] has been found to be effective in patients who have kidney stones [caused by certain conditions]. We have followed 22 patients with kidney stones who were treated with intermediate doses of pyridoxine for eight months to six years (average 2.3

years). None has shown any neurological complication . . . and we have decided to continue this treatment in our patients."

Finally, from St. Thomas's Hospital Medical School in London: "In a series of 630 women taking 80–200 mg. vitamin B_6 daily for premenstrual syndrome who were studied by various members of this department in 1976–1983, only minimal side effects were noted and certainly no neuropathy [nerve damage] was seen."

Also from England, however, comes a report that 40 percent of women taking 50 to 300 mg. B_6 daily for premenstrual syndrome showed symptoms of nervous system problems. The evidence? Complaints of burning, shooting, tingling pains, clumsiness, numbness, and loss of coordination. Nonetheless, it does not sound to me as though the severity of these symptoms approached those experienced by the seven patients of Dr. Schaumburg's who had been taking 2,000 to 6,000 mg. daily.

THE 500 MG. SURPRISE

The B_6 debate is continuing, and the story of the nerve damage syndrome is still unfolding. Regardless of who is right about the safety of moderate doses, though, it seemed at first that major disability from too much vitamin B_6 would be reserved for those taking extremely large doses: 2,000 mg. or more. But not long after Dr. Schaumburg published details of the seven cases of nerve damage resulting from such high doses, a new patient was at his door. And she had been taking much, much less vitamin B_6 than the others.

Here is her story, excerpted from a letter to the editor by Dr. Schaumburg and Alan Berger, M.D.

A 34-year-old woman sought medical attention because of progressive difficulty in walking. Three years previously, she had begun daily ingestion of a multivitamin containing 200 mg. of vitamin B_6. Two years later, she increased her daily intake to 500 mg., which was supplemented by an additional 300 mg. no more than once per week.

One month before presentation [for medical care] she began to have the sensation of electric shocks shoot-

ing down her spine upon [flexing her] neck . . . afterward, progressive unsteadiness [when walking] occurred, which was worse when she walked in the dark. She had progressive numbness in both feet . . . She was unable to walk without assistance. A diagnosis of multiple sclerosis was proposed.

But it wasn't multiple sclerosis at all! The doctors performed various tests of her sensory abilities, such as the capability to detect temperature, vibration, and pinpricks. The results: abnormal. The verdict: another case of the nerve damage syndrome from vitamin B$_6$.

A month after visiting the doctor, she stopped taking vitamin B$_6$. Her symptoms started to improve. Happily, she continued to improve as months went by.

While her improvement was reason to cheer, the facts of the case were not. This woman had developed a serious case of toxicity from 500 mg. of B$_6$ daily—much less than previous victims had taken. And she probably wasn't alone.

Richard Podell, M.D., of New Providence, New Jersey, reports one of his patients, too, developed the same symptoms linked to B$_6$ overdose. This man also took only 500 mg. a day, but for eight years rather than one. Says Dr. Podell, "His symptoms improved after several months off the vitamin regimen and deteriorated again when (unknown to me) he went back on it. When he stopped again, improvement was less rapid."

The doctor is worried, he says, for if 500 mg. or less can cause an overdose, "then tens, perhaps hundreds of thousands of individuals are potentially at risk."

HOW MUCH IS TOO MUCH

Side effects from vitamin B$_6$ do occur, as we will discuss shortly. But the syndrome of impaired senses and nerve damage is the most severe and, therefore, the key issue in B$_6$ toxicity. So setting guidelines for its use centers on the levels that might lead to the nerve damage syndrome.

If you want a safe dose of vitamin B$_6$, my recommendation is 50 mg. or less. But as I usually say, many people can tolerate higher doses. My current thinking is that doses in the 50 to 200 mg. range will be well tolerated by many. While 200 to 400 mg. will probably cause no problems for some, I feel that such levels call for regular follow-up by your doctor.

At 500 mg. and higher, of course, there is a risk of toxicity to some people, and a very high risk at doses in the thousands of milligrams. Keep in mind that the risk is not just of a medical problem, but of one that may disable severely and require many months for recovery.

It is precisely this long recovery period that concerns me greatly. None of the other vitamins that we have talked about so far have been linked to symptoms that take so long to subside. There's also the fact that permanent damage has not been completely ruled out in some of the victims who had been taking 2,000 mg. or more.

Recommended Dietary Allowances for Vitamin B$_6$

Group/Age	Mg.
Infants 0–6 mon.	0.3
Infants 6–12 mon.	0.6
Children 1–3 yr.	0.9
Children 4–6 yr.	1.3
Children 7–10 yr.	1.6
Males 11–14 yr.	1.8
Males 15–18 yr.	2.0
Males 19–50 yr.	2.2
Males 51+ yr.	2.2
Females 11–14 yr.	1.8
Females 15–50 yr.	2.0
Females 51+ yr.	2.0
Pregnant women	2.4–2.6
Nursing women	2.3–2.5

Note: The U.S. RDA for vitamin B$_6$ is 2 mg.

One final matter: the issue of your body becoming dependent on B$_6$ supplements. One group of researchers has reported that 200 mg. daily for one month created a dependency in the people studied. But quite a few other studies mention no such effect. So, in my mind, this is an idea that will require more convincing evidence.

THE STAR SYSTEM SHINES ON VITAMIN B$_6$

As I have just pointed out, the nerve damage syndrome is the most severe, but not the only consequence of taking too much B$_6$. So let's take a look at the other possibilities that may affect you.

Side effects—Nausea, headache, and fatigue are the main side effects of vitamin B$_6$. In a study of schizophrenic patients (also taking drugs to control their illness), the following effects were noted in one of ten patients who took 75 mg. of vitamin B$_6$ daily:

- Dizziness
- Nausea and vomiting
- Rapid heartbeat
- Skin rash
- Weight gain

Two of the ten developed flushing of the skin.

Acute ailments—I can report no known acute ailments from vitamin B$_6$. Occasionally, people may be allergic or hypersensitive to it, but such isolated cases of unusual sensitivity don't qualify as toxic reactions. Incidentally, two allergic reactions to the vitamin B$_6$ in a hair care product and a skin cream also have been reported.

Long-term problems—As I have said, the nerve damage syndrome is the key issue here. In the best of all worlds, everyone would take B$_6$ so sensibly that this syndrome would never occur. But some people may be unusually sensitive or unaware of the problem, so that knowing the symptoms of the nerve damage syndrome are also important. I call these symptoms the four ifs, and here they are:

• If you have a burning, tingling, or crawling sensation on your skin
• If you have trouble walking, reaching for objects, or using your fingers (to type, for example)
• If your ability to sense vibration or the position of your limbs seems impaired
• If your sense of temperature and touch, such as a pinprick, seems decreased

If any of these things happen to you, *stop taking the B$_6$ and see your doctor.*

Two other findings have been reported from high doses of vitamin B$_6$: decreased amounts of another B vitamin, folic acid, in the blood and increased amounts of an enzyme called AST or SGOT in the blood. A number of drugs and conditions can raise the AST level. How common or troublesome these effects are is unclear.

Conflicting combinations—Mysteries never cease in medicine, and more than once, B$_6$ has been the culprit. One doctor noticed that two of his patients whose Parkinson's disease seemed under control with the drug levodopa (L-dopa) suddenly relapsed. The cause: nausea-control medication containing B$_6$. It's clear that vitamin B$_6$ can strip levodopa of its healing properties, so this is a combination that doesn't mix. (Actually, small amounts of B$_6$ may be acceptable, but the textbooks say supplements containing more than 5 mg. are out.)

Be sure to talk with your doctor, then, if you take levodopa or have Parkinson's disease. The doctor can add another compound to the regimen that prevents B$_6$ from interfering with the levodopa.

If you are taking phenobarbital or phenytoin (better known by the brand name, Dilantin), take B$_6$ only on doctor's orders. Moderate doses of vitamin B$_6$ can sharply reduce the amount of the drug in your blood, interfering with treatment. Are you wondering about how much? Let me give you an example: In one study, 200 mg. of B$_6$ taken daily for one month *halved* the amount of these needed drugs in the bloodstream.

Vitamin B$_6$ also interacts with the following drugs, and your need for the vitamin may actually increase if you take them:

- Birth control pills
- Cycloserine (brand name Seromycin), an antibiotic
- Hydralazine, an ingredient in certain drugs used to lower blood pressure (including Apresazide, Apresoline, Rezide, Ser-Ap-Es, Serpasil-Apresoline, and Unipres)
- Isoniazid or INH, the antituberculosis drug
- Penicillamine (brand names Cuprimine and Depen), which is not a type of penicillin, but a drug used in rare genetic diseases and in severe cases of rheumatoid arthritis

Hidden consequences—Vitamin B$_6$ can cause a false positive reading in a laboratory test for urobilogen. This test helps evaluate liver health.

Finally, nursing mothers will want to avoid high doses of vitamin B$_6$. There is a report that substantial doses, such as 200 mg., may interfere with the mother's secretion of breast milk. Whether or not this effect is confirmed, it seems foolish for a nursing mother to take this much unless absolutely necessary.

A PARTING PERSPECTIVE

The story of B$_6$ may seem like one of two extremes: the promise of relief from various conditions on the one hand and the hazards of serious toxicity on the other. But despite the harrowing experiences of some victims, I believe those who feel helped by B$_6$ can continue to take it safely by following sensible guidelines for its use.

I am committed to keeping an open mind to both the benefits and hazards. I hope that you are, too.

C O O K I N G
for Vitamin B$_6$

TROPICAL BANANA DELIGHT

(Makes 2 servings)

Vitamin B$_6$: 0.47 mg. per serving
Calories: 199 per serving

1 cup plain low-fat yogurt
½ cup unsweetened
    pineapple juice
½ cup skim milk
1 medium banana, sliced
2 teaspoons honey

Place all ingredients in a blender and process until smooth.
Serve immediately.

AVOCADO AND GREEN CHILI SOUP

(Makes 4 servings)

Vitamin B$_6$: 0.34 mg. per serving
Calories: 220 per serving

1 cup plain low-fat
    yogurt
2 avocados, peeled and
    mashed (about 1½
    cups)
1½ cups chicken stock
4 ounces mild green
    chilies (about ⅓
    cup) or 1 tablespoon
    chopped jalapeño
    pepper
3 scallions, minced
¼ teaspoon grated lime
    rind
¼ teaspoon ground
    cumin
½ teaspoon ground
    coriander
    freshly ground black
    pepper

Combine all ingredients except pepper in a food processor or
blender and process until well blended. Add pepper to taste.
Serve at room temperature or slightly chilled.

C O O K I N G
for Vitamin B₆—*continued*

VARIATION: This soup can be turned into a dip or sandwich spread by omitting the chicken stock and substituting 2 cups of plain low-fat yogurt.

NATURALLY DELICIOUS CHICKEN NUGGETS

(Makes 4 servings)

Vitamin B₆: 0.42 mg. per serving
Calories: 183 per serving

Serve these with rice or stir-fried vegetables, or wrap them in tender lettuce leaves and eat by hand.

1	pound lean ground chicken breast	1	clove garlic, minced
1	tablespoon honey	1	cup chicken stock
½	teaspoon soy sauce	¼	cup minced fresh chives
1	egg, lightly beaten	1	thin slice fresh ginger
1½	tablespoons cornstarch	2	cloves garlic, mashed
2	tablespoons minced fresh parsley		

In a medium-size bowl, combine the chicken, honey, soy sauce, egg, cornstarch, parsley, and minced garlic. Shape mixture into 1-inch balls and set aside.

In a 10-inch skillet, combine the chicken stock, chives, ginger, and mashed garlic and bring to a boil. Add the chicken nuggets, reduce heat to a simmer and braise, stirring frequently, for 5 to 6 minutes, or until nuggets are cooked through. Serve immediately.

Vitamin B$_6$ Content
of Selected Supplements

Dosage is one tablet or capsule unless otherwise indicated.

Supplement	Manufacturer	Mg.
Abdec Baby Drops (per 0.6 ml.)	Parke-Davis	1.00
Abdec Kapseal	Parke-Davis	1.50
Abdol with Minerals	Parke-Davis	0.50
Abron	O'Neal, Jones & Feldman	4.00
Allbee C-800	Robins	25.00
Allbee C-800 plus Iron	Robins	25.00
Allbee-T	Robins	10.00
Allbee with C	Robins	5.00
AVP Natal	A.V.P.	10.00
B6-Plus	Anabolic	50.00
B-C-Bid Capsules	Geriatric Pharm.	5.00
B-Complex Capsules	North American	0.10
B Complex Tablets	Squibb	0.90
Becomco	O'Neal, Jones & Feldman	3.00
Belfer	O'Neal, Jones & Feldman	2.00
Beminal 500	Ayerst	10.00
Beminal Forte with Vitamin C	Ayerst	3.00
Brewers Yeast	North American	0.01
Bugs Bunny	Miles	1.05
Bugs Bunny Plus Iron	Miles	1.05
Bugs Bunny with Extra C	Miles	1.05
Cal-M	Anabolic	45.00
Cal-Prenal	North American	1.00
C-B Bone Capsules	USV	1.50
Cebefortis	Upjohn	1.00
Cebetinic	Upjohn	0.50
Centrum	Lederle	3.00
Cherri-B Liquid (per 0.6 ml.)	North American	0.09
Chew-Vite	North American	1.00
Cluvisol 130	Ayerst	0.50
Cluvisol Syrup (per tsp.)	Ayerst	0.60
Dayalets	Abbott	2.00
Dayalets plus Iron	Abbott	2.00
Engram-HP	Squibb	2.50

Supplements—*continued*

Supplement	Manufacturer	Mg.
Feminins	Mead Johnson	25.00
Femiron with Vitamins	J.B. Williams	2.00
Filibon Tablets	Lederle	2.00
Flintstones	Miles	1.05
Flintstones Plus Iron	Miles	1.05
Flintstones with Extra C	Miles	1.05
Folbesyn	Lederle	3.00
Ganatrex (per 0.6 ml.)	Merrell Dow	2.00
Geralix Liquid (per tbsp.)	North American	0.70
Geriamic	North American	0.50
Gerilets	Abbott	3.00
Geriplex-FS Liquid (per 2 tbsp.)	Parke-Davis	1.00
Geritinic	Geriatric Pharm.	0.10
Geritol Junior Liquid (per tsp.)	J.B. Williams	1.00
Geritol Junior Tablets	J.B. Williams	1.00
Geritol Liquid (per tsp.)	J.B. Williams	1.00
Geritol Tablets	J.B. Williams	0.50
Gerix Elixir (per 2 tbsp.)	Abbott	1.64
Gerizyme (per tbsp.)	Upjohn	1.00
Gevrabon (per 2 tbsp.)	Lederle	1.00
Gevral	Lederle	2.00
Gevral Protein	Lederle	0.22
Gevral T Capsules	Lederle	3.00
Gevrite	Lederle	2.00
Hi-Bee Plus	North American	5.00
Hi-Bee W/C Capsules	North American	5.00
Iberet	Abbott	5.00
Iberet-500	Abbott	5.00
Iberet-500 Oral Solution (per tsp.)	Abbott	1.25
Iberet Oral Solution (per 0.6 ml.)	Abbott	1.25
Iberol	Abbott	1.50
Incremin with Iron Syrup (per tsp.)	Lederle	5.00
Lederplex Capsules	Lederle	0.20
Lederplex Liquid (per tsp.)	Lederle	0.25
Lederplex Tablets	Lederle	0.10

(continued)

Supplements—continued

Supplement	Manufacturer	Mg.
Lipoflavonoid Capsules	Cooper Vision Pharm.	0.33
Lipotriad Capsules	Cooper Vision Pharm.	0.33
Lipotriad Liquid (per tsp.)	Cooper Vision Pharm.	1.00
Livitamin Capsules	Beecham Labs	3.00
Livitamin Chewable	Beecham Labs	3.00
Livitamin Liquid (per tbsp.)	Beecham Labs	3.00
Lufa Capsules	USV	2.00
Methischol Capsules	USV	2.00
Multicebrin	Lilly	1.20
Multiple Vitamins	North American	1.00
Multiple Vitamins with Iron	North American	1.00
Multivitamins	Rowell	0.50
Myadec	Parke-Davis	5.00
Natabec	Parke-Davis	3.00
Natalins Tablets	Mead Johnson	4.00
Norlac	Rowell	4.00
Obron-6	Pfipharmecs	8.20
One-A-Day	Miles	2.00
One-A-Day Core C 500	Miles	2.00
One-A-Day Plus Iron	Miles	2.00
One-A-Day Vitamins Plus Minerals	Miles	2.00
Optilets-500	Abbott	5.00
Optilets-M-500	Abbott	5.00
Orexin Softabs	Stuart	5.00
Os-Cal Forte	Marion	2.00
Os-Cal Plus	Marion	0.50
Paladec (per tsp.)	Parke-Davis	1.00
Paladec with Minerals	Parke-Davis	1.00
Panuitex	O'Neal, Jones & Feldman	3.00
Peritinic	Lederle	7.50
Poly-Vi-Sol Chewable	Mead Johnson	1.05
Poly-Vi-Sol Drops (per 0.6 ml.)	Mead Johnson	0.40
Poly-Vi-Sol with Iron Chewable	Mead Johnson	1.05
Poly-Vi-Sol with Iron Drops (per 0.6 ml.)	Mead Johnson	0.40
Probec-T	Stuart	5.00
Roeribec	Pfipharmecs	8.20
Rogenic	O'Neal, Jones & Feldman	6.00

Supplements—*continued*

Supplement	Manufacturer	Mg.
Simiron Plus	Merrell Dow	1.00
S.S.S. Tablets	S.S.S.	0.50
Stresscaps Capsules	Lederle	2.00
Stresstabs 600	Lederle	5.00
Stresstabs 600 with Iron	Lederle	25.00
Stresstabs 600 with Zinc	Lederle	10.00
Stuart Formula	Stuart	2.00
Stuart Hematinic Liquid (per tsp.)	Stuart	0.50
Stuartinic	Stuart	1.00
Stuart Prenatal	Stuart	4.00
Super Plenamins	Rexall	1.00
Surbex	Abbott	2.50
Surbex 750 with Iron	Abbott	25.00
Surbex 750 with Zinc	Abbott	20.00
Surbex-T	Abbott	5.00
Surbex with C	Abbott	2.50
Thera-Combex H-P Kapseals	Parke-Davis	10.00
Theragran	Squibb	4.10
Theragran Liquid (per tsp.)	Squibb	4.10
Theragran-M	Squibb	4.10
Theragran-Z	Squibb	4.10
Therapeutic Vitamins	North American	5.00
Thera-Spancap	North American	6.00
Thex Forte	Medtech	5.00
Tonebec	A.V.P.	5.00
Tri-B-Plex	Anabolic	25.00
Unicap	Upjohn	2.00
Unicap Chewable	Upjohn	2.00
Unicap T	Upjohn	6.00
Vi-Aqua	USV	0.50
Vicon-C	Glaxo	5.00
Vicon Iron	Glaxo	5.00
Vicon Plus	Glaxo	2.00
Vigran	Squibb	2.00
Vigran Chewable	Squibb	0.70
Vigran plus Iron	Squibb	2.00
Vio-Bec	Rowell	25.00
Vio-Geric	Rowell	2.40

(continued)

Supplements—*continued*

Supplement	Manufacturer	Mg.
Vi-Penta Multivitamin Drops (per 0.6 ml.)	Roche	1.00
Vitagett	North American	1.50
Vita-Kaps Tablets	Abbott	1.00
Vita-Kaps-M Tablets	Abbott	1.00
Vitamin-Mineral Capsules	North American	1.00
Viterra	Pfipharmecs	0.82
Viterra High Potency	Pfipharmecs	1.60
Z-Bec	Robins	10.00
Zymacap Capsules	Upjohn	3.00
Zymalixir Syrup (per tsp.)	Upjohn	0.50
Zymasyrup (per tsp.)	Upjohn	0.50

Source: Adapted from the American Pharmaceutical Association, *Handbook of Nonprescription Drugs,* 7th ed. (1982), 240–57.

Note: This chart is intended only as a guide. Vitamin formulations change periodically; always read product labels for accurate and up-to-date information on their nutrient levels.

8

Folic Acid

When it came to folic acid supplements, the late nutritionist Adelle Davis felt she couldn't buy American. Government policy kept the folic acid content of supplements too low, she wrote in her book *Let's Eat Right to Keep Fit*, so she imported her supplements from Canada, where higher-potency tablets could be found. And she suggested that Americans should write to Washington demanding that high-potency folic acid be made available in the United States.

But that was in 1970, before we knew about folic acid what we know now: that high doses of this B vitamin can interfere with your body's ability to absorb zinc. Certainly Adelle Davis valued zinc as much as she did folic acid, and her position might have been different were she writing *Let's Eat Right to Keep Fit* today.

So, let's cut right to the heart of folic acid issues and decide how to maximize your chances of holding on to your fair share of both folic acid and zinc.

THE ZINC LINK

This is definitely not a matter of folate (another name for folic acid) being toxic in and of itself, a topic we will talk about shortly. Rather, the issue is whether, for all its talents, folic acid adversely affects your body's ability to absorb and/or retain zinc, a vital mineral.

Here's what sounded the recent alarm. A preliminary but very well designed study found that a supplement of 400 micrograms (mcg.) of folic acid added to a diet already containing 150 mcg. caused men to excrete greater amounts of zinc than when no supplement was given. The amount of zinc in the men's diets varied from low (25 to 50 percent of the Recommended Dietary Allowance) to high (twice the recommended allowance).

Clearly, folic acid did not block zinc absorption completely. Rather, it seemed to interfere only partially, resulting in less zinc absorption. That's a far cry from *stopping* zinc absorption.

So we have a case where taking in more folate meant that more zinc was excreted. The opposite, though, also has occurred. Other work has found the amount of zinc in the blood to increase during folic acid deficiency. This makes it more probable that the interaction seen in the first study is real.

The trick, then, is to find the right balance between folic acid and zinc. We'll talk about doing just that later in this chapter, but first I want to tell you a bit about how the vitamin works on its own.

TALES OF TOXICITY?

Here's a familiar story. As one of the water-soluble B vitamins, folic acid was always thought nontoxic. The wisdom of nutritionists held that any excess would simply be excreted, and quite quickly at that.

But a 1970 report in *Lancet*, a major British medical journal, took the health community by surprise. Four scientists had been looking at how high doses of folic acid affected vitamin B_{12} nutrition, but announced that they had abandoned the study because of unexpected side effects from the folate.

The subjects had been 14 healthy adults, and they were taking 15,000 mcg. of folic acid daily. After a month, according to the researchers, most of the subjects were complaining of effects

Folate: The Vital Facts

As a nutrient, folic acid is extremely important. It is absolutely essential for healthy blood, for a healthy pregnancy, and for metabolism of proteins. Without it, normal growth is impossible.

So critical is this nutrient that key signs of deficiency can appear after about 100 days of a diet containing too little. Too little folic acid causes a type of anemia, with early symptoms of fatigue, loss of appetite, and pallor. Inflammation of the tongue—often experienced as a burning sensation—is another telltale sign.

Most frequently, victims of folic acid deficiency are alcoholics or those suffering from any of the various malabsorption syndromes. Recent research also suggests that folate deficiency may be more of a problem among elderly Americans than previously realized.

The most exciting fact about folic acid is this: Researchers are now studying whether it can help prevent cancer. In the first round of tests, folic acid helped prevent the breaking of genetic material that is probably a key step in the cancer process. Research now in progress is looking at whether folic acid can turn around precancerous conditions of the lung and cervix. What a breakthrough it will be if folate proves capable of stopping or reversing these changes that may be omens of future cancer!

so severe as to be interfering with their work. Only one had no complaints; the rest reported a variety of digestive and nervous system effects. To quote from the report:

> Eight complained of gastrointestinal disturbances —anorexia, nausea, abdominal [bloating] and discomfort . . . Two slept more deeply and dreamed less, one had difficulty waking in the morning, and six complained of varying degrees of insomnia either waking intermittently throughout the night or an hour or two before their usual time . . . Seven said they had vivid anxiety dreams

> ... *Two dreamed in colour for the first time to their recollection. One had nightmares in the first week but slept normally thereafter ... Eight complained of malaise and irritability. In five it was noted [first] by relatives or friends.*

To make the case more convincing, the subjects reported that the symptoms vanished within three weeks of stopping the folate supplements. So it looked like a pretty good case against high doses of the vitamin.

But little is accepted in nutrition until duplicated by others. The intense interest sparked by this report led others in the field to conduct tests of their own in hopes of confirming these adverse effects. But no one truly did. A better designed experiment using the same dose of folate found no effects on sleep, vigor, anxiety, ability to concentrate, or digestive function.

Another study involved patients having Parkinson's disease. Only 3 of the 18 patients complained of side effects from the same high dose of folate. One told of a buzzing sensation in his ears, another felt jittery, and one other had trouble sleeping. And in still another study, initial results showed no ill effects from 15,000 mcg. taken daily for up to a year.

A HEALTHY SKEPTICISM

The record shows that, more often than not, enormous doses of folate do not cause side effects or toxic reactions. This is not to insist that no one has suffered adverse effects. But how much concern this deserves is debatable in light of the enormous doses studied. Each of the four studies we have just reviewed involved daily doses of 15,000 mcg., or about 40 times the U.S. Recommended Daily Allowance (U.S. RDA). Of course, some people react to far lower doses than most, making it conceivable that the side effects reported by some will occur at lower doses. Nonetheless, the chances of such ill effects occurring seem small at the dosages that most supplement users take.

Some observers, though, are skeptical about these claims of side effects. The original report prompted letters to the editor suggesting, among other things, that the ill effects might have resulted from contamination of the folate supplements or from the power of suggestion, since most of the complaints were subjective ones, not documented with hard facts.

When faced with conflicting findings, scientists favor the study with the better design. And since the best study showed no toxic effects from folate, most scientists would probably accept this conclusion until someone could show otherwise. The effect of folate on zinc, of course, is a separate issue that doesn't fall under the category of toxicity.

ALLERGIES AND EPILEPSY

As you might have guessed, folate may produce special effects in special conditions. In some cases, it clearly does; in others, the possibility exists but remains to be firmly documented.

Allergy to folate is extremely rare, but a few cases are on record. One man, 36-year-old Benjamin, for instance, started to itch after taking 1,000 mcg. of folic acid. The supplement was discontinued, then retried a few months later. Benjamin developed fever, itching, pain, chills, and hives. A skin test similar to the ones allergists use revealed him to be allergic to folic acid.

I have found five other reports of folate allergy, which I think make clear that it does happen, but only on rare occasions.

More common, though, are serious reactions to folate in epileptics. Folate interacts with several of the drugs used in treating epilepsy, so decisions about folic acid supplements should be left to your doctor if you have this condition.

Finally, two cases of high-dose folate affecting psychotic illnesses are on record. Take the case of Samuel, a 30-year-old schizophrenic man treated with 3,000 mcg. of folic acid daily. He was also taking several prescription drugs. Two weeks after starting him on folate, his doctors noticed a change in his behavior. "He gradually became irritable, hostile, aggressive, and combative," they reported.

Samuel's doctors gradually reduced his folate dosage, then stopped the supplement entirely. His excited demeanor improved. Next, the doctors noticed that another patient with schizophrenia reacted similarly to a prescribed folate supplement of only 1,000 mcg. Based on these two cases, the doctors raised concern that folate might affect the course of schizophrenia.

The Diet Detective Searches for Folic Acid

The benefits of folate and reports about deficiencies in the elderly have many concerned about their folate intake. And, of course, the best decision about supplement use considers first how much is in your diet. So, take this quiz as you did the others, giving yourself the number of points specified for each of the foods you ate yesterday or today.

1 point
½ grapefruit
1 cup chopped dates
1 cup strawberries
1 cup iceberg lettuce
1 cup lentils
1 tablespoon wheat germ

2 points
⅓ cup almonds
⅓ cup cashews
2 tablespoons peanut
  butter
1 medium banana
1 cup raw carrots
1 cup raw or frozen green
  beans
1 cup raw or frozen wax
  beans
1 medium potato
1 cup pearled barley
1 egg white

3 points
1 cup canned grapefruit
  juice
1 cup frozen brussels
  sprouts
1 cup raw cabbage
1 cup raw kale
1 tomato
1 cup frozen lima beans
1 cup canned beans in
  tomato sauce
⅓ cup peanuts
⅓ cup all-bran cereal

4 points
1 orange
1 cup raw asparagus
1 cup broccoli
1 cup frozen peas

MASKED DANGER

Whether folate is toxic or a serious threat to your zinc nutrition, one can argue for hours. But on another count, there also can be no argument about folate's ability to do physical harm.

5 points
1 cup raw broccoli
1 cup frozen cauliflower
1 cup romaine lettuce
1 cup raw spinach
1 cup sweet potato

6 points
1 cup pinto beans
1 cup raw beets

7 points
1 cup orange juice
1 cup canned black-eyed
  peas

8 points
4 ounces beef liver

9 points
½ cup raw soybeans

10 points
1 cup canned chick-peas
1 cup spinach

13 points
4 ounces chicken liver

16 points
1 tablespoon brewer's
  yeast

Scoring

Add up your points. Multiply the total by 5. The result is an estimate of the percent of the U.S. RDA for folic acid that you are getting in your diet. If you scored 15 points, for example, multiply 15 by 5 for a score of 75 percent of the U.S. RDA.

As is the case for vitamin B_6, facts about folic acid in many foods are unavailable. As you no doubt noticed, this is especially true for cooked foods; often, information for only the uncooked item can be found. Therefore, this quiz probably overlooks some of the folate in your diet. But if your score is substantially below the U.S. RDA—by a third or more—chances are your diet falls short of the allowance.

The danger falls under the category of hidden consequences—in this case, your doctor's ability to spot the vitamin B_{12} deficiency that can lead to permanent nerve damage. Here's the story of a near miss, reported to the *New England Journal of Medicine* by Max Katz, M.D.

We recently saw a 48-year-old man in whom self-medication with large quantities of folic acid in a multivitamin preparation could have been disastrous. One year before admission he noted anorexia and fatigue and became progressively weak and pale. He subsequently had several episodes of dizziness with nausea, and noted the onset of ankle swelling. He also became extremely depressed. A week before admission [to the hospital], on the advice of a friend, he went to a health food shop, bought some special vitamin pills [containing 8,000 mcg. of folic acid] and began to take them with marked amelioration of his symptoms.

The symptoms, unfortunately, had been caused by pernicious anemia, a disorder marked by inability to absorb vitamin B_{12}. Large doses of folic acid can mask this condition by hiding the signs of anemia from the doctor. Only because this patient had been taking folate for just a week before seeing his doctor did the signs of the anemia survive long enough for a correct diagnosis.

This patient went home fully recovered and remained "entirely well" because his condition was diagnosed in time and treated properly with vitamin B_{12}. But what could have happened is every bit as important. Had the anemia been masked by the folate supplement, the B_{12} deficiency would have gone unchecked, leading to irreversible nerve damage.

That's enough to scare anyone, and government policy on folic acid centers on this concern that high doses—perhaps 1,000 mcg. or more—might mask the anemia and B_{12} deficiency. Food manufacturers, for instance, may add no more than 400 mcg. of folic acid to a serving of food.

What are your chances of developing B_{12} deficiency? The condition is actually quite rare. Victims are usually those with pernicious anemia, a condition that prevents B_{12} from being absorbed in the stomach. Strict vegetarians are considered at risk, since there is no proof positive that plant foods provide B_{12}.

Should we all avoid folate supplements because of this rare but potentially irreversible condition? That's a tough question that, as far as I can see, has never been laid to rest. But were the danger great, folate supplements would be available only by prescription, and food companies would be prohibited from using it at all. So I suspect that once more, finding a low-risk level, not banning the supplement entirely, is the way to go.

THE STAR SYSTEM SHINES ON FOLIC ACID

Folic acid is unusual in that its most serious adverse effects are hidden consequences rather than toxic reactions. Here is a wrap-up on all counts.

Side effects—Reported, but somewhat unconfirmed side effects from extremely high doses of folate are nervous symptoms (excitability, sleep changes, impaired concentration) and digestive disturbances. These appear to be extremely rare. No such problems have been reported at modest doses of 1,000 mcg. or less.

Acute ailments—A handful of people have proved hypersensitive to folic acid and react to it quickly with rash, itching, hives, and other signs of allergy. Aside from these exceedingly rare reactions, no immediate toxic effects are on record.

Long-term problems—It is difficult to decide whether the digestive and nervous complaints occasionally reported in one or two studies should be considered side effects or toxic reactions. I suspect that more doctors would view them as side effects, but if intense enough, these symptoms might be considered a toxic reaction. Regardless, the risk of these reactions seems remote.

Conflicting combinations—The facts here are much clearer. Folic acid can interfere with the work of anticonvulsant drugs, so those who take them should take the vitamin only as prescribed by their doctors.

That's all as far as folate interfering with desired effects of drugs. Quite a few drugs, though, may interfere with folate nutrition by decreasing the amount in the blood. In this category are certain members of the following categories:

- Antibacterial drugs
- Anticancer drugs, such as methotrexate
- Anticonvulsant drugs

- Antituberculosis drugs
- Barbiturates
- Birth control pills
- Cortisone
- Sulfa drugs

Short-term use of these drugs may not pose any risk to folate nutrition, but if you take them long-term, your doctor may want to check on the folate level in your blood.

Alcohol, by the way, also interferes with folate nutrition by causing your body to excrete more of it. More likely than not, this should be of concern only to heavy drinkers.

Hidden consequences—Of all of the vitamins, folic acid poses the most potential harm in this category. It can mask symptoms of B_{12} deficiency, which left untreated can lead to permanent nerve damage. The possible effect of folic acid on zinc nutrition is another hidden consequence.

As far as laboratory tests go, folic acid may interfere with a correct reading in the acetaminophen screen test. This is a urine test to detect the aspirin substitutes, better known by such trade names as Tylenol.

HOW MUCH IS TOO MUCH

Most of us will never develop B_{12} deficiency, experience folate allergy, or take enough folic acid to risk toxic effects. So deciding whether to take a supplement, and if so, how much to take, rests on the folate-zinc interaction.

Those who see this issue in black-and-white see evidence that folate impairs zinc absorption and therefore condemn folate supplements. I disagree wholeheartedly with this approach. To me, the issue is whether folate impairs zinc enough to be cause for concern, and if so, how much folate is necessary to inflict significant damage. Or, as the scientist would say, what is the *magnitude* of this effect and how significant is it from a practical standpoint?

I have looked very closely at the results of the key study on folate and zinc. I feel that the researchers did not show that the magnitude of a 400 mcg. supplement is alarming. The supplement caused the amount of zinc in the men's blood to fall by a few milligrams (mg.), but these slightly reduced zinc levels remained within the normal range, except when zinc deficiency was deliberately created by feeding the men a diet almost free of zinc. The folate hardly can be blamed for the abnormally low zinc levels in this case.

Nonetheless, I don't recommend exceeding the 400 mcg. level without precautions: occasional measurement of blood zinc or attention to zinc intake. On a supplement regimen of 400 mcg. folate and 30 mg. zinc, the men had plenty of zinc in their blood, for instance. So when intakes of both were high, the inhibiting effect of folate on zinc absorption was a matter of academic, not practical, significance.

Prenatal vitamins often contain higher levels of folate than my suggested limit of 400 mcg., and with good reason. Folate needs increase quite a bit during pregnancy, with the recommended allowance doubling to 800 mcg. Such a supplement level is fine during this time. In addition to prenatal vitamins, folate supplements containing 800 mcg. also are widely available. Those who

Recommended Dietary Allowances for Folic Acid (Folate)

Group/Age	Mcg.
Infants 0–6 mon.	30
Infants 6–12 mon.	45
Children 1–3 yr.	100
Children 4–6 yr.	200
Children 7–10 yr.	300
Males 11–50 yr.	400
Males 51+ yr.	400
Females 11–50 yr.	400
Females 51+ yr.	400
Pregnant women	800
Nursing women	500

Note: The U.S. RDA for folic acid is 400 mcg.

take them would be well advised to insure a zinc intake of at least 15 mg. per day (the U.S. RDA).

If you have any reason to believe that you might have undiagnosed pernicious anemia or B_{12} deficiency, check on the possibility before taking folic acid, particularly in excess of 1,000 mcg. a day.

Aside from the zinc issue and anemia-masking issues, folate seems to have little potential to cause trouble in healthy people. In fact, several university researchers studying benefits of folate are giving people levels of 5,000 to 10,000 mcg. daily. Such regimens must pass the close scrutiny of professors charged with protecting the welfare of human subjects. The willingness to experiment with such high levels, even in these short-term studies, shows confidence in the relative safety of folate.

If you have to take high doses of folate for a medical reason, you can do so without major fear. Just be sure to pay attention to zinc and be alert for the rare side effects that a handful of people have reported.

C O O K I N G
for Folate

OATMEAL À L'ORANGE

(Makes 2 servings)

Folic acid: 63 mcg. per serving
Calories: 214 per serving

2 oranges	1 teaspoon maple syrup
orange juice, as needed	¼ cup plain low-fat yogurt
½ cup quick-cooking oats	pinch of cinnamon
2 tablespoons raisins, chopped	

Halve and seed the oranges and scoop the pulp and juice into a measuring cup. Add enough extra orange juice to make 1 cup. Set the shells aside.

C   O   O   K   I   N   G
for Folate—*continued*

In a small saucepan, combine the pulp, juice, oats, raisins, and syrup and bring to a boil, stirring constantly. Reduce the heat and simmer, continuing to stir until all liquid is absorbed, about 2 to 3 minutes. Scoop the oatmeal into the shells and top with yogurt and cinnamon.

FRUITED CHICKEN LIVERS SALAD

(Makes 4 servings)

Folic acid: 945 mcg. per serving
Calories: 308 per serving

1   tablespoon grated
     orange rind
1   cup orange juice
1   cup water
1   bay leaf
     freshly ground black
     pepper
1   pound chicken livers
1   orange, peeled,
     sectioned, seeded,
     and each section
     quartered

6   black mission figs,
     quartered
¼   cup chopped walnuts
1   cup watercress, stems
     removed
2   tablespoons orange
     juice
1   teaspoon walnut oil
     dash of nutmeg
     freshly ground black
     pepper

In a large saucepan, combine the orange rind, 1 cup orange juice, water, bay leaf, and pepper and bring to a boil. Add the chicken livers, reduce the heat to a simmer, cover and poach for 10 minutes. Remove the livers from poaching liquid and allow to cool.

In a medium-size serving bowl, combine the orange pieces, figs, walnuts, and watercress. Slice livers in half and add.

(continued)

C O O K I N G
for Folate—*continued*

In a small bowl, whisk together the 2 tablespoons orange juice, walnut oil, nutmeg, and pepper. Sprinkle over salad and toss to coat all ingredients. Serve immediately.

CHICK-PEA SOUP

(Makes 4 servings)

Folic acid: 83 mcg. per serving
Calories: 164 per serving

Roasting the onions before using them gives you a full-flavored soup without the addition of salt.

2 medium-size onions, peeled, quartered, and roasted*	1½ cups chicken stock
2 to 3 cloves garlic juice of 2 lemons	1 cup skim milk plain low-fat yogurt, for garnish
1 tablespoon tahini	sprigs of fresh mint, for garnish
1½ cups cooked chick-peas	

In the bowl of a food processor, combine the onions with the garlic, lemon juice, tahini, chick-peas, stock, and skim milk and process until smooth. Heat gently before serving. Garnish with yogurt and mint.

*To roast onions, place them in a lightly oiled glass baking dish in a preheated 350°F oven for 45 minutes.

VARIATION: To make hummus, a traditional Arabic dip, omit the stock and skim milk. Serve it cold with raw vegetables or use it as a sandwich spread.

Folic Acid Content
of Selected Supplements

Dosage is one tablet or capsule unless otherwise indicated.

Supplement	Manufacturer	Mcg.
Abdol with Minerals	Parke-Davis	100
Abron	O'Neal, Jones & Feldman	400
Allbee C-800 plus Iron	Robins	400
Bugs Bunny	Miles	300
Bugs Bunny Plus Iron	Miles	300
Bugs Bunny with Extra C	Miles	300
Cal-Prenal	North American	100
Cebefortis	Upjohn	2
Centrum	Lederle	400
Dayalets	Abbott	400
Dayalets plus Iron	Abbott	400
Engram-HP	Squibb	800
Feminins	Mead Johnson	100
Femiron with Vitamins	J.B. Williams	100
Ferritrinsic	Upjohn	33
Filibon Tablets	Lederle	400
Flintstones	Miles	300
Flintstones Plus Iron	Miles	300
Flintstones with Extra C	Miles	300
Folbesyn	Lederle	400
Gerilets	Abbott	400
Gevral	Lederle	400
Gevral T Capsules	Lederle	400
Lederplex Capsules	Lederle	3
Livitamin Chewable	Beecham Labs	5
Myadec	Parke-Davis	400
Natalins Tablets	Mead Johnson	800
Norlac	Rowell	400
One-A-Day	Miles	400
One-A-Day Core C 500	Miles	400
One-A-Day Plus Iron	Miles	400
One-A-Day Vitamins Plus Minerals	Miles	400
Peritinic	Lederle	50
Poly-Vi-Sol Chewable	Mead Johnson	300

(continued)

Supplements—*continued*

Supplement	Manufacturer	Mcg.
Poly-Vi-Sol with Iron Chewable	Mead Johnson	300
Simiron Plus	Merrell Dow	100
Stresstabs 600 with Iron	Lederle	400
Stresstabs 600 with Zinc	Lederle	400
Stuart Formula	Stuart	400
Stuart Prenatal	Stuart	800
Surbex 750 with Iron	Abbott	400
Surbex 750 with Zinc	Abbott	400
Tri-B-Plex	Anabolic	200
Unicap	Upjohn	400
Unicap Chewable	Upjohn	400
Unicap T	Upjohn	400
Vigran	Squibb	400
Vigran Chewable	Squibb	200
Vigran plus Iron	Squibb	400
Vio-Geric	Rowell	400
Zymacap Capsules	Upjohn	400

Source: Adapted from the American Pharmaceutical Association, *Handbook of Nonprescription Drugs*, 7th ed. (1982), 240–57.

Note: This chart is intended only as a guide. Vitamin formulations change periodically; always read product labels for accurate and up-to-date information on their nutrient levels.

————9

Vitamin B$_{12}$

When it comes to B vitamins, B$_{12}$ is in a class by itself. Unlike other B vitamins, which are used up quickly and need to be replaced, B$_{12}$ is guarded preciously by the body. It's called upon to do its work, then reabsorbed for later use. How nice to see a vitamin recycled!

But how safe is this last-discovered of the B vitamins? I'm not going to keep you in suspense—B$_{12}$ seems to be as safe as its first-discovered cousin thiamine. But like thiamine, it's not without its quirks.

B$_{12}$ BASICS

Nutritionists think of B$_{12}$ mostly in conjunction with its role in treating pernicious anemia, a blood disorder that can lead to nerve damage. But B$_{12}$ is a versatile vitamin that does more than alleviate anemia. It also serves as an "ingredient" used along the way to manufacture blood and other body cells, as well as the covering of nerve fibers. Finally, at a very basic level, it helps the body to metabolize carbohydrates and fats.

Vitamin B_{12} is absorbed principally in the stomach. A substance there called intrinsic factor allows the absorption to take place. That is why people who don't secrete intrinsic factor or who undergo removal of the stomach are frequent victims of vitamin B_{12} deficiency.

Because vitamin B_{12} is recycled in the body, you don't have to meet your Recommended Dietary Allowance (RDA) every day in order to have adequate B_{12} nutrition. In fact, it can take years of inadequate intake before B_{12} deficiency develops. The body's efficiency at holding on to it (and perhaps other unknown factors) must be why.

THE TOUGHEST TEST

It was a group of Swedish scientists who put B_{12} safety to the toughest challenge. Their subjects were 64 patients whose health was monitored for as long as five years on B_{12} therapy. Both the short-term and long-term safety of the vitamin were put to the test.

The results were remarkable. A single dose of up to 100,000 micrograms (mcg.) produced no ill effects in the patients studied. Such a test dose is astronomical by any standards; after all, the RDA for adults is a mere 3 mcg.

In the long-term studies, subjects took 500 to 1,000 mcg. of vitamin B_{12} daily, for as long as five years. Again, this was an extraordinarily high dose. And was anyone harmed? Apparently not. No signs of toxicity or side effects were reported, and the Swedish doctors say that this type of treatment is used widely in their country in the treatment of pernicious anemia with no known untoward effects.

THE ALLERGY CONNECTION

There is one area that prevents B_{12} from having a clean slate—allergy. As is true of certain other vitamins, however, allergies to vitamin B_{12} occur but are extremely rare. I have found only a few reported cases of true allergy to B_{12} tablets. Almost always the allergy results from injected B_{12}, not oral supplements. In one case, the allergy actually may have been caused by the person getting B_{12} shots before changing to the supplements. Here is what happened, in the words of C. N. Ugwu and F. J. Gibbons, M.D., the experts who reported this case of allergy to injection:

An 89-year-old lady (Miss L. F.) with no significant past medical illness or history of allergy was found to be anemic six years ago by her general practitioner. The diagnosis of pernicious anemia was made and she received B$_{12}$ injections . . . She remained well and exhibited no adverse reactions.

Five years later she developed symptoms of malaise, vomiting, and collapse one hour after injections. Hypersensitivity reaction to B$_{12}$ injections was suspected by her G.P. and various batches of [injectable] B$_{12}$ preparations and halving of the dosage were tried.

However, these reactions were getting progressively worse, and the District Nurse who was administering the injections subsequently became alarmed and refused subsequently to give the injections.

From here the detective work began. Miss L. F. was admitted to the hospital where, through meticulous investigation, her allergy to vitamin B$_{12}$ injections was confirmed. Naturally, the doctors ordered that the injections be stopped. Instead, the doctor

(continued on page 160)

Recommended Dietary Allowances for Vitamin B$_{12}$

Group/Age	Mcg.
Infants 0–6 mon.	0.5
Infants 6–12 mon.	1.5
Children 1–3 yr.	2.0
Children 4–6 yr.	2.5
Males 7+ yr.	3.0
Females 7+ yr.	3.0
Pregnant and nursing women	4.0

Note: The U.S. RDA for vitamin B$_{12}$ is 6 mcg.

The Diet Detective
Searches for Vitamin B$_{12}$

Some people are convinced that their diets are deficient in everything. But, with the exception of strict vegetarians who eat no animal products at all, inadequate B$_{12}$ intake is unlikely among Americans.

Vitamin B$_{12}$ abounds in the typical American diet. Surveys have found that the customary intake of vitamin B$_{12}$ varies from one and a half to five times the RDA, depending on income. Consider, for instance, that a hamburger and milkshake in a fast-food restaurant would almost satisfy the dietary allowance. The vitamin is plentiful in the United States, simply because we eat so many animal products, and that is where B$_{12}$ resides.

To get an idea of your B$_{12}$ intake, just check off the foods below that you ate yesterday or today, then follow the directions at the end for scoring.

1 point
1 ounce whole milk
   mozzarella cheese

2 points
4 ounces tuna
4 ounces chicken
2 links pork sausage
1 ounce American cheese
1 ounce cheddar cheese
1 ounce natural brick
   cheese
1 ounce part-skim
   mozzarella cheese
1 ice cream sandwich

3 points
1 ounce Swiss cheese
4 ounces turkey

4 points
1 frankfurter
2 slices all-meat bologna
4 ounces ham
4 ounces lobster
1 cup ice cream

5 points
1 cup cottage cheese
2 ounces (4 thin slices)
   salami
4 ounces pork roast

6 points
1 cup milk
1 milk shake (1 cup
   homemade or 1 fast-
   food)
1 cup ice milk

8 points
4 ounces haddock fillet

10 points
4 ounces halibut fillet

11 points
4 ounces veal

13 points
1 3-ounce hamburger patty

15 points
4 ounces beef

17 points
4 ounces lamb

51 points
4 ounces salmon

53 points
2 ounces liverwurst

60 points
4 ounces canned herring

132 points
4 ounces canned oysters

147 points
4 ounces chicken liver

546 points
4 ounces beef liver

Scoring

Add up your total points. Multiply the total by 5. The result is an estimate of the percent of the U.S. RDA for vitamin B₁₂ that you took in on the day in question. I'll bet that for most of you, the results were quite a surprise. And of course if you ate liver yesterday, well, your vitamin B₁₂ intake was sky-high.

Of course, not every food with a substantial B₁₂ content is listed. Such a list would go on for pages, as the vitamin occurs in virtually all animal protein foods. You can compensate for this, though, with a little ingenuity. If, for instance, you ate a cheese that is not listed, simply give yourself the number of points for the cheese above that it most closely resembles. Then you will have an even better estimate of how much B₁₂ you're feeding your body.

prescribed B_{12} tablets, 50 mcg. daily, for Miss L. F. "She has remained on this treatment for the last four months and has showed no adverse reactions whatsoever," reported her doctor. "Her serum B_{12} level is being monitored and has remained well within the normal range."

That's a story with a happy ending. Sadly enough, some years ago, one man died from a B_{12} injection.

I read of another case, however, where the patient was allergic to both the shots and the oral tablets. Her reactions always involved hives, and on some occasions she also suffered flushing, dizziness, headache, and difficult breathing. Fortunately, her doctors were able to tailor a treatment for her pernicious anemia that didn't require her to take B_{12} shots or tablets.

THE SKIN PROTESTS

Three kinds of skin problems, none of them serious, have been attributed to vitamin B_{12}:

• A swelling and crusting of skin around the lips, attributed to the victim's allergy to the cobalt in vitamin B_{12}
• Eruptions of itchy, inflamed, scaling skin that doctors refer to as eczema
• A type of acne that develops rapidly after B_{12} injections

How frequent are these reactions? From what I can see, they are rarer than rare, and the acne may occur only with injected B_{12}, not with tablets. The first two of these reactions, incidentally, were believed to be allergies. As I have said earlier, allergic reactions are not the same as toxicity. Whether the acne is an allergic response is unknown.

VEGETARIANISM: HOW RISKY?

According to food chemists, vitamin B_{12} occurs only in animal foods. Owing to this belief, it has become standard for nutritionists to recommend vitamin B_{12} supplementation to the strict vegetarians who shun not only meat, but also eggs and dairy products.

Yet those who have studied the matter have remarked that B_{12} deficiency develops in strict vegetarians much less often than would be expected. As a result, some nutritionists now speculate that certain vegetable foods may contain B$_{12}$-producing bacteria that provide strict vegetarians with at least some small amount of the vitamin.

The possibility is exciting. But I am with those who are not quite ready to consider this a confirmed fact. I am also concerned with research that has found abnormal EEG readings (a test of brain function) among some strict vegetarians. So I do advise strict vegetarians to take a B$_{12}$ supplement of about 3 mcg. daily. These supplements, incidentally, are generally prepared by bacterial action and do not contain any animal products that would compromise the vegetarian ethic.

THE STAR SYSTEM SHINES ON VITAMIN B$_{12}$

Now for a wrap-up of what can only be considered a very reassuring history.

Side effects—Skin problems such as lip crusting and eczema have turned up in a handful of individuals. Both were considered allergic reactions and do not indicate that B$_{12}$ has any known toxic potential. Acne may follow B$_{12}$ injections; whether it can occur from high doses of oral B$_{12}$ is unknown. It hasn't yet.

Acute ailments—No immediate toxic reactions to oral B$_{12}$ have been reported, even after single doses as high as 100,000 mcg. Acute allergic reactions, particularly to B$_{12}$ injections, do occur in sensitive people. These reactions can be serious to life-threatening for those affected. However, their occurrence does not indicate any potential for harm among those who are not allergic to the vitamin.

Long-term problems—Again the story is similar to that of acute ailments. Allergic reactions may occur after long-term use of vitamin B$_{12}$ tablets, but toxic reactions have not been reported at doses as high as 1,000 mcg. daily for three to five years.

Conflicting combinations—Vitamin B$_{12}$ does not interfere with the action of any drugs. However, the reverse happens;

certain drugs reduce absorption or retention of the vitamin. Among the culprits are certain members of the following categories: anticonvulsants, antituberculosis drugs, and cholesterol-lowering drugs. The anticancer drug methotrexate, and colchicine, a drug used to treat gout, also may affect B_{12} adversely. But because B_{12} deficiency often requires three to five years to develop, short-term use of these drugs does not necessarily call for a B_{12} supplement. Talk it over with your doctor if you are concerned.

Alcohol doesn't agree with many nutrients, and B_{12} is one of them. Heavy use of alcohol can have serious effects on B_{12} nutrition.

Hidden consequences—There are no reports of vitamin B_{12} interfering with accurate readings in laboratory tests, with one exception. A test for intrinsic factor antibodies, used to determine whether a patient can absorb vitamin B_{12}, may turn out a false reading if B_{12} is taken before the test.

Now for the matter of masking signs of other diseases. You know, for example, that folic acid can mask the signs of B_{12} deficiency. The reverse may also be true. According to the American Society of Hospital Pharmacists, vitamin B_{12} can mask signs of folate deficiency at doses of 10 mcg. or more. I actually have not read any reports of this occurring, though, so I am not sure that it happens very often. Of course, if you don't have the anemia caused by folic acid, this should not worry you.

A SIGH OF RELIEF

I end my story about vitamin B_{12} with a sigh of relief, for two reasons. The first reassuring fact is that Americans as a group are taking in more than enough B_{12} from their diets. The second is that I have little reason to suspect that those who take B_{12} supplements orally will be harmed, even at very high doses. As vitamins go, B_{12} simply is one of the safest.

C O O K I N G
for Vitamin B$_{12}$

PINEAPPLE-APRICOT BREAKFAST CHEESE

(Makes 1½ cups)

Vitamin B$_{12}$: 0.07 mcg. per tablespoon
Calories: 8½ calories per tablespoon

Breakfast cheese can replace high-fat, high-calorie butter on your morning toast or muffin.

½ cup dried pineapple, tightly packed	1 cup low-fat cottage cheese
½ cup dried apricots, tightly packed	pinch of ginger
	pinch of cinnamon
	¼ teaspoon vanilla extract

In the bowl of a food processor, mince the pineapple and apricots. Add the cottage cheese, ginger, cinnamon, and vanilla and blend until mixture is the consistency of cream cheese. Refrigerate.

NOTE: The cheese will keep, covered and refrigerated, for about 1 week.

CLASSIC CLAM SAUCE FOR PASTA OR FISH

(Makes approximately 1 cup)

Vitamin B$_{12}$: 16 mcg. per ¼ cup
Calories: 103 per ¼ cup

2 dozen littleneck clams	1 cup chicken stock
2 teaspoons flour	¼ cup milk
1 teaspoon olive oil	1 teaspoon dijon-style mustard
2 cloves garlic, minced	
3 bay leaves	pinch of dried thyme

(continued)

C   O   O   K   I   N   G
for Vitamin B₁₂—*continued*

Steam clams in 1 inch of water in a heavy, deep pot for 6 to 10 minutes or just until clams open. Cool and mince. Toss clams with flour and set aside.

In a large no-stick skillet, heat the olive oil. Add the garlic and bay leaves and sauté for several minutes. Add the stock, milk, mustard, and thyme and whisk frequently until the sauce is reduced by half. Add clams and heat for about 1 minute or until sauce thickens. Remove bay leaves. Serve immediately over pasta or fish.

SALMON TERIYAKI

(Makes 4 servings)

Vitamin B₁₂: 4 mcg. per serving
Calories: 255 per serving

1 tablespoon soy sauce	½ teaspoon grated fresh
1 tablespoon mirin (sweet	ginger
rice vinegar) or 2½	dash of sesame oil
teaspoons rice	1 pound salmon fillets,
vinegar plus ½	cut into 4 pieces
teaspoon honey	

In a shallow glass baking dish, make a marinade by combining the soy sauce, mirin or vinegar-honey mixture, ginger, and sesame oil. Roll the salmon in the marinade to coat. Let it sit for 20 minutes, turning the fish after 10 minutes. Reserve the marinade.

Spray a no-stick skillet with no-stick spray and cook the salmon over low to medium heat for about 3 minutes. Flip and cook for 3 more minutes, adding reserved marinade after 2 minutes. Serve immediately after 2 minutes.

Vitamin B$_{12}$ Content
of Selected Supplements

Dosage is one tablet or capsule unless otherwise indicated.

Supplement	Manufacturer	Mcg.
Abdec Kapseal	Parke-Davis	2.00
Abdol with Minerals	Parke-Davis	1.00
Abron	O'Neal, Jones & Feldman	12.00
Allbee C-800	Robins	12.00
Allbee C-800 plus Iron	Robins	12.00
Allbee-T	Robins	5.00
B12-Plus	Anabolic	250.00
B-C-Bid Capsules	Geriatric Pharm.	5.00
B Complex Tablets	Squibb	2.00
Belfer	O'Neal, Jones & Feldman	10.00
Beminal 500	Ayerst	5.00
Beminal Forte with Vitamin C	Ayerst	2.50
Beta-Vite Liquid (per tsp.)	North American	25.00
Beta-Vite with Iron Liquid (per tsp.)	North American	25.00
Bugs Bunny	Miles	4.50
Bugs Bunny Plus Iron	Miles	4.50
Bugs Bunny with Extra C	Miles	4.50
Cal-Prenal	North American	2.00
C-B Bone Capsules	USV	5.00
Cebefortis	Upjohn	5.00
Cebetinic	Upjohn	5.00
Centrum	Lederle	9.00
Chew-Vite	North American	1.00
Cluvisol 130	Ayerst	2.50
Cluvisol Syrup (per tsp.)	Ayerst	2.00
Dayalets	Abbott	6.00
Dayalets plus Iron	Abbott	6.00
Engram-HP	Squibb	8.00
Feminins	Mead Johnson	10.00
Femiron with Vitamins	J.B. Williams	5.00
Feostim	O'Neal, Jones & Feldman	5.00
Filibon Tablets	Lederle	6.00
Flintstones	Miles	4.50
Flintstones Plus Iron	Miles	4.50
Flintstones with Extra C	Miles	4.50

(continued)

Supplements—continued

Supplement	Manufacturer	Mcg.
Folbesyn	Lederle	9.00
Ganatrex (per 0.6 ml.)	Merrell Dow	6.00
Geriamic	North American	3.00
Gerilets	Abbott	9.00
Geriplex	Parke-Davis	2.00
Geriplex-FS Kapseals	Parke-Davis	2.00
Geriplex-FS Liquid (per 2 tbsp.)	Parke-Davis	5.00
Geritinic	Geriatric Pharm.	5.00
Geritol Junior Liquid (per tsp.)	J.B. Williams	3.00
Geritol Junior Tablets	J.B. Williams	2.50
Geritol Liquid (per tsp.)	J.B. Williams	3.00
Geritol Tablets	J.B. Williams	3.00
Gerix Elixir (per 2 tbsp.)	Abbott	6.00
Gerizyme (per tbsp.)	Upjohn	3.30
Gevrabon (per 2 tbsp.)	Lederle	1.00
Gevral	Lederle	6.00
Gevral Protein	Lederle	0.87
Gevral T Capsules	Lederle	9.00
Golden Bounty B Complex with Vitamin C	Squibb	25.00
Iberet	Abbott	25.00
Iberet-500	Abbott	25.00
Iberet-500 Oral Solution (per tsp.)	Abbott	6.25
Iberet Oral Solution (per 0.6 ml.)	Abbott	6.25
Iberol	Abbott	12.50
Incremin with Iron Syrup (per tsp.)	Lederle	25.00
Lederplex Capsules	Lederle	1.00
Lederplex Liquid (per tsp.)	Lederle	6.25
Lederplex Tablets	Lederle	1.00
Lipoflavonoid Capsules	Cooper Vision Pharm.	1.67
Lipotriad Capsules	Cooper Vision Pharm.	1.67
Lipotriad Liquid (per tsp.)	Cooper Vision Pharm.	5.00
Livitamin Capsules	Beecham Labs	5.00
Livitamin Chewable	Beecham Labs	3.00
Livitamin Liquid (per tbsp.)	Beecham Labs	5.00
Lufa Capsules	USV	1.00
Methischol Capsules	USV	2.00

Supplements—*continued*

Supplement	Manufacturer	Mcg.
Mucoplex	ICN	5.00
Multicebrin	Lilly	3.00
Multiple Vitamins	North American	1.00
Multiple Vitamins with Iron	North American	1.00
Multivitamins	Rowell	2.00
Myadec	Parke-Davis	6.00
Natabec	Parke-Davis	5.00
Natalins Tablets	Mead Johnson	8.00
Norlac	Rowell	8.00
Obron-6	Pfipharmecs	2.00
One-A-Day	Miles	6.00
One-A-Day Core C 500	Miles	6.00
One-A-Day Plus Iron	Miles	6.00
One-A-Day Vitamins Plus Minerals	Miles	6.00
Optilets-500	Abbott	12.00
Optilets-M-500	Abbott	12.00
Orexin Softabs	Stuart	25.00
Os-Cal Forte	Marion	1.60
Os-Cal Plus	Marion	0.03
Paladec (per tsp.)	Parke-Davis	5.00
Paladec with Minerals	Parke-Davis	5.00
Panuitex	O'Neal, Jones & Feldman	2.00
Peritinic	Lederle	50.00
Poly-Vi-Sol Chewable	Mead Johnson	4.50
Poly-Vi-Sol with Iron Chewable	Mead Johnson	4.50
Probec-T	Stuart	5.00
Roeribec	Pfipharmecs	4.00
Rogenic	O'Neal, Jones & Feldman	25.00
Simiron Plus	Merrell Dow	3.33
S.S.S. Tablets	S.S.S.	1.50
S.S.S. Tonic (per tbsp.)	S.S.S.	0.20
Stresscaps Capsules	Lederle	4.00
Stresstabs 600	Lederle	12.00
Stresstabs 600 with Iron	Lederle	12.00
Stresstabs 600 with Zinc	Lederle	25.00
Stuart Formula	Stuart	6.00
Stuartinic	Stuart	25.00
Stuart Prenatal	Stuart	8.00

(continued)

Supplements—*continued*

Supplement	Manufacturer	Mcg.
Super Plenamins	Rexall	1.50
Surbex	Abbott	5.00
Surbex 750 with Iron	Abbott	12.00
Surbex 750 with Zinc	Abbott	12.00
Surbex-T	Abbott	10.00
Surbex with C	Abbott	5.00
Thera-Combex H-P Kapseals	Parke-Davis	5.00
Theragran	Squibb	5.00
Theragran Liquid (per tsp.)	Squibb	5.00
Theragran-M	Squibb	5.00
Theragran-Z	Squibb	5.00
Therapeutic Vitamins	North American	5.00
Thera-Spancap	North American	6.00
Tonebec	A.V.P.	3.00
Tri-B-Plex	Anabolic	12.50
Unicap	Upjohn	6.00
Unicap Chewable	Upjohn	6.00
Unicap T	Upjohn	18.00
Vi-Aqua	USV	1.00
Vigran	Squibb	6.00
Vigran Chewable	Squibb	3.00
Vigran plus Iron	Squibb	6.00
Vio-Geric	Rowell	6.00
Vitagett	North American	2.50
Vita-Kaps Tablets	Abbott	3.00
Vita-Kaps-M Tablets	Abbott	3.00
Vitamin-Mineral Capsules	North American	2.00
Viterra	Pfipharmecs	2.00
Viterra High Potency	Pfipharmecs	5.00
Z-Bec	Robins	6.00
Zymacap Capsules	Upjohn	9.00
Zymalixir Syrup (per tsp.)	Upjohn	2.00
Zymasyrup (per tsp.)	Upjohn	3.00

Source: Adapted from the American Pharmaceutical Association, *Handbook of Nonprescription Drugs*, 7th ed. (1982), 240–57.

Note: This chart is intended only as a guide. Vitamin formulations change periodically; always read product labels for accurate and up-to-date information on their nutrient levels.

10
The Rest of the B's

Ask a nutrition-minded friend for the first word that comes to mind when you say "B vitamins," and you'll get a variety of answers. But I'm certain neither biotin, inositol, pantothenic acid, nor choline is likely to be among them.

These four are the quiet members of the B family—the ones mentioned much less frequently than leaders like thiamine and riboflavin. There is a reason for what you might call a lack of attention to these four nutrients. It seems that under normal circumstances, we can manufacture our own supply of them. For this reason, the four are sometimes referred to as "conditional B vitamins." Conditional, of course, because under some circumstances, the body may fail to make them and need food or supplements to supply them.

Two of these substances—choline and inositol—are conditional for another reason. A controversy has been raging for some time as to whether these two actually qualify for the vitamin label. In 1974, for instance, the committee issuing the Recommended Dietary Allowances (RDA) considered choline to be a vitamin. Six

169

years later, its 1980 revision insisted that choline cannot be considered a vitamin. Look in nutrition textbooks and you will find more signs of the debate; some list inositol and/or choline as vitamins, but others do not. The majority of nutritionists, I think, believe that neither are vitamins under the strict definition of the term. But one or both may nonetheless serve a useful nutritional need.

Vitamins or not, I think the safety of choline and inositol deserves a look. Ditto for pantothenic acid and biotin, considered vitamins by every nutritionist I know. But because there is so little information about all four of these vitamins, I will discuss them as a group, rather than one by one.

THE ROLES THEY PLAY

Biotin plays a central role in your health. It helps the body metabolize its three sources of fuel: proteins, carbohydrates, and fats. Pantothenic acid, also known as pantothenate, has these roles and more; the body uses it in the process of making a variety of important substances, including certain hormones.

Like pantothenic acid, choline, too, is one of the body's raw ingredients. It's part of a substance called acetylcholine that plays referee in the brain and nervous system, regulating a variety of body functions. Choline also helps in carrying fats throughout the bloodstream. Every cell in the body contains components derived from choline. And it wears still another label—lipotropic factor. These factors are believed to help prevent fat from being deposited in body organs. Inositol may be one as well.

Inositol is found in virtually every cell of the body. The heart, brain, and muscles of the skeleton contain notably large amounts, but the reason for this remains a mystery. One can only suspect that its presence in such important places, however, signals a valuable role in maintaining good health.

FROM DUTIES TO DEFICIENCIES

Deficiencies of biotin and pantothenic acid are rare among people eating normal mixed diets. Only two situations have been associated with biotin deficiency: tube feeding and high intake of raw eggs. In the raw state, eggs contain a substance, avidin, that prevents biotin absorption. Cooking destroys avidin. So, since we usually eat our eggs cooked, biotin deficiency is extremely rare.

Nutritionists believe that pantothenic acid deficiency almost never occurs naturally. But there has been an exception to this rule. Some of the prisoners of war held by the Japanese during World War II developed a condition known as "burning feet" syndrome. It seemed that pantothenic acid, but not other B vitamins, alleviated the condition.

Of course, malnutrition in itself might be expected to cause a deficiency of pantothenate. But the only other deficiencies on the books were created deliberately in volunteers who agreed to take a substance that antagonizes the vitamin. Naturally, doing this created a pantothenic acid deficiency. After a few weeks, the volunteers complained of such symptoms as headache, tiredness, insomnia, cramps, vomiting, diarrhea, tingling sensations in the hands and feet, and difficult coordination.

As for choline and inositol, no deficiency syndrome exists; that is, no one has ever found a choline or inositol deficiency among adults. But without all the answers in, the American Academy of Pediatrics recommends that choline and inositol be added to infant formulas made without milk so that the products contain the same levels found in milk-based formulas. The needs of infants and young children, after all, may be different from those of adults.

Deficiencies of these four nutrients—however rare or unknown they may be—is only one side of their unique story. Over the years, many have wondered if taking amounts greater than we normally get through foods or those our bodies manufacture on their own could actually benefit a host of medical conditions. From these inquiries, we have learned some reassuring facts and important lessons.

SIDE EFFECTS? SOMETIMES

Half of this story is a very short one. For two of the group—biotin and inositol—no side effects or toxic reactions have been reported. That makes it impossible to set a maximum safe or recommended dose for either one.

That leaves pantothenic acid and choline. At doses of panto-

(continued on page 174)

The Diet Detective
Searches for Pantothenate

Here's a quiz that I'll bet you have never taken—one that estimates the pantothenic acid content of your diet. As you might guess, finding facts about pantothenic acid in food takes some hunting, and the tables that exist are not complete. But based on what is known, you can get an idea of how your diet fares.

You are familiar already with how to take these tests, but this time scoring will be a little different, so be sure to read the scoring section that follows the food listings.

You won't find quizzes for the other three B's—biotin, choline, and inositol. The reason? I am still waiting for someone to measure levels of these nutrients in our staple foods.

1 point
1 cup canned apricots
3 raw apricots
¼ cup chopped dates
1 cup grapefruit juice
1 orange
1 cup orange juice
1 cup red kidney beans
1 cup raw carrots
1 cup canned corn
1 cup frozen lima beans
1 tomato
1 cup oatmeal
1 cup chick-peas
4 ounces roast beef
4 ounces lean roast lamb
1 ounce Camembert
  cheese
1 ounce mozzarella cheese

2 points
½ grapefruit
1 cup strawberries

1 cup canned asparagus
1 cup frozen brussels
  sprouts
1 cup frozen cauliflower
1 cup frozen corn
1 cup chopped celery
1 cup frozen kale
1 cup frozen peas
1 potato, baked in skin
10 French fries (4 inches
  long)
1 cup canned tomato
⅓ cup pecans
¼ cup sunflower seeds
⅓ cup all-bran cereal
1 ounce blue cheese
1 cup ice cream
1 cup crabmeat
4 ounces flounder
4 ounces canned salmon
4 ounces turkey

3 points
1 cup raw asparagus
1 cup raw broccoli
1 cup raw cauliflower
1 cup canned sweet potato
⅓ cup roasted peanuts
1 cup lentils
1 cup soybeans
1 cup milk (skim, low-fat,
   or whole)
1 cup yogurt
1 egg
4 ounces lobster
1 tablespoon brewer's
   yeast

4 points
1 cup raw brussels sprouts
4 ounces smoked herring

6 points
1 cup broccoli
1 cup raw kale

11 points
1 avocado

13 points
½ cup chicken liver

14 points
4 ounces beef liver

Scoring

Add up your total points. Multiply the total by 5. If you scored 12 points, for example, multiply 12 by 5 for a score of 60. Since there aren't as yet any RDA for pantothenic acid, the score you have is not a percentage of a recommended intake. But you can translate the score into milligrams of pantothenic acid to be compared with a "safe and adequate" range that has been defined.

Use the table below to convert your score to the approximate number of milligrams of pantothenic acid that you took in on the day in question. How does your score compare to the estimated "safe and adequate" range of 4 to 7 mg. daily for an adult?

Points	Pantothenic Acid (mg.)	Points	Pantothenic Acid (mg.)
20	1.2	90	5.4
30	1.8	100	6.0
40	2.4	110	6.6
50	3.0	120	7.2
60	3.6	130	7.8
70	4.2	140	8.4
80	4.8	150	9.0

thenate ranging in the area of 10,000 to 20,000 milligrams (mg.) daily, "occasional diarrhea and water retention" have been reported, according to one report. Here are highlights from a few others:

- No side effects at doses of 1,000 to 2,000 mg. daily for six months.
- Transient nausea—but no other adverse effects—at doses up to 10,000 mg. daily of a related form of pantothenic acid (pantothenyl alcohol) taken daily for as long as three years.
- Headache, sleepiness, depression, memory loss, flatulence, and abdominal pain in 4 of 19 patients taking 100 mg. pantothenic acid daily. The other 15 patients had no complaints. Ironically, subjects who were receiving a placebo instead of pantothenic acid also complained of headache and gastrointestinal upsets.

These reports make clear that the majority of those treated with pantothenic acid suffered no ill effects. When you consider also that in all of these studies but one, doses were well over a thousand times the suggested range, you probably will agree pantothenic acid deserves its current status as a very, very safe vitamin. Of course, no one has tested doses such as these taken for a lifetime, so using these enormous amounts for decades is not guaranteed to be safe.

COLOR CHOLINE DIFFERENT

Of the four subjects of this chapter, choline has the most colorful profile. For starters, there's its smell. "Choline imparts an odor of dead fish to the breath and body," says the standard pharmaceutical handbook. And the fishy odor is but one of the facts you should know about.

Doctors have tried treating several brain disorders with a form of choline called choline chloride. Choline supplements available without prescription derive their choline from other sources—choline bitartrate or choline dihydrogen citrate. But these forms of choline must be considered to have potentially similar side effects as choline chloride until proven otherwise.

Here are some of the findings regarding side effects, or lack of side effects, in studies done so far:

- A study lasting about six weeks reports, "On only the highest dose of choline chloride [roughly 16,000 mg. a day] five [of seven]

patients developed a slight 'fishy odor' and one developed mild diarrhea. There were no other side effects." Other dose levels tested amounted to roughly 4,000 and 8,000 mg. a day.
• In another six-week study, 1 of 16 patients taking 3,000 to 6,000 mg. choline chloride daily developed headache on the 3,000 mg. dose. No other side effects were reported.
• In another short-term study that assessed mental, but not physical effects of doses up to 20,000 mg. daily, scientists reported, "Patients were more depressed during choline chloride administration." Other aspects of mental health were not affected.

You may be wondering if there were any apparent benefits from the chloride during these studies. For a few patients, the answer was yes. Selected patients suffering from disordered control of their body movements, a condition known as tardive dyskinesia, did seem to benefit from the choline treatment. This disorder is an unfortunate risk associated with long-term use of antipsychotic drugs, and promising treatments for it attract much interest.

But as I have always said, anything that confers benefits almost surely brings risks. Choline is no exception, for one of the problems mentioned above is not a mere side effect, but a serious adverse reaction. I am referring to the problem of depression, and it deserves a closer look.

DEPRESSIONS THAT DEEPENED

I would like to share with you two stories that convey the potential for high-dose choline to aggravate depression. Both were reported to the medical journal *Lancet* by Carol Tamminga, M.D., and coworkers at the University of Chicago.

The first case involved 29-year-old Douglas, who developed a movement disorder after receiving antipsychotic drugs for three years. The doctors hoped that choline might help him, but they ran into an unexpected problem. Here is Doug's story, in the words of his doctors.

> He received oral choline for the proposed treatment of his movement disorder, beginning at 3 grams [3,000 mg.] a day, increasing to 9 grams [9,000 mg.] over 1½ weeks. His [depressive] symptom development paralleled the dose increase until, at 9 g [9,000 mg.], he became

*highly agitated, paranoid, and even more severely de-
pressed, with feelings of worthlessness and hopelessness.
Choline was withdrawn and restarted two weeks later.
The patient's mood changes were carefully observed.
When the choline was increased to 9 g [9,000 mg.] per
day, he again developed feelings of hopelessness, worthlessness, paranoia, and suicidal thoughts . . . At that dose
level he made an unsuccessful suicide attempt. After the
drug [choline] was stopped, the symptoms remitted over
4–5 days.*

The doctors' experience with Douglas also occurred with
Rose, aged 57. She, too, suffered from tardive dyskinesia, the
inability to stop involuntary movements of her body. Her story, as
told by her doctors, follows:

*She began on 3 g [3,000 mg.] per day of choline,
increasing to 9 g [9,000 mg.] over two weeks. Although
choline produced a modest reduction of her dyskinesia
symptoms, she developed severe depressive symptoms
. . . accompanied by delusional talk of death, hopelessness, and despair. She began to talk of dying and never
leaving hospital. After drug [choline] withdrawal, the
weakness and the depressive delusional talk remitted
over 7–8 days.*

Other doctors who have treated patients with choline report
mixed results on the depression issue. In one study of five patients, for instance, two were more depressed during choline
treatment, while two others were less so.

Making sense of this handful of cases and scattered results
may seem impossible, but I am willing to wager that the depressive reactions of some patients were no fluke. I think this because
of strong clues that a quartet of chemicals in the brain can influence depression. The body uses choline to make one of these
chemicals, acetylcholine. Certainly high doses of choline might
stimulate formation of acetylcholine. That, in turn, could alter the
usual balance of the brain chemicals in a way that triggers depression.

These reactions, of course, involve very large doses of choline—in the thousands of milligrams or tens of thousands of

Counting on Choline

As best as I can determine, nutritionists have measured the choline content in only a handful of foods. This is far too few, in my opinion, to make a quiz that would give even a rough estimate of your choline intake. Here is the next best thing: A chart for your reference if you are interested in food sources of choline.

Food	Amount	Choline (mg.)
Avocado	½ small	14
Beans, green	1 cup	18
Beef rib, lean	4 ounces	94
Bologna	1 slice (1 ounce)	17
Bran	1 tablespoon	13
Brewer's yeast	1 tablespoon	24
Cabbage, raw	1 cup	16
Carrot, raw	1 medium	11
Cashews	1 ounce	37
Egg	1 medium	242
Frankfurter	1	29
Lamb, leg of, untrimmed	4 ounces	95
Lentils, raw	½ cup	212
Milk, whole	1 cup	49
Molasses	1 tablespoon	17
Rice, brown	1 cup	218
Rice, long-grain white	1 cup	147
Rice, white	1 cup	89
Soybeans	½ cup	328
Tomato sauce	½ cup	25
Turnip greens, from frozen	1 cup	45
Wheat germ	1 tablespoon	28

milligrams. Moreover, the patients had a history of some type of mental illness or brain disorder. Would a dose in the 500 to 1,000 mg. range, for instance, worsen depression or bring on depressive symptoms in these patients? In healthy people? No one has the information to answer that question. (Incidentally, whether the fishy odor will occur at such lower doses is likewise unknown.)

What to do when so little is known? First, accept that no one can say with any certainty whether choline will be free of depressive or other side effects. Second, rest assured that so far, the adverse reactions have disappeared after discontinuing choline. Therefore, be alert for possible symptoms if you do embark on a supplement program containing substantial amounts of choline

Recommended Intakes for the Other B's

Recommended Dietary Allowances for pantothenic acid, biotin, choline, or inositol have not been defined. However, a range considered to be "safe and adequate" has been issued by the Food and Nutrition Board for biotin and pantothenic acid. They appear below. Even though there are no RDA for these substances, the FDA has issued U.S. RDA.

As for choline, the committee that establishes the dietary allowances says only that, "The average intake from foods ordinarily consumed (400 to 900 mg. a day) is apparently adequate for health but should not be equated with a dietary requirement."

Group/Age	Biotin (mcg.)	Pantothenic Acid (mg.)
Infants 0–6 mon.	35	2
Infants 6–12 mon.	50	3
Children 1–3 yr.	65	3
Children 4–6 yr.	85	3–4
Children 7–10 yr.	120	4–5
Males 11+ yr.	100–200	4–7
Females 11+ yr.	100–200	4–7

Note: The U.S. RDA for biotin is 300 mcg. The U.S. RDA for pantothenic acid is 10 mg.

and stop if you experience untoward effects.

Though, as I say, I have no basis for judging the potential of choline to aggravate depression in doses lower than those tested, my instincts tell me that anyone who is depressed or has a history of depression ought to be very cautious. Looking through supplement catalogs, I often see choline supplements that provide 500 to 650 mg. per tablet. Would I advise a depressed person that there is no harm in taking such a daily dose? Not on your life, though the risk is probably small. Do I worry about the 20 mg. or so of choline in some multivitamin supplements? No, I don't. As the chart on page 177 shows, quite a few foods contain more than that.

THE LECITHIN ALTERNATIVE

You may already know that there's more than one way to add choline to your diet. Instead of choline tablets, you can choose the popular alternative, lecithin, available in both capsule and granule form.

One group of choline researchers has already decided to favor lecithin. To its credit, it doesn't cause the fishy odor problem. Also, their patients expressed a preference for sprinkling the granules on their food rather than taking choline powder. But as far as I am concerned choline is choline, and the choline in lecithin may be just as capable of aggravating depression as choline in other forms.

The choline content of lecithin granules may vary from product to product, but the ones I have seen contain about 2,000 mg. of choline per tablespoon, again, a level that calls for being alert for depressive symptoms. Capsules generally contain much smaller amounts of lecithin. Therefore, their choline content is likely to be fairly low, for choline is but one of lecithin's constituents. But check your labels to be sure.

THE STAR SYSTEM SHINES ON THE REST OF THE B'S

Now for the final portrait of the four members of this chapter. Perhaps I should call it a sketch rather than a portrait, in light of how little research has been done. Regardless, the facts are generally favorable.

Side effects—For biotin and inositol, a simple "none." And for pantothenic acid, almost none—possibly headaches and gastrointestinal upset among a few users. As for choline, it can give the body and breath a very unpleasant odor.

Acute ailments—Be it choline, inositol, pantothenic acid, or biotin, immediate reactions to oral doses have never been reported. However, the depression that developed over a one-to-two-week period with choline deserves prominent mention.

Long-term problems—Call this the unknown territory. I cannot find any reports of problems that developed after long-term use for any of the four. But, then again, I can hardly find any studies of long-term use, period. In the words of a group of scientists evaluating choline safety for the Food and Drug Administration, "No long-term toxicity studies of choline, or studies of its carcinogenic, mutagenic, or terategenic potential have come to [our] attention." Nor to mine.

I have found one long-term study for pantothenic acid and inositol, each showing no side effects. For pantothenic acid, the dose was up to 10,000 mg. of a related form of the vitamin for up to three years. For inositol, the dose ranged from 1,000 to 3,000 mg. daily for up to a year.

Conflicting combinations—In light of the link between depression and choline, I would consider choline and antidepressant drugs to be an unadvisable partnership. Choline may also interact with the potent painkiller morphine. How much of each is required to become troublesome is not clear.

I didn't find anything in this category for inositol, biotin, or pantothenic acid.

Hidden consequences—None of these four substances are known to mask any condition or disease. As for interfering with accurate readings in laboratory tests, all but inositol have clean records. Inositol may affect readings for ketones in the urine, and possibly one method of measuring urinary phosphate.

TURN THE PAGE TO CONTROVERSY

We have now finished our look at all members of the B complex. The next vitamin is one often packaged with the B's, but when the subject is safety, it is in a class by itself. No other vitamin has been more talked about, exalted, or assailed. The C in its name seems to stand for controversy, and it's next, in chapter 11.

C O O K I N G
for Pantothenic Acid

MEXICAN BLACKENED SALMON

(Makes 4 servings)

Pantothenic acid: 0.56 mg. per serving
Calories: 269 per serving

Blackening fish is a wonderful cooking method that leaves fish crisp on the outside and moist and tender inside. It will, however, cause some smoke so it's best cooked near a window with a fan or outside on a hot grill.

1	teaspoon cumin seed	1	pound salmon fillet, no thicker than ½ inch, cut into 4 pieces
1	teaspoon coriander seed		
1	2-inch dried chili pepper	1½	teaspoons olive oil
1	teaspoon dried oregano		

Heat a large cast-iron frying pan on high (or on a charcoal grill close to the coals) until it begins to turn white. This will take about 10 minutes.

In a spice grinder or mortar, crush the cumin seed, coriander seed and chili pepper. Add the oregano and set aside.

Rub the salmon with the olive oil. Then rub in the spice mixture so that each piece of salmon is well coated. Place each piece in the skillet and cook for 2 minutes on each side.

C O O K I N G
for Pantothenic Acid—continued

BEST-FOR-BREAKFAST FRUIT SALAD

(Makes 8 servings)

Pantothenic acid: 0.85 mg. per serving
Calories: 152 per serving

1 honeydew melon, peeled and cut into 1-inch chunks (about 8 cups)
2 avocados, peeled and cut into 1-inch chunks
½ teaspoon grated lime rind
juice of 2 limes (about ⅓ cup)
1 tablespoon minced fresh mint or 1½ teaspoons dried mint
½ cup plain low-fat yogurt

Combine all the ingredients in a large bowl and toss until well coated with the yogurt. Serve immediately on chilled plates.

BROCCOLI POPOVERS

(Makes 6 popovers)

Pantothenic acid: 0.71 mg. per popover
Calories: 139 per popover

1⅓ cups minced broccoli
½ cup whole wheat pastry flour
½ cup unbleached flour
1 cup buttermilk
1 tablespoon safflower oil
2 eggs, beaten

Preheat oven to 450°F.
    Place the broccoli in a fine mesh strainer and blanch it by pouring boiling water over it for about 5 seconds. Pat dry and set aside to drain.

C O O K I N G
for Pantothenic Acid—continued

In a medium-size bowl, combine the flours, buttermilk, oil, eggs, and drained broccoli, using as few strokes as possible—20 is ideal. (A large rubber spatula works well for this type of mixing.)

Oil 6 popover pans. Fill each ⅔ full and bake for 20 minutes. Reduce the oven heat to 350°F and bake for 20 to 25 minutes more. Remove the popovers from the pans and poke a hole in the bottom of each to allow steam to escape. Serve warm.

NOTE: If you don't have popover pans, muffin tins or custard cups are acceptable. However, if they're not deeper than they are wide (as popover pans are), the popovers may not pop over.

C O O K I N G
for Choline

ROASTED SOY NUTS

(Makes 2 cups)

Choline: 82 mg. per ¼ cup
Calories: 63 per ¼ cup

These are a great snack, but don't rule them out for lunch. Sprinkle them on tossed salads, add them to chicken, egg, and tuna salads, or use them to garnish soups.

1   cup dried soybeans
1½ teaspoons soy sauce
1   teaspoon chili powder

Soak the soybeans in water overnight. Check them periodically to make sure the water level is high enough to cover all

(continued)

C O O K I N G
for Choline—*continued*

the beans. Add more if necessary.

Drain the beans, pat them dry, and toss them with the soy sauce and chili powder. Spread them in a single layer on a jelly roll pan. Use 2 pans if necessary.

Roast the beans for about 1 hour at 300°F, stirring them once after 30 minutes. Let the beans cool before storing them in a screw-top glass jar or a Ziploc bag.

MOROCCAN EGGS WITH COUSCOUS

(Makes 4 servings)

Choline: minimum 242 mg. per serving*
Calories: 330 per serving

1   cup chicken stock or
        water
1   cup couscous†
½   cup minced onion
1   teaspoon safflower oil
1   small zucchini, cut into
        2-inch julienne strips
        (about ¾ cup)

¼   cup minced fresh
        parsley
4   eggs, beaten
¼   cup pine nuts, toasted
        generous dash of
        freshly grated
        nutmeg

In a medium-size saucepan, bring the stock or water and couscous to a boil, stirring frequently. Remove from heat, cover, and set aside.

In a no-stick sauté pan, sauté the onion in the oil for about 10 minutes. Add the zucchini and parsley and sauté for 1 minute more. Add the onion mixture to the couscous and toss to combine.

In the same no-stick sauté pan, cook the eggs until they are set and still creamy. Add them and the pine nuts to the couscous. Sprinkle with nutmeg. Toss gently and serve.

C   O   O   K   I   N   G
for Choline—*continued*

*Data not available for all ingredients.

†Available at specialty food stores.

NOTE: Add extra choline and crunch by sprinkling toasted wheat germ over each serving.

PEANUTTY RICE PILAF

(Makes 4 servings)

Choline: 56 mg. per serving*
Calories: 346 per serving

1 cup arborio or other
   short grain rice
1 teaspoon olive oil
2 cloves garlic, minced
1 thin slice fresh ginger,
   minced
¼ cup minced celery
   leaves
½ teaspoon dried
   rosemary, crushed
½ teaspoon dried lovage,
   crushed, or diced
   celery leaf
3 bay leaves
3 cups chicken stock
½ cup minced sweet red
   pepper
½ cup chopped roasted
   peanuts
¼ cup grated Parmesan
   cheese

Preheat oven to 350°F.

In a flameproof dish, combine the rice, olive oil, garlic, ginger, celery leaves, rosemary, lovage, and bay leaves. Place on medium heat and sauté, stirring constantly, for about 5 minutes. Add the stock and pepper and bring to a boil. Remove from heat, cover, and bake for 15 to 20 minutes. Uncover and stir. Bake uncovered for an additional 10 minutes. Remove from heat and add peanuts and Parmesan, stirring well to combine. Serve immediately.

*Data not available for all ingredients.

Pantothenic Acid Content
of Selected Supplements

Dosage is one tablet or capsule unless otherwise indicated.

Supplement	Manufacturer	Mg.
Abdec Baby Drops (per 0.6 ml.)	Parke-Davis	5.0
Abdec Kapseal	Parke-Davis	10.0
Abdol with Minerals	Parke-Davis	2.5
Allbee C-800	Robins	25.0
Allbee C-800 plus Iron	Robins	25.0
Allbee-T	Robins	23.0
Allbee with C	Robins	10.0
B-Complex Capsules	North American	1.0
C-B Bone Capsules	USV	8.0
Cebefortis	Upjohn	10.0
Centrum	Lederle	10.0
Cherri-B Liquid (per 0.6 ml.)	North American	0.1
Cluvisol Syrup (per tsp.)	Ayerst	3.0
Feminins	Mead Johnson	10.0
Femiron with Vitamins	J.B. Williams	10.0
Geriamic	North American	2.0
Gerilets	Abbott	15.0
Geritinic	Geriatric Pharm.	1.0
Geritol Junior Liquid (per tsp.)	J.B. Williams	4.0
Geritol Junior Tablets	J.B. Williams	2.0
Geritol Liquid (per tsp.)	J.B. Williams	4.0
Geritol Tablets	J.B. Williams	2.0
Gerizyme (per tbsp.)	Upjohn	3.3
Gevrabon (per 2 tbsp.)	Lederle	10.0
Gevral Protein	Lederle	2.2
Hi-Bee Plus	North American	20.0
Hi-Bee W/C Capsules	North American	10.0
Iberet	Abbott	10.0
Iberet-500	Abbott	10.0
Iberet-500 Oral Solution (per tsp.)	Abbott	2.5
Iberet Oral Solution (per 0.6 ml.)	Abbott	2.5
Iberol	Abbott	3.0
Lederplex Liquid (per tsp.)	Lederle	2.5

Supplements—*continued*

Supplement	Manufacturer	Mg.
Lederplex Tablets	Lederle	3.0
Lipoflavonoid Capsules	Cooper Vision Pharm.	0.3
Lipotriad Capsules	Cooper Vision Pharm.	0.3
Lipotriad Liquid (per tsp.)	Cooper Vision Pharm.	1.0
Livitamin Capsules	Beecham Labs	2.0
Livitamin Liquid (per tbsp.)	Beecham Labs	2.0
Lufa Capsules	USV	1.0
Methischol Capsules	USV	2.0
Multiple Vitamins	North American	1.0
Multiple Vitamins with Iron	North American	1.0
Multivitamins	Rowell	5.0
Myadec	Parke-Davis	20.0
Obron-6	Pfipharmecs	0.9
One-A-Day Vitamins Plus Minerals	Miles	10.0
Optilets-500	Abbott	20.0
Optilets-M-500	Abbott	20.0
Paladec (per tsp.)	Parke-Davis	5.0
Paladec with Minerals	Parke-Davis	5.0
Panuitex	O'Neal, Jones & Feldman	5.0
Peritinic	Lederle	15.0
Probec-T	Stuart	20.0
Roeribec	Pfipharmecs	18.0
Stresscaps Capsules	Lederle	20.0
Stresstabs 600	Lederle	20.0
Stresstabs 600 with Iron	Lederle	20.0
Stresstabs 600 with Zinc	Lederle	25.0
Stuart Hematinic Liquid (per tsp.)	Stuart	1.4
Stuartinic	Stuart	10.0
Surbex	Abbott	10.0
Surbex 750 with Iron	Abbott	20.0
Surbex 750 with Zinc	Abbott	20.0
Surbex-T	Abbott	20.0
Surbex with C	Abbott	10.0
Thera-Combex H-P Kapseals	Parke-Davis	18.4
Theragran	Squibb	21.4
Theragran Liquid (per tsp.)	Squibb	18.4
Theragran-M	Squibb	20.0

(continued)

Supplements—continued

Supplement	Manufacturer	Mg.
Theragran-Z	Squibb	18.4
Therapeutic Vitamins	North American	20.0
Thera-Spancap	North American	6.0
Thex Forte	Medtech	10.0
Tonebec	A.V.P.	10.0
Tri-B-Plex	Anabolic	50.0
Unicap T	Upjohn	10.0
Vi-Aqua	USV	5.0
Vicon-C	Glaxo	20.0
Vicon Iron	Glaxo	10.0
Vicon Plus	Glaxo	10.0
Vio-Bec	Rowell	40.0
Vi-Penta Multivitamin Drops (per 0.6 ml.)	Roche	10.0
Vitagett	North American	5.0
Vitamin-Mineral Capsules	North American	2.0
Viterra	Pfipharmecs	4.6
Viterra High Potency	Pfipharmecs	4.6
Z-Bec	Robins	25.0
Zymacap Capsules	Upjohn	15.0
Zymasyrup (per tsp.)	Upjohn	3.0

Source: Adapted from the American Pharmaceutical Association, *Handbook of Nonprescription Drugs*, 7th ed. (1982), 240–57.

Note: This chart is intended only as a guide. Vitamin formulations change periodically; always read product labels for accurate and up-to-date information on their nutrient levels.

11
Vitamin C

I have to admit it—there's something special about C. While new vitamin products come and go within a few months or years, C's popularity endures. For almost two decades, it has been an undisputed bestseller, with about one-third of vitamin users buying C as a single-nutrient supplement, apart from any multiple vitamin they might take. And when Linus Pauling first published his book *Vitamin C and the Common Cold*, C became so popular that some pharmacies couldn't even keep it on the shelf!

What makes it so popular, no one knows for sure. But I suspect that some users are seeking the traditional benefits of vitamin C, while others are after the newly discovered ones. The wisest vitamin users, however, are probably on the lookout for both.

ROLES TO REMEMBER

You've probably heard a lot about the new areas of vitamin C research in the newspaper or on the television news. Its potential to prevent cancer or alleviate colds seems to have taken the limelight, making its traditional functions all but forgotten.

Yet vitamin C (ascorbic acid) plays many traditional roles—much more so than some of the other vitamins whose jobs are fewer and narrower.

Among its varied, but often forgotten, duties are:

- Absorption of iron
- Fighting infection
- Formation of collagen, a substance essential to the health of body tissues
- Formation of the brain chemicals, norepinephrine and serotonin
- Metabolism of folic acid, a B vitamin
- Metabolizing proteins
- Wound healing

When vitamin C intake is so inadequate that some of the above functions cannot take place, deficiency symptoms occur that ultimately result in the well-known but now rare disease called scurvy. Loss of appetite, irritability, and weight loss are early signs of deficiency. As the problem progresses, pain during movement and tenderness in the limbs almost always occur. Bleeding into tissues may follow, along with certain types of anemia.

Of course, it has long been known that 10 milligrams (mg.) of vitamin C—one-sixth the Recommended Dietary Allowance (RDA) for adults—will prevent scurvy in most people. But today, people aren't worried about scurvy. They take their vitamin C because they want relief from colds and reduced risk of cancer. (If you have read my book *Foods That Fight Cancer*, you know I am sold on vitamin C's role in cancer prevention.) And as a result of these sought-after benefits, supplements of 500 mg., 1,000 mg., and more are common. So the issue, quite simply, is whether doses such as these are safe.

GENERALLY RECOGNIZED AS SAFE

Certainly vitamin C has its detractors, but they are few. Most authorities grant that barring certain health conditions (which we'll discuss shortly) or consuming very large doses, vitamin C is very safe. Some quotes from experts illustrate my point:

*Consensus from individual studies and several re-
view articles is that consumption of supplemental vitamin C leads to no significant adverse health effects to
humans in general.*

Mary Ann Sestili
National Cancer Institute

*[W]e have seen no symptomatic evidence of toxicity
resulting from doses of up to 2,000 mg. daily over three to
four months in healthy persons. [This] does not mean
that this dose level is necessarily safe for longer periods,
particularly in individuals with preexisting disease, or
that the occasional individual might not show some unusual and undesirable reaction.*

Terence Anderson
University of Toronto

*A substantial number of short-term experiments
with human subjects ingesting 1 to 4 grams [1,000 to
4,000 mg.] of ascorbate [ascorbic acid] daily have generally not revealed any harmful effects.*

Select Committee on GRAS Substances
for the Food and Drug Adminstration

Ascorbic acid is a cheap and safe drug.

Human Nutrition and Dietetics
(7th edition)

But the story does not end here, as you surely know. Detractors charge that high doses of vitamin C are guilty of a long list of
health problems. In a 1979 editorial, the medical journal *Lancet*
listed the following concerns:

- Destruction of vitamin B_{12}
- Interference with anticlotting drugs
- Kidney stones
- Scurvy after high doses are taken, then stopped

The editorial also mentioned some "unconfirmed reports"
that vitamin C might enhance the toxicity of certain metals,
diminish the ability to adjust rapidly to a rise in altitude, and
interact with other drugs.

(continued on page 196)

The Diet Detective Searches for Vitamin C

Vitamin C abounds in the American food supply—at least in theory. The U.S. Department of Agriculture estimates that the average American diet contains about 125 mg. of vitamin C per day—about double the current recommended (and hotly disputed) allowance.

But the USDA figures don't account for vitamin C in food thrown away (after all, who could account accurately for that?). Nor does the USDA adjust for vitamin C that is lost as a result of the vitamin's supersensitive personality. Chop it, heat it, expose it to oxygen, and vitamin C literally self-destructs. Not all at once, of course. But as the chopped pepper sits in the bin at the salad bar, it is slowly losing its vitamin C. Ditto for the sliced strawberries in the refrigerator waiting for their place on some shortcake. And not to mention the potential harm to C-rich vegetables cooking in a pot of water. The longer you cook them and the more water you use, the less vitamin C emerges.

I offer this little preamble so that as you take the following vitamin C quiz, you are aware that it does not account for vitamin C lost in consumer preparation of the foods listed. Food industry losses are already factored in, though, as the vitamin C measurements are done on foods after they're packaged for consumer use.

In the scoring section, I will give you some tips on estimating how much of your daily C might be lost to "the elements," as I call the destructive factors.

The rules of the game, of course, are the same as for previous quizzes—base your intake on what you ate yesterday or today.

1 point

½ cup dried apricots
½ cup dried pears
1 large apple
10 sweet cherries
1 cup cranberry sauce
1 cup limeade
1 medium peach
1 cup canned peaches
1 pear

1 pomegranate
1 cup eggplant
1 large carrot
1 tablespoon chopped
  parsley

2 points
3 fresh apricots
1 cup canned apricots
1 medium banana
1 cup canned sour cherries
1 cup grape juice
½ cup dried peaches
1 artichoke
1 cup beets
1 cup raw or cooked
  carrots
1 cup yellow corn,
  creamed or plain
1 ear of corn
10 French fries
1 cup hash brown potatoes
1 cup romaine lettuce
⅔ cup any of the following
  cereals:
  Golden Grahams, Honey
  Bran, Special K, Team,
  or Wheaties
1 cup Rice Chex cereal

3 points
1 cup blueberries
1 cup lemonade
1 nectarine
1 cup canned pineapple
  chunks

1 cup green beans
1 cup mixed vegetables
½ cup tomato puree
1 cup stewed tomatoes
1 cup parsnips
1 cup rhubarb, sweetened
1 cup wax beans
1 cup sliced zucchini
1 cup most children's
  ready-to-eat cereals
⅓ cup Bran Buds or 100%
  bran cereal
⅔ cup Bran Chex,
  Cracklin' Oat Bran, or
  Wheat Chex cereal
1 cup Corn Chex, Honey
  Nut Cheerios, or Kix
  cereal
4 Frosted Mini-Wheats

4 points
1 cup fresh pineapple
1 cup beet greens
1 cup bok choy
10 pods okra
1 cup peas
1 boiled potato
1 cup summer squash
1 sweet potato
⅔ cup Buc Wheats cereal

5 points
1 avocado
1 cup blackberries
½ cup frozen mixed fruit

(continued)

The Diet Detective—
Vitamin C *(continued)*

1 tangerine
½ package frozen
   raspberries, sweetened,
   10-ounce package
¹⁄₁₆ watermelon
1 baked potato
1 cup raw spinach
1 medium tomato
1 cup winter squash
¾ cup (one 6-ounce can)
   vegetable juice cocktail
1 cup Kaboom cereal

6 points
1 cup apricot nectar
¹⁄₁₀ honeydew melon
1 plaintain
1 cup asparagus
1 cup raw green cabbage
1 cup mashed sweet potato
1 cup sauerkraut
1 cup turnips

7 points
1 cup tomato juice
⅔ cup Total or Corn Total
   cereal
1 cup canned tomatoes
1 cup raw red cabbage
½ grapefruit

8 points
1 cup green cabbage
1 cup spinach

9 points
⅔ cup Product 19 cereal

10 points
1 cup mango chunks

11 points
1 orange
1 cup mustard greens
1 cup turnip greens

12 points
1 cup cauliflower

13 points
1 cup sweetened grapefruit
   juice
1 cup papaya chunks
1 cup unsweetened
   pineapple juice
½ package frozen
   strawberries, 10-ounce
   package
⅔ cup Most cereal

14 points
1 cup cranberry juice
   cocktail
1 cup unsweetened
   grapefruit juice

15 points
1 cup fresh strawberries
½ cantaloupe
1 cup raw cauliflower

16 points
1 cup grapefruit juice from
   frozen concentrate

17 points
1 cup canned orange juice

20 points
1 cup Awake
1 cup Orange Plus
1 cup orange juice from
   concentrate

21 points
1 cup fresh orange juice
1 cup kale

23 points
1 cup broccoli
1 cup brussels sprouts

24 points
1 cup collard greens

Scoring

Add your total points. Multiply the total by 10. The result is an estimate of the percent of the U.S. RDA for vitamin C that you took in on the day in question. For instance, if you scored 13 points, as the average American would, multiply 13 by 10 for a score of 130 percent of the U.S. RDA.

Of course, a significant amount of vitamin C is lost during consumer preparation of food, particularly from fruits and vegetables. For that reason, I advise you to do something with this score that I haven't recommended for other nutrients: Reduce it to account for losses that nutritionists know will happen. Such an adjustment can only be a rough guess as to how much vitamin C was lost from your food, for it depends on how much you cook, chop, or keep foods before eating. But as a rough allowance, I suggest reducing your score by 25 percent. That means that a score of 100 percent falls to 75 percent of the U.S. RDA; a score of 150 percent falls to 113 percent of the U.S. RDA; and a score of 200 percent falls to 150 percent of the U.S. RDA.

Of course, you can minimize losses by chopping foods coarsely rather than dicing; microwaving or steaming instead of cooking in water; and keeping cooking time to a minimum. Even with the noblest of efforts, though, some vitamin C will be lost. That's just its nature.

And if this collection of charges isn't enough, others have accused vitamin C of lowering fertility, interfering with accurate laboratory readings, and accelerating loss of calcium and other minerals from the bones. The latter charge is based solely on research in animals using extremely high doses.

Can the critics support their charges with solid facts? You'll find out as you read on.

THE HIDDEN HAZARD

Anyone who pays attention to the issues surrounding vitamin C supplementation knows that a deafening amount of noise has been made about its safety in medical journals. Strangely enough, the doctors making the noise have paid no attention to the one issue that probably affects the greatest number of people. It's one that has changed my personal vitamin C habits for good.

It all began when a young woman, Elise, found herself suffering from a problem called dental erosion, a condition in which the top surface of the teeth—the enamel—is worn away. Elise sought advice from John L. Giunta, D.M.D., of the Tufts University School of Medicine in Boston. Here is her story, as the doctor reported it to the *Journal of the American Dental Association*:

> A 30-year-old female had requested a second opinion about whether her teeth were eroded and what might be the probable cause. Her dentist had informed her that she had severe dental erosion that required restoration by full crowns on at least 12 teeth. She wanted to know the cause so that the process might be halted before proceeding with restorative dentistry. Currently her teeth were painful to brush and she had been told to use a desensitizing toothpaste... When questioned about pills, she admitted taking vitamin supplements including chewable vitamin C tablets. The examination showed the patient to be healthy. [Dental] examination showed that there were several posterior teeth with deficient tooth structure ... [Certain surfaces and cusps] were missing on the premolars and on the first molars.

Dr. Giunta repeated the diagnosis of severe dental erosion given by the first dentist. He told Elise that her daily chewing of multiple vitamin C tablets was probably a major cause of her severe dental erosion. She did not believe him, he said, so he set out to convince her otherwise. Rolling up his sleeves and getting to work, Dr. Giunta first compared the acidity of his own saliva with that of three brands of chewable vitamin C tablets. The tablets were roughly three times as acid. Next, he allowed an extracted tooth to sit in a solution of water and an acerola-C wafer—a popular source of chewable vitamin C. Within a few days the tooth enamel became chalky and some of it could be scraped away. The process worsened over the next few days.

Of course, Elise's teeth were not exposed to acerola-C around the clock, as was the tooth in the experiment. Naturally, the loss of tooth enamel would take longer when teeth are exposed to the chewable C for only a part of the day. But another dentist who has seen the problem firsthand says that the chewable C can take its toll in a matter of months.

I used to chew acerola-C tablets myself, preferring their distinctive taste to the dull routine of swallowing a tablet. Now I forgo the pleasure and am back to the old swallow method. And according to Dr. Giunta, Elise, too, has abandoned chewable vitamin C.

CONCERN ABOUT KIDNEYS

As I remember, the opening rounds of the great C debate began with warnings of dire damage to kidneys. You see, nutritionists long had known that some of the vitamin C in the body breaks down to oxalic acid, also known as oxalate. Oxalic acid also occurs in certain foods. And in kidney stones.

Doctors are sure that kidney stones containing oxalic acid result from high levels of oxalate in the urine. With kidney stones considered one of the most excruciating of disorders, and vitamin C's link to oxalate formation, opponents of vitamin C seized the opportunity to argue that high doses of vitamin C might have very painful consequences.

Fortunately, investigations were launched into the effect of vitamin C supplements on the amount of oxalic acid in the urine. The results were both surprising and reassuring. Some people did excrete far more oxalic acid after taking a high dose of vitamin C. But in others, the oxalic acid content of the urine hardly changed at all, despite a great increase in C intake. And regardless of one's tendency to turn or not to turn vitamin C into oxalate, major increases occurred only at very high doses.

Where does the danger zone begin? The best evidence available says at 4,000 mg. a day. Lesser amounts have not been shown to have much effect on oxalic acid. Moreover, most would also agree that this concern does not apply to everyone, but only to those whose bodies overproduce oxalic acid. And such people are prone to kidney stones, even without C supplements. By all appearances, they are a small minority.

So, does this mean the rest of us can handle moderately high doses of vitamin C without fear of kidney stones? Consider, for instance, a case reported by Eduard Poser, M.D., about a patient for whom he had prescribed 4,000 mg. daily of vitamin C for four months. Here's an excerpt from the doctor's letter published in the *New England Journal of Medicine.*

> A chemist at the University of Chicago who was in his mid-thirties experienced diminished visual acuity ... Blood, urine, and physical examinations were found to be normal. Since there is no specific therapy for this condition, large amounts of ascorbic acid were suggested. Following this suggestion, he took 4 grams [4,000 mg.] daily. Four months later, his visual acuity had increased from 20/40 to 20/20 ... He was advised to discontinue the ascorbic acid ... However, he was afraid to do so and kept on taking the same amount [4,000 mg.] for 13 years, after which I lost contact with him. During all this time he had experienced no clinical symptoms of [excessive oxalic acid production or kidney stones]. This is an exceptional case.

Exceptional, yes, for few people can offer 13 years' experience with such a large dose of vitamin C. But other testimonies like this one have appeared in medical journals, offering a degree of reassurance about the kidneys' ability to process vitamin C safely.

HAS ANYONE SEEN A STONE?

Impressed with safety stories such as Dr. Poser's, skeptics claim that the link between C and kidney stones is simply theory—until people who have been taking high doses actually suffer kidney stones. Some advocates of high-dose C maintain that not a single such stone has been reported. But they are wrong.

I have found eight cases of such kidney stones reported in the medical literature, of which seven are quite believable. The circumstances varied. In five cases, for instance, the victims had a history of stones that later became inactive. A period of taking lots of vitamin C (4,000 mg. or more daily) seemed to reactivate their stone-forming problem. Another case developed after a 1,000 mg. dose of vitamin C was taken daily for several months.

Seven may not seem like many and I can imagine that dozens more may have occurred but gone unreported to medical journals. Not that the doctors are delinquent here; they generally report cases that are unusual. But kidney stones in patients taking vitamin C would strike few doctors as unique given the uproar that has taken place over the issue during the last 15 years.

To sum up the matter of kidney stones, I think the risk is real for those predisposed to overproduction of oxalic acid and/or development of kidney stones. If you are one of them, do yourself a favor by leaving the vitamin C decision to your doctor. And if you don't know whether you are one of them, keep your vitamin C intake below the 4,000 mg. level known to give oxalate production a boost.

People who already have serious kidney disease (not simply stones) or kidney failure are at special risk. In these patients, large doses of vitamin C have been followed by severe kidney damage, worsening of oxalate overproduction, and even death. These cases hardly apply to the general population. But they illustrate that sometimes, in the very ill, a lot of C is more than the kidneys can handle.

THE B$_{12}$ BROUHAHA

Some would call it a real possibility requiring more research. More would probably say that it was, as the saying goes, a tempest in a teapot. At issue? The charge, dating back a decade, that high doses of vitamin C can destroy the body's stores of vitamin B$_{12}$.

The opening salvo was fired a decade ago when two researchers assembled some laboratory equipment to mimic digestion. They "fed" their mechanical setup some standard foods, along with supplemental vitamin C. Their results showed a decrease in the vitamin B_{12} content of the food, and the finger was wagged at vitamin C.

But there is a more accurate way to find out what vitamin C does to B_{12} in the human body. It's to test humans. After all, measuring vitamin B_{12} in the blood of people who take supplemental C is simple enough. Fortunately, a few researchers have done just that. Here is what they found:

• Not one of ten patients in a veterans hospital who had received 4,000 mg. daily of vitamin C for at least 11 months had abnormal B_{12} levels.
• Only 3 of 90 subjects tested in a Cleveland hospital who had been taking 500 mg. or more of vitamin C daily had below-normal levels of B_{12} in their blood. These three had all been taking at least 3,000 mg. daily and were 50 to 60 years old. Whether age might have been a factor here, I wonder, but cannot say.

If you think like I do, you will find these results with humans much more convincing than the original evidence cooked up in a simulated situation. And for the record, a second group of scientists later charged that the B_{12} was destroyed in this original laboratory experiment because of the technical method used, not because vitamin C poses a great potential to destroy B_{12}.

What I cannot help but think of, though, is how generously Americans partake of B_{12}. In chapter 9, I pointed out that Americans take in plenty of the vitamin and that our bodies have an amazing ability to conserve it well. So even if vitamin C were to destroy some of it (not that I am fully convinced that it does), I suspect that most of us would retain more than enough to stay healthy. Moreover, another report says that vitamin C can damage only one of the four principal types of B_{12}.

At moderate doses, then, such as 500 mg. or less, it seems highly unlikely that a healthy adult would suffer any harm to his or her B_{12} nutrition. Better evidence will have to come along before I think otherwise.

All this skepticism does not mean I'm letting vitamin C off the hook completely, though. There is evidence that it interferes with another nutrient, and I don't think the matter is one to take lightly. I'll tell you about it next.

THE COPPER SNATCHER?

This is a tale that reminds me of the folate-zinc connection that I discussed in chapter 8. First because the story involves a vitamin that antagonizes a trace mineral. And second because I base my concern primarily on just one study, something I generally don't do. Again, this is an exception because I consider the study itself impressive.

Recently, nutritionists at Oregon State University asked 13 men to take 500 mg. of supplemental vitamin C with every meal—a total of 1,500 mg. of additional C per day. Over the course of two months, indicators of their copper nutrition fell continuously. By "indicators," I mean the amount of copper in the men's blood and also the amount of a copper-bearing protein that carries most of this mineral in the blood. Sure enough, when the men stopped taking the vitamin C supplements, their signs of copper nutrition improved.

What does all this mean? Perhaps that vitamin C interfered with the absorption of copper. More important, I think, is whether the vitamin C reduced levels of copper to abnormal levels. Fortunately, the answer is no, but barely so. After two months, the average blood copper level was at the bottom of the normal range.

This study poses the possibility that higher doses of vitamin C might push blood copper to undesirably low levels. And if the average level was at the bottom of the normal range in the study group, that means that some of the men had below-normal levels. (Later in this chapter, I will talk more about applying these findings when deciding how much supplemental C to take.)

Finally, take note of one important fact here. All of the subjects in this study were male. The effect of vitamin C on copper nutrition in females may differ because a woman's estrogen hormones affect copper nutrition. As a result, how vitamin C would affect copper in women is unknown. I hope it won't be long before we have some answers—as well as some more results for men that will either confirm or refute the vitamin C/copper connection.

THE IRON DILEMMA

Until calcium recently forced it to step aside, iron was the superstar mineral for health. Nutritionists have long considered

Recommended Dietary Allowances for Vitamin C

Listed below are the RDA for vitamin C set by the National Academy of Sciences' Food and Nutrition Board. As you may know, many scoff at these allowances, which are based on traditional roles such as preventing the deficiency disease scurvy. Newer roles for vitamin C—such as its role in cancer prevention—have yet to be considered in formulating the allowances.

Because I am convinced that vitamin C plays an important role in cancer prevention, I consider these allowances too low. Yet in 1985, scientists on the RDA committee sought to lower them further on grounds that the RDA should only reflect levels needed to prevent nutritional deficiency diseases. An uproar broke out, and the president of the National Academy of Sciences chose not to release their proposed report. He instead formed a new committee charged with applying broader issues in setting the recommended allowances.

Whether this new group will raise the allowances in

iron a problem nutrient in the United States, mostly for women of childbearing age who lose iron each month during menstruation. Adding to the concern was the fact that some of these women also consume diets notoriously low in iron. As a result, vitamin manufacturers began offering multiple vitamins that also contain iron, and supplements containing only iron became widely available.

Putting a nutrient into the body is one thing, but having it absorbed is another. That is where vitamin C lends a hand. It enhances iron absorption—an important accomplishment for two reasons. First, the body absorbs only a small fraction of the iron taken in. Second, despite nutritionists' best efforts in trying to sell us on the importance of the mineral, some people still take in too little iron. So it only makes sense then that the next best thing to an adequate iron intake is something to enhance absorption of whatever iron is available. However, it's not good sense for all people.

their upcoming RDA report, one can only guess. I do think, however, that we will see a major change in attitudes about vitamin C within a decade. Meanwhile, surveys have found, as have I, that many people are choosing to exceed the RDA in their supplement program.

Group/Age	Mg.
Infants 0–12 mon.	35
Children 1–10 yr.	45
Males 11–14 yr.	50
Males 15+ yr.	60
Females 11–14 yr.	50
Females 15+ yr.	60
Pregnant women	80
Nursing women	100

Note: The U.S. RDA for vitamin C is 60 mg.

If nutrition has a single case where one man's meat is another man's poison, this is it. While most of us can put vitamin C's iron-enhancing effects to good use, some people need to avoid it. They already have too much iron in their bodies, an excess that can cause serious health problems and even death. Their condition is called hemochromatosis, or simply iron overload, and it runs in the family.

Needless to say, if you have hemochromatosis, you should be avoiding vitamin C supplements unless prescribed by your doctor. You probably have been told as much already. In fact, if one of your relatives has hemochromatosis, you should be tested before taking high doses of vitamin C. An odd bronze pigment or discoloration of the skin is a common symptom, and cirrhosis of the liver and disease of the heart muscle are sometimes found upon physical examination if the condition has progressed.

There is a very sad story in the medical literature of a 29-year-old man who had undiagnosed hemochromatosis. He had been taking 1,000 mg. of vitamin C daily and drinking a vitamin C-fortified beverage for about a year when he became so ill that he was admitted to the hospital. He died only eight days later, and the doctors could not help but speculate that the vitamin C had accelerated the course of his disease. The doctors promptly tested the man's six siblings, two of whom proved to have hemochromatosis also.

Iron overload can result from conditions other than hemochromatosis. When it does, vitamin C supplementation is again taboo except as prescribed by a doctor. Some other conditions that can be associated with iron overload include:

- Folic acid deficiency, especially as a result of alcoholism
- Leukemia (a cancer of the blood)
- Polycythemia (an increase in total cell mass of the blood)
- Thalassemia (a hereditary form of anemia)

Large amounts of vitamin C may be harmful in these conditions not only because of increased iron absorption, but also due to unfavorable effects on blood and other body tissues occurring in those with these disorders.

MORE CAUTIONS
FOR SPECIAL CONDITIONS

I would have to say that vitamin C's potential to cause harm to people with certain special conditions concerns me very much. Consider, for instance, the story of Anita, a woman in her 40s who had sickle cell disease. This condition is marked by frequent infections and periodic, painful "crises" that can require hospital treatment.

Her doctor, Mervyn Goldstein, M.D., reported that she "managed to get through her life with few crises until this year, when it appeared that every minor illness precipitated a sickle cell crisis worthy of her hospitalization. She recently asked advice about a developing cold. I gave the usual recommendations, and casually mentioned that she should not use high doses of ascorbic acid. I was surprised (and so was Dr. Goldstein) to hear that prior to each recent crisis she had administered just such doses to 'ward off symptoms.' "

Needless to say, Anita stopped taking vitamin C, and, not surprisingly, she had no further crises. Apparently, vitamin C affected her blood cells in a way that increased the risk of sickle cell crises.

Similarly, vitamin C has been linked to potential problems in people who have a condition called G-6PD deficiency. Those affected can have a variety of health problems ranging from a blood disorder (hemolytic anemia) that can cause attacks of pain, chills, and fever, to liver disease. Certain drugs, and in some people, fava beans, can trigger the attacks, and the evidence so far shows that high doses of vitamin C probably interact at this point in a way that makes matters worse.

This condition occurs in about 10 percent of American black males; fewer black women and Caucasians are affected. Screening tests are widely available, and those diagnosed with the disorder should consult their physician about use of vitamin C supplements.

One more note about special conditions. With a name like ascorbic acid, vitamin C is obviously acidic. This resulted in a problem for one young woman who had a motor disorder in her esophagus that delayed food and drugs from reaching her stomach. A single 500 mg. tablet of vitamin C apparently lodged in her esophagus long enough to cause severe inflammation.

C ADDICTION: REAL OR RIDICULOUS?

Anyone who has followed the vitamin C controversy has heard critics charge that large doses may lead to dependency, resulting in deficiency disease if the high dose is later stopped. The most widely used term for this is "rebound scurvy." I dislike the term, because, in my mind, scurvy refers to vitamin C deficiency that has progressed beyond the early warning symptoms. So I prefer to call the condition vitamin C withdrawal syndrome.

Such a withdrawal syndrome may exist, I grant you, but critics certainly cannot charge that it happens very often. I can almost count on one hand the number of cases in adults that I found in medical journals. However remote, it *can* happen and the following case reported by three Kansas City dentists to the *Journal of Periodontology* deserves mention. An excerpt from their report:

A 49-year-old male was originally accepted for dental care at the university clinic on January 19, 1979 ... January 22, 1980, the patient was seen again with sore gums.

Upon further inquiry, the patient admitted taking megadosage of AA [ascorbic acid] (1,000 mg. per day) plus additional multiple vitamins and a health food diet for over 1 year. The soreness started suddenly, about 1 and 1½ weeks after stopping the AA megadosage ... After other [conditions producing bleeding] were ruled out, the possibility was considered that the patient's problems were related to his AA [ascorbic acid] levels. The patient was therefore instructed to resume the full megadosage of AA immediately, and 1 week later he reported by phone that he was free of symptoms.

In the spirit of true scientific detective work, the process was repeated a few weeks later; the patient stopped vitamin C again, and his gum problems reappeared. Convinced that the patient was suffering from a vitamin C withdrawal syndrome, the dentists asked him to resume the 1,000 mg. dose, then lower it gradually to 100 mg. over the course of seven weeks.

The treatment worked! The symptoms never returned.

WHY WITHDRAWAL?

As I noted, reports of withdrawal syndromes such as this one are extremely rare. But when it does occur, a sensible explanation for it exists. Research at the University of California has shown that at the 2,000 mg. level of supplementation, the body breaks down and/or excretes vitamin C more rapidly. If this higher-speed process becomes a habit and continues after a high intake ends, the body could dispose of too much of its vitamin C. The result, of course, would be signs of deficiency.

But victims of such a syndrome remain extremely hard to find. The reason, perhaps, is that vitamin C users who stop their high doses still may be taking in enough from food and/or a multiple vitamin to prevent a withdrawal syndrome. Another explanation might be that they were not taking as much supplemental vitamin C (2,000 mg. daily) as was used in the test study.

This issue has been a favorite of vitamin C critics. My own feeling is that, in addition to exaggerating the likelihood of the withdrawal syndrome, critics ignore the ease of treatment and expectation of full recovery for those affected. So unless a victim of this rare syndrome foolishly ignores the symptoms and allows the disease to progress to a full-blown case of scurvy, I don't see this as grounds to preach against the use of vitamin C. It is hard to imagine that supplement users, who tend to be health conscious, would not seek medical attention if the painful symptoms of vitamin C deficiency were to develop.

If you do take a high dose of vitamin C for some time, and later stop abruptly, simply be alert for the possible symptoms of deficiency described at the beginning of this chapter under the heading "Roles to Remember." In the unlikely event that such signs occur, do the only sensible thing: See a doctor.

THE GREAT UNKNOWN

Nutrition and medicine are full of maybe's, and that is how I feel about an assortment of issues that have been raised about vitamin C safety. Maybe there is a problem for some people on these points; maybe not. Only future research will tell, but here are some of the concerns that you may be hearing more about in coming years:

EFFECT ON FERTILITY. If vitamin C helps fight the mucus buildup of colds, does it reduce mucus in the cervix, where it is needed to allow conception? M. H. Briggs, M.D., posed this question in the medical journal *Lancet* and received 15 replies about fertility in women taking vitamin C supplements. Nine of the women, who were taking 400 to 1,000 mg., had conceived without difficulty, but five who had been taking 2,000 mg. or more for 6 to 17 months had infertility problems. Two of them became pregnant within 3 months of stopping supplemental vitamins.

Based on these limited facts, the doctor suggested that doses of 2,000 mg. or more may reduce fertility in some women. On a related matter, I would like to point out that pregnancy is not a good time to experiment with high doses of vitamin C. There is no assurance of safety for the mother or infant.

EFFECTS ON DETOXIFICATION. Here is an issue that I hesitate to even mention, because I think it is (at most) relevant only to extremely high doses of vitamin C. But since you may hear about it elsewhere, I feel I should give you the facts and my perspective.

At issue, based on only one study, is whether vitamin C will use up the body's supply of cysteine, an amino acid. Cysteine is believed to play a role in detoxification of certain drugs and perhaps smoking-related substances. The research in question showed that 3,000 mg. of vitamin C did lower cysteine levels. However, the cysteine supply was hardly depleted, making me wonder if this is worth worrying over, especially at doses near or below the test level.

EFFECTS ON RESISTANCE TO HIGH ALTITUDES. At high altitudes, we can encounter less oxygen, and the body's ability to adapt to this change is called high-altitude resistance. It's a fascinating subject, but one that applies mainly to people whose working conditions expose them to sudden or temporary changes in the oxygen supply. Pilots and mountain climbers are good examples.

A small, but well-conducted study found that 3,000 mg. of vitamin C taken for about a week reduced the high-altitude resistance of three test subjects. Other test subjects received 2,000 mg. and were unaffected. Those affected, though, regained their normal resistance upon stopping the high dose of vitamin C.

EFFECT ON BACTERIA-FIGHTING BY WHITE BLOOD CELLS. In subjects taking 2,000 mg. of vitamin C for several weeks, the infection-fighting activity of white blood cells exposed to one common type of bacteria was reduced. A dose of 200 mg. had no such effect, and antibacteria activity was restored to original levels after the 2,000 mg. dose of vitamin C was withdrawn.

Again, this is simply a preliminary finding. Incidentally, it does not apply to the issue of vitamin C and colds. Viruses, not bacteria, cause the common cold.

THE STAR SYSTEM SHINES ON VITAMIN C

We have looked at safety issues, and I think found vitamin C to be a rather safe substance for healthy people. However, it may have more potential to cause hidden consequences than any other vitamin. For many of us, this may be its chief (or only) danger.

In this section, then, I will not only summarize the safety facts that you've read so far, but also tell you about side effects, drug interactions, and hidden consequences of vitamin C that have not yet been mentioned. Here we go.

Side effects—Side effects from vitamin C are rare and, of course, more likely to occur with increasing dosages. According to the American Society of Hospital Pharmacists, the following have been reported: abdominal cramps, fatigue, flushing, headache, heartburn, insomnia, nausea, sleepiness, and vomiting. Those who develop heartburn or sour stomach after taking vitamin C in its most common form—ascorbic acid—may tolerate without trouble calcium or sodium ascorbate instead. Both are related forms of ascorbic acid that have vitamin C activity.

Perhaps the most common side effect of vitamin C is diarrhea, usually not a problem unless the dose is 1,000 mg. or more.

Acute ailments—No acute reactions to vitamin C are known, with the exception of a handful of allergic reactions. Most of these involved vitamin C injections; again, such allergic reactions are not the same as toxic reactions.

Long-term problems—Kidney stones, aggravation of gout, and vitamin C withdrawal syndrome are possible, but rare. If vitamin C is taken in chewable form, damage to tooth surfaces may be a much greater risk than these other disorders. Reduction in blood copper levels is another possible problem that I consider more likely than kidney damage or C withdrawal. Risk to those with iron overload, history of thrombosis, and diabetes is of enough concern that use of supplemental C should be discussed with a doctor.

Other potential risks discussed under the heading "The Great Unknown" remain possible, but speculative as of this writing.

Conflicting combinations—It works both ways with vitamin C; the vitamin may interfere with the work of certain drugs, and yet certain drugs may interfere with it. In the latter case, of course, the body's need for the vitamin could increase.

The most controversial of claims involves the antiblood-clotting drug called warfarin (brand names: Coumarin, Panwarfin). Some research shows that vitamin C reduces the effectiveness of the drug; another study found no "clinically significant" effect after doses ranging from 3,000 to 10,000 mg. of vitamin C were given for a week. The amount of warfarin in these subjects' blood dropped slightly while taking vitamin C, but the researchers called the decline too small to interfere with the drug's effectiveness. My own feeling is that warfarin users should be cautious, as this study only measured short-term effects. Be careful also with a related drug, dicoumarol.

Vitamin C may possibly reduce the effectiveness of two other classes of drugs. The first are amphetamines, a type rarely used these days. The other group, tricyclic antidepressants, are, to the contrary, widely used. The tricyclic category includes more than a half dozen different drugs, some marketed under more than one brand name or as combination pills containing both a tranquilizer and an antidepressant. Here is a list of both generic and brand name tricyclics:

- Amitriptyline (Elavil, Endep, Etrafron, Limbitrol, Triavil)
- Amoxapine (Asendin)
- Desipramine (Norpramin, Pertofrane)
- Doxepin (Adapin, Sinequan)
- Imipramine (Tofranil)
- Nortriptyline (Aventyl, Pamelor)
- Protriptyline (Vivactil)
- Trimipramine (Surmontil)

I wouldn't worry about the vitamin C in a multiple vitamin if using these drugs, but would shy away from an intake of more than 200 mg. for now. Of course, if you want to take more vitamin C and your doctor is willing, you can compare a period of taking a sizable dose of vitamin C with a period of not doing so; see if you notice any difference in your medication's effect. I offer this suggestion only because the effect of vitamin C here is still not well established and needs further study.

As for drugs that may increase the need for vitamin C (not the vitamin's fault, of course), the following have been named: barbiturates, birth control pills, cortisones, levodopa, phenacetin, salicylates, sulfonamides, and tetracycline. Of course, the issue is essentially long-term use of these drugs—not a brief treatment with them. Researchers are also trying to pin down an apparent interaction between the most common of these drugs—aspirin—

and vitamin C; it seems that large doses of aspirin cause more vitamin C to be excreted.

What qualifies as a large dose of aspirin? In one study, the aspirin dosage was equivalent to about eight daily for a week. So if you take two a week for an occasional headache, I doubt you need to be concerned.

Needless to say, vitamin C also conflicts with the special conditions discussed earlier.

Hidden consequences—If you have ever used a colon cancer test kit, you know that high doses of vitamin C can cause false readings in laboratory tests. The list of lab tests that can be affected by high concentrations of vitamin C in the blood or urine is fairly long. Tests that are interpreted based on color are among those affected. I have compiled the following list of the most common tests that may be affected, depending on the method used to conduct the test.

- Blood bilirubin (a test of liver health)
- Blood glucose (sugar)
- Creatinine (a test of kidney function)
- LDH (a general test of health)
- Occult blood test for colon cancer
- SGOT (a test of liver health)
- Uric acid (a test for gout)
- Urinary glucose (sugar)

Because high doses of vitamin C might give false readings in tests such as these, doctors are concerned that conditions such as liver disease and gout might go undiagnosed as a result. However, I have not read of this actually happening to anyone.

I wish I could tell you the dosage required to cause false readings, but this depends not so much on what you take in, but how much your body keeps in the blood or excretes in the urine. This, of course, will vary among people taking the same dosage. Moreover, two people might take the same supplement, but have as much as a 500 mg. difference in their dietary intake of vitamin C. That makes the issue one of total C intake, not simply supplement dosage.

For the bilirubin test, however, I did find one reassuring report. It is estimated that at a dose of 2,400 mg. of vitamin C, about 6 percent of the bilirubin level would be masked. That is a much higher dose than the 500 or even 1,000 mg. that many people take, and not nearly as serious a misreading as I had feared from the warnings I have heard. Raise the vitamin C dosage to 10,000 mg., though, and an estimated 25 percent of the bilirubin would go undetected. That is not good.

For those who want to play it safest, stopping all but a multiple vitamin for about a week before lab tests sounds like a good idea to me. If you don't agree, do inform the doctor or lab of your current vitamin C intake at test time.

HOW MUCH IS TOO MUCH

"How much vitamin C should I take?" I would say that, as a nutritionist, no other question is asked of me more frequently. Deciding how to answer has been tough, despite months spent reading and thinking about everything I could find on vitamin C safety.

An expert committee of independent scientists charged with reviewing vitamin C safety for the federal government has already concluded that many people can consume large doses short-term—in the range of 1,000 to 4,000 mg. for a few months. But I think of a supplement program as long-term. So, the question is: Are such high levels safe over the course of many years?

I suspect that for some people they are. I am troubled, though, about approving long-term doses of these levels. Why? Because a time-honored tradition in medicine has not been factored in. I am referring to a principle called the margin of safety. You already may be familiar with it, but if not, let me explain.

Researchers studying a certain chemical will first determine at what level it begins to become hazardous. Depending on the type of chemical, they might follow a standard procedure that calls for dividing this minimum hazardous level by 100. That greatly reduced level would become the maximum level for public exposure to insure a margin of safety. Clearly, this is the "better safe than sorry" approach. Though it might seem extreme, I believe it has served our nation's health well.

I am not about to propose such a large margin of safety for vitamin C. Doing so could no doubt cause deficiency in some people, and the substance is too safe for the "divide by 100" approach. But considering all issues I have told you about in this chapter and wanting some margin of safety, I think of 500 mg. as a good, safe dose. If you argue with me long enough, you might get me up to 1,000 mg., depending on your body weight, but I wouldn't make it as an across-the-board recommendation.

As for taking more than 1,000 mg. for long periods, I would recommend a periodic test of blood copper. Of all the people who have told me of taking huge doses of vitamin C safely for many years, not one has considered that some problems, such as a low copper level, might go unnoticed.

I do not like to see 2,000 mg. or more taken long-term unless prescribed for a therapeutic purpose and accompanied by medical follow-up.

But despite any reservations expressed, I feel that all things considered, vitamin C remains one of the safest items that you can buy over-the-counter in a drugstore. Just take a sensible dose and honor my final request: Please don't chew it.

C O O K I N G
for Vitamin C

GREAT GREENS

(Makes 4 servings)

Vitamin C: 49 mg. per serving
Calories: 83 per serving

1¾ pounds collard greens, stems and center ribs removed	½ pound plum tomatoes, peeled and chopped (drain if using canned)
¼ pound spinach, stems removed	¼ cup minced fresh parsley
1 tablespoon olive oil	
1 large onion, thinly sliced	¼ teaspoon dried marjoram
1 clove garlic, minced	1 tablespoon red wine vinegar

Steam the collard greens until tender, about 10 minutes. Drain well. Chop. Steam the spinach 2 minutes. Drain well. Chop.

(continued)

C O O K I N G
for Vitamin C—continued

In a medium-size skillet, heat the oil over medium-low heat. Add the onion and garlic and sauté until soft, about 7 minutes. Add the tomatoes, parsley, marjoram, and vinegar. Cover and cook 5 minutes. Add greens and heat through, 1 to 2 minutes. Serve immediately.

NOTE: For extra vitamin C, serve as a topping over baked potatoes.

FRUIT 'N SWEET PEPPER SALAD

(Makes 4 servings)

Vitamin C: 141 mg. per serving
Calories: 122 per serving

3 cups diced cantaloupe
1 pint strawberries, hulled
     and halved
     lengthwise
1 cup diced papaya
1 small green pepper, cut
     into julienne strips
3 tablespoons fresh lime
     juice

1 teaspoon finely grated
     lime rind
2 teaspoons honey
2 tablespoons chopped
     toasted walnuts*

In a large bowl, combine the cantaloupe, strawberries, papaya, and green pepper. Chill well.

In a small bowl, stir together the lime juice, rind, and honey. Pour over the fruit and toss. Chill for 30 minutes.

Sprinkle with walnuts. Serve immediately.

*Toast chopped walnuts until golden in a small frying pan on medium heat.

VARIATION: Add 1½ cups cooked diced turkey or chicken.

C O O K I N G
for Vitamin C—continued

OPAL ORANGE SUNRISE

(Makes 4 servings)

Vitamin C: 78 mg. per serving
Calories: 105 per serving

2 cups freshly squeezed orange juice, chilled	4 teaspoons honey
⅔ cup freshly squeezed grapefruit juice, chilled	½ cup skim milk
	¼ teaspoon ground nutmeg

Stir together juices and honey in a medium-size bowl.
In a medium-size bowl, whip the skim milk and nutmeg with an electric beater. Slowly beat in the juice mixture. Pour into chilled glasses and serve immediately.

Vitamin C Content
of Selected Supplements

Dosage is one tablet or capsule unless otherwise indicated.

Supplement	Manufacturer	Mg.
Abdec Baby Drops (per 0.6 ml.)	Parke-Davis	50
Abdec Kapseal	Parke-Davis	75
Abdol with Minerals	Parke-Davis	50
Abron	O'Neal, Jones & Feldman	100
Allbee C-800	Robins	800
Allbee C-800 plus Iron	Robins	800
Allbee-T	Robins	500
Allbee with C	Robins	300
AVP Natal	A.V.P.	100
B-C-Bid Capsules	Geriatric Pharm.	300

(continued)

Supplements—*continued*

Supplement	Manufacturer	Mg.
Belfer	O'Neal, Jones & Feldman	50
Beminal 500	Ayerst	500
Beminal Forte with Vitamin C	Ayerst	250
Bugs Bunny	Miles	60
Bugs Bunny Plus Iron	Miles	60
Bugs Bunny with Extra C	Miles	250
Cal-Prenal	North American	50
C-B Bone Capsules	USV	250
Cebefortis	Upjohn	150
Cebetinic	Upjohn	25
Cecon Solution (per 0.6 ml.)	Abbott	60
Centrum	Lederle	90
Cetane (timed release)	O'Neal, Jones & Feldman	500
Cevid-Bid	Geriatric Pharm.	500
Ce-Vi-Sol Drops (per 0.6 ml.)	Mead Johnson	35
Chew-Vite	North American	50
Cluvisol 130	Ayerst	150
Cluvisol Syrup (per tsp.)	Ayerst	15
Cod Liver Oil Tablets with Vitamin A	Schering	50
Dayalets	Abbott	60
Dayalets plus Iron	Abbott	60
Di-Cal D with Vitamin C Capsules	Abbott	15
Dura-C 500 Graduals	Amfre-Grant	500
Engram-HP	Squibb	60
Feminins	Mead Johnson	200
Femiron with Vitamins	J.B. Williams	60
Feostim	O'Neal, Jones & Feldman	20
Ferritrinsic	Upjohn	50
Filibon Tablets	Lederle	60
Flintstones	Miles	60
Flintstones Plus Iron	Miles	60
Flintstones with Extra C	Miles	250
Folbesyn	Lederle	180
Ganatrex (per 0.6 ml.)	Merrell Dow	60
Geriamic	North American	75
Gerilets	Abbott	90
Geriplex	Parke-Davis	50
Geriplex-FS Kapseals	Parke-Davis	50

Supplements—*continued*

Supplement	Manufacturer	Mg.
Geritinic	Geriatric Pharm.	60
Geritol Junior Tablets	J.B. Williams	30
Geritol Tablets	J.B. Williams	75
Gest	O'Neal, Jones & Feldman	30
Gevral	Lederle	60
Gevral Protein	Lederle	22
Gevral T Capsules	Lederle	90
Gevrite	Lederle	60
Golden Bounty B Complex with Vitamin C	Squibb	100
Hi-Bee Plus	North American	300
Hi-Bee W/C Capsules	North American	300
Iberet	Abbott	150
Iberet-500	Abbott	500
Iberet-500 Oral Solution (per tsp.)	Abbott	125
Iberet Oral Solution (per 0.6 ml.)	Abbott	38
Iberol	Abbott	75
K-Forte Potassium w/Vit. C (25)	O'Connor	25
K-Forte Potassium w/Vit. C Chewable (10)	O'Connor	10
Lipoflavonoid Capsules	Cooper Vision Pharm.	100
Livitamin Capsules	Beecham Labs	100
Livitamin Chewable	Beecham Labs	100
Multicebrin	Lilly	75
Multiple Vitamins	North American	50
Multiple Vitamins with Iron	North American	50
Multivitamins	Rowell	50
Myadec	Parke-Davis	250
Natabec	Parke-Davis	50
Natalins Tablets	Mead Johnson	90
Norlac	Rowell	90
Nutra-Cal	Anabolic	8
Obron-6	Pfipharmecs	50
One-A-Day	Miles	60
One-A-Day Core C 500	Miles	500
One-A-Day Plus Iron	Miles	60
One-A-Day Vitamins Plus Minerals	Miles	50

(continued)

Supplements—*continued*

Supplement	Manufacturer	Mg.
Optilets-500	Abbott	500
Optilets-M-500	Abbott	500
Os-Cal Forte	Marion	50
Os-Cal Plus	Marion	33
Paladec (per tsp.)	Parke-Davis	50
Paladec with Minerals	Parke-Davis	50
Panuitex	O'Neal, Jones & Feldman	100
Peritinic	Lederle	200
Poly-Vi-Sol Chewable	Mead Johnson	60
Poly-Vi-Sol Drops (per 0.6 ml.)	Mead Johnson	35
Poly-Vi-Sol with Iron Chewable	Mead Johnson	60
Poly-Vi-Sol with Iron Drops (per 0.6 ml.)	Mead Johnson	35
Probec-T	Stuart	600
Roeribec	Pfipharmecs	500
Rogenic	O'Neal, Jones & Feldman	100
Selenace	Anabolic	250
Simiron Plus	Merrell Dow	50
Spancap C Capsules	North American	500
S.S.S. Tablets	S.S.S.	75
Stresscaps Capsules	Lederle	300
Stresstabs 600	Lederle	600
Stresstabs 600 with Iron	Lederle	600
Stresstabs 600 with Zinc	Lederle	600
Stuart Formula	Stuart	60
Stuartinic	Stuart	525
Stuart Prenatal	Stuart	60
Super Plenamins	Rexall	56
Surbex 750 with Iron	Abbott	750
Surbex 750 with Zinc	Abbott	750
Surbex-T	Abbott	500
Surbex with C	Abbott	250
Tega-C Caps	Ortega	500
Tega-C Syrup (per tsp.)	Ortega	500
Thera-Combex H-P Kapseals	Parke-Davis	500
Theragran	Squibb	200
Theragran Liquid (per tsp.)	Squibb	200
Theragran-M	Squibb	200
Theragran-Z	Squibb	200

Supplements—*continued*

Supplement	Manufacturer	Mg.
Therapeutic Vitamins	North American	200
Thera-Spancap	North American	150
Thex Forte	Medtech	500
Tonebec	A.V.P.	300
Tri-Vi-Sol Chewable	Mead Johnson	60
Tri-Vi-Sol Drops (per 1 ml.)	Mead Johnson	35
Tri-Vi-Sol with Iron Drops (per 1 ml.)	Mead Johnson	35
Unicap	Upjohn	60
Unicap Chewable	Upjohn	60
Unicap T	Upjohn	300
Vi-Aqua	USV	50
Vicon-C	Glaxo	300
Vicon Iron	Glaxo	300
Vicon Plus	Glaxo	150
Vigran	Squibb	60
Vigran Chewable	Squibb	40
Vigran plus Iron	Squibb	60
Vio-Bec	Rowell	500
Vio-Geric	Rowell	60
Vi-Penta Infant Drops (per 0.6 ml.)	Roche	50
Vi-Penta Multivitamin Drops (per 0.6 ml.)	Roche	50
Vitagett	North American	50
Vita-Kaps-M Tablets	Abbott	50
Vita-Kaps Tablets	Abbott	50
Vitamin-Mineral Capsules	North American	50
Viterra	Pfipharmecs	520
Viterra High Potency	Pfipharmecs	150
Vi-Zac	Glaxo	500
Z-Bec	Robins	600
Zymacap Capsules	Upjohn	90
Zymasyrup (per tsp.)	Upjohn	60

Source: Adapted from the American Pharmaceutical Association, *Handbook of Nonprescription Drugs*, 7th ed. (1982), 240–57.

Note: This chart is intended only as a guide. Vitamin formulations change periodically; always read product labels for accurate and up-to-date information on their nutrient levels.

12
Vitamin D

If there were a dubious distinction award for supplements, vitamin D would win hands down. You probably think I am joking, especially if you can remember back to the days when rickets, the vitamin D deficiency disease, was rampant. How can a vitamin that cured a plague qualify for a not-so-honorable award? Read on and you'll find out.

Simply stated, vitamin D is the most toxic of the vitamins, with the potential to do damage at levels not much higher than the Recommended Dietary Allowances (RDA). That's usually not so for other vitamins. And to make matters worse, the damage from too much vitamin D can be irreparable under certain unfortunate circumstances.

For reasons that I cannot explain, some of the most important aspects of vitamin D safety have received precious little coverage in the news media. So if you take vitamin D, it's to your own good that you read this chapter very carefully.

WHAT D DOES

With an introduction like that one, you may have the idea that I am really down on vitamin D. I would like to clear up any impression to that effect right now. After all, vitamin D plays a key role in calcium nutrition—the subject of my most recent book, *The Calcium Bible*.

Basically, vitamin D has one role in nutrition, and it is a most important one. A hormone as well as a vitamin, D regulates the metabolism of two minerals: calcium and phosphorus. When this regulatory function goes awry due to too little vitamin D, the result is one of the two vitamin D deficiency diseases. Both can have serious effects on bone health.

The formal names for the vitamin D deficiency syndromes depend on the victim's age. In children, the condition is called rickets—a familiar term, I am sure. In adults, the condition is referred to as osteomalacia. A major factor in the diseases is that inadequate vitamin D prevents the body from absorbing enough calcium. And without enough calcium, bones are in trouble.

Nutritionists have long hailed the importance of vitamin D for good calcium absorption. Until recently, however, the bones and teeth were considered the beneficiaries of good calcium absorption. Then, in 1985, impressive research came along linking both vitamin D and the calcium it helps to absorb to reduced risk of colon cancer. Extra calcium seems to tie up troublemakers in the digestive tract, preventing them from causing damage to the colon wall that can lead to colon cancer.

Residents of Florida, for instance, have a much lower risk of colon cancer than those living in northern climates. It's a good bet that better vitamin D nutrition, thanks to the sunshine factor discussed below, explains the difference. But the amount of vitamin D needed to confer the benefit appears to be modest. There's no reason for taking high doses.

Vitamin D comes in several forms: some natural, some synthetic. For practical purposes, only two need mention: vitamin D_2 (ergocalciferol) and vitamin D_3 (cholecalciferol). If you're up on vitamin D, you know that the D_2 form is synthetic, made in the laboratory from yeast or other fungi. Vitamin D_3 is the form that occurs naturally in certain foods and is made by our skin when exposed to the sun. More on that in a second.

Which form of vitamin D is most effective? It's a draw. Either one will do the job, and as far as nutritionists can tell, both forms are equally effective.

THE SUNSHINE FACTOR

Nutritionists have always held vitamin D to be unique because food is not our primary source of it. Sunlight is. Exposure to sunlight starts a manufacturing process within us that provides most of us with more vitamin D than an ordinary diet would. The process is not complicated. Sunlight activates a compound in the skin (7-dehydrocholesterol), which the liver and kidneys convert to the active form of vitamin D. I am always asked if, in today's indoor world, we are spending enough time in the sun to meet our vitamin D needs. Some people even ask how much skin must be exposed to the sun in order to make enough vitamin D.

I wish the answer were simple. It isn't. How much vitamin D you will make on exposure to sunlight depends on the time of day, for starters. The noon sun provides much more of the ultraviolet radiation needed to stimulate the skin than does the setting sun. If your skin is fair, it is more cooperative with the process than dark skin, which lets in less of the sun's D-making rays. If you live in the country, away from the city's pollution, you will also have more success.

Some hard facts are at hand, however, from a recent study at Tufts University, just outside of Boston. With only arms, hands, and face bared to the noonday sun, the average white adult living in Boston needed a twice-weekly session in the sun lasting 10 to 15 minutes to make recommended levels of vitamin D.

As for soaking up the sun's rays inside your home or office by raising the blinds or opening the curtains, forget it. It can't happen. Window glass screens out ultraviolet light, which activates the D-forming process.

AGE AND EXCESSES

Nutritionists long believed that the body's ability to make vitamin D from sunshine did not vary with age. Today, that notion is rapidly losing adherents.

New research makes it almost certain that this ability does decline with age. The Tufts University researchers found that an 80-year-old's skin makes only half as much vitamin D as that of a 20-year-old. The meaning is clear: The elderly either need more time in the sun or another source of vitamin D. As you read on,

Recommended Dietary Allowances for Vitamin D

In 1974, pregnant and nursing women were the only adults with vitamin D allowances. The needs of other adults, said the RDA committee, could be met by exposure to sunlight. The RDA chart showed only a blank space under vitamin D for adults age 23 and older.

In the 1980 revision of the RDAs, the tables turned without explanation. The spaces were no longer blank, but filled in with the recommended allowances listed below. I don't know what caused the change of heart. However, the committee did mention that sunlight may be inadequate in some climates and that chronic air pollution in certain areas may prevent beneficial rays of sun from reaching the skin.

As you can see, there are no differences in current allowances according to sex. Whether that might change in a few years, as concern mounts over osteoporosis in American women, one can only guess.

Group/Age	I.U.
Infants 0–12 mon.	400
Children 1–10 yr.	400
Males 11–18 yr.	400
Males 19–22 yr.	300
Males 23+	200
Females 11–18 yr.	400
Females 19–22 yr.	300
Females 23+	200
Pregnant and nursing women	
18 yr. or less	600
19–22 yr.	500
23+ yr.	400

Note: The U.S. RDA for vitamin D is 400 I.U.

you'll learn about the alternatives and how much of them to use.

People often ask me if they can get too much vitamin D from exposure to the sun. As far as we know, the answer is no. Excessive exposure to sunlight does have its risks (skin cancer and premature aging are the most noteworthy), but overdosing on vitamin D is not one of them. However, overuse of supplemental vitamin D is a different story.

TWO CLASSIC CASES

The first case of vitamin D overdose dates back to 1929, and the first death from the condition was recorded in 1930. Numerous cases have been reported since, but this 1977 report affecting both a boy and his mother particularly caught my attention. Their story was told to the *Illinois Medical Journal* by Takaki Hirano, M.D., and his colleagues. An excerpt from their report:

> *A 13-year-old black male was admitted to the Department of Pediatrics of the Cook County Hospital because of nausea, vomiting, weight loss, and abdominal pain. Anorexia [loss of appetite] began three weeks prior to admission, followed by vomiting which was associated with vague intermittent abdominal pain. During the week prior to admission, he started to have severe nausea with frequent [vomiting] and was unable to attend school. He lost [11 pounds] of weight during this period. Muscle weakness and frequency of urination were noted.*
>
> *The child's 35-year-old mother was admitted simultaneously, with severe abdominal pain, anorexia, vomiting, and weight loss of two weeks' duration.*
>
> *The patient [Jon] was thin, moderately dehydrated, and appeared chronically ill.*

Both Jon and his mother had too much calcium in their blood—a symptom never ignored by doctors. That, combined with symptoms that were classic signs of vitamin D overdose, led the doctors to suspect overuse of vitamin D supplements. But Jon's mother repeatedly denied use of any vitamin D supplements.

Later, she gave doctors her own theory about the cause of her own and her son's illness: a condensed milk product that the family had been using for six weeks. She suspected the milk because the family dog had died after drinking it.

The condensed milk proved to be a product used commercially—by the food industry—to fortify milk. Never intended for consumer use, it had an intense concentration of vitamin D. The manufacturer's instructions called for using 5 ounces—a little more than a half cup—to fortify 175,000 quarts of milk! The doctors calculated that Jon, his mother, and other family members might have been taking in as much as 180,000 International Units (I.U.) daily of vitamin D from drinking the milk directly.

Said the doctors, "It was not clear how and where this material [the highly fortified milk] had been obtained, although they claimed that it was a gift from one of their friends who worked at a warehouse company."

HIGH CALCIUM DANGER

Both Jon and his mother had one or more of the symptoms that now have become classic signs of vitamin D overdose: loss of appetite, nausea and vomiting, abdominal pain, and excessive urination. Excessive thirst and headaches are also classic symptoms.

The underlying cause of some of these symptoms is too much calcium in the blood. Because vitamin D promotes calcium absorption, excessive intake of vitamin D leads to excessive amounts of calcium in the blood and urine.

Too much calcium in the blood—officially known as hypercalcemia—is a serious medical condition. The consequences magnify as the amount of calcium in the blood increases. If the blood calcium becomes severely elevated, muscles may weaken, and symptoms such as confusion, delirium, and coma can occur. At the highest of levels, shock and death may occur. Rarely, however, does vitamin D overdose get that far.

The most common sites affected by high blood calcium caused by excessive vitamin D intake are the bones and the kidneys. Other organs can be affected, but the kidneys are usually of greatest concern.

It's an irony of bone health that a healthy vitamin D intake strengthens bones, while an excessive intake weakens them. When too much vitamin D is taken in, the bones may let too much of their calcium leach into the blood. The bones become weaker and risk fracturing; the blood calcium level increases, possibly into the danger zone. Between the excess of calcium in the blood and the urine, the kidneys may be hit particularly hard.

KIDNEY COMPLAINTS

Vitamin D overdose can affect kidney health in more ways than one. Left untreated, excess calcium from the condition may be deposited within the kidneys themselves. And if high blood calcium reaches a severe state, the kidneys may fail completely, unable to cope with the burden of so much calcium in the blood.

In an effort to remove excess calcium, the kidneys may direct it into the urine for excretion. This may occur with no ill effects; but in other cases, the stage may be set for the development of kidney stones.

In chapter 11, we talked about kidney stones containing oxalate, a breakdown product of vitamin C. Kidney stones may also contain calcium. In fact, calcium is found in 90 percent of kidney stones diagnosed in the United States. So it makes sense that overdoing a nutrient that increases calcium absorption could spell trouble.

W. H. Taylor, M.D., put this possibility to the test. He surveyed supplementation habits in patients with kidney stones and those who had no stones. Among his most notable findings:

• The average daily dose of supplemental vitamin D was higher in patients with kidney stones than in those free of stones.
• The highest dosages of supplemental vitamin D were found among kidney stone patients for whom doctors could find no other basis for stone development. (Some patients have conditions that predispose them to stones.)
• The first kidney stone developed within two years of starting on supplemental vitamin D in 80 percent of those patients who had no prior history of such stones.
• The average dose of supplemental vitamin D was 1,254 I.U. daily in patients for whom no cause for the kidney stone could be found.

I found these findings sobering. The research was done in England, however, and I have to keep in mind that differences between the British and American diet might be involved with vitamin D and the risk of kidney stones. And no one has tried to confirm Dr. Taylor's findings. But one cannot argue with the notion that through its effect on calcium metabolism, vitamin D might be involved in kidney stones. So I take the results here seriously.

When we talk later about "How Much Is Too Much," we'll apply these findings to choosing a supplement dosage and monitoring its safety. Those predisposed to kidney stones, however, should have a doctor's approval before taking supplemental vitamin D. This same advice goes for those with chronic infection of the urinary tract, high urinary calcium levels, and hyperparathyroidism.

HOW OVERDOSES ARE TREATED

The outcome of vitamin D overdose runs the gamut of possibilities. Some cases clear up after two weeks or less of treatment. Other cases have required a few months to clear. In one very odd case, full recovery took two years. Of course, extreme cases may lead to permanent kidney damage or calcification in other organs, such as the lungs or stomach.

But generally speaking, doctors can treat vitamin D overdose effectively. Two measures are obvious: Stop the supplement and go on a low-calcium diet during treatment. The doctor may also want the patient to avoid exposure to sunlight and to force fluids.

The cortisone drugs have gained a major role in treatment because of their ability to restore normal blood calcium levels. In some cases, blood calcium has returned to normal within a few days or weeks of cortisone therapy. If the kidneys are not functioning fully, or an underlying condition exists, treatment can be expected to take longer.

The most important step, aside from preventing overdoses from happening, is to nip the problem in the bud through early treatment. Diagnosis is rarely complicated.

THE SENSITIVITY FACTOR

People vary enormously in their sensitivity to vitamin D. One has only to look at the case of Jon and his mother, discussed earlier.

Eight other members of their family also drank the same vitamin D concentrate without becoming ill.

The doctors who treated Jon and his mother noted that some people will develop high blood calcium at levels of only 10 times the RDA; others succumb to toxicity only at levels 100 times the recommended allowance. Take a recent study of 63 elderly patients. Two of them developed high blood calcium on a daily dose of 2,000 I.U. of vitamin D—just 10 times the current RDA for adults.

This difference in sensitivity is such that some succumb to vitamin D toxicity within a few weeks; others not for years or more than a decade.

Despite the great variation, I think some numbers are possible. In the hypersensitive, vitamin D toxicity might develop at levels as low as 1,000 I.U. for an infant and 2,000 for an adult. Most cases, however, involve much higher doses, ranging from 25,000 I.U. to 1,000,000 I.U. daily in adults.

Unfortunately, there is no foolproof way of knowing who is very sensitive and who is resistant among the general population. There is one type of sensitive person, however, who can be spotted right away: Those who have a special condition predisposing to high blood calcium. I'll tell you who they are next.

CAUTION FOR SPECIAL CONDITIONS

In reading through all the cases of vitamin D overdose that I could find in the literature, I noticed something that I hadn't anticipated. Many of the victims already had underlying health problems in which calcium metabolism was disturbed.

Here is a selected list of conditions that could be predisposing factors in vitamin D overdose:

- Addison's disease
- All types of cancer
- Hyperthyroidism
- Milk-alkali syndrome
- Osteoporosis that results from being bedridden (not to be confused with the kind affecting the average woman with bone loss)
- Sarcoidosis, a condition characterized by abnormal tissue growth on the organs
- Therapy with diuretics ("water pills") of the diazide class

- Tumors producing parathyroid hormones
- Vitamin A overdose

Why should these factors be so critical? Perhaps our bodies have a vitamin D thermostat that regulates the way we activate the vitamin. When more D is not needed, the thermostat might slow or stop the process that turns our vitamin D into its most active form. But people with special conditions might have something awry with this thermostat, hence the large percentage of overdose victims with underlying disorders.

In addition, those who have two special conditions—gout and rheumatoid arthritis—may develop complications from vitamin D overdose that have not been observed when overdose occurs in people without these two conditions. Several doctors have reported accumulation of calcium around already damaged joints and the skin above them only in patients having these two conditions combined with vitamin D overdose.

If you have any of the conditions mentioned in this section, you should be sure to consult with your doctor before taking a vitamin D supplement.

TAKE SPECIAL CARE WITH CHILDREN

Children, and especially infants, are more sensitive to vitamin D than adults. In infants, a rare disorder called "idiopathic hypercalcemia" long has been linked to overuse of vitamin D. In its mild form, infants suffer slowing of growth, a condition that usually can be treated successfully. But in the more severe form, infants suffer failure to thrive, "elfin" facial appearance, kidney malfunction, and severe mental retardation.

There is no reason to fear this condition in infants taking vitamin D supplementation in normal amounts—400 I.U. per day. Many authorities have favored such supplementation out of concern that infants have little exposure to sunlight. In fact, the vitamin D deficiency disease rickets, once common in the United States, is rare today because infants receive sensible amounts of supplemental vitamin D in some form.

Increasing the dosage of vitamin D greatly, however, cannot be recommended except as prescribed by a doctor. An occasional infant may be so sensitive to vitamin D that problems can develop on as little as 1,000 I.U. a day. Admittedly, however, most toxic reactions in infants have involved much higher doses.

HEART HEALTH: THE NEW ISSUE

Take it from me, most of what you have read so far is old news. Some of our knowledge about the effects of too much vitamin D goes back a half century. More recently, however, nutritionists have seen preliminary evidence that a high intake of vitamin D may be a potential threat to heart health. And in this case "high intake" is not the 25,000 to 1,000,000 I.U. intake that has caused cases like that of Jon and his mother that you read about earlier.

This time, we are talking about the possibility that intakes slightly above 1,000 I.U. may have unwanted effects. The evidence comes from only a handful of studies, but is nonetheless worthy of attention.

The first topic is the blood cholesterol level, one of the greatest risk factors for heart disease. The healthful range for blood cholesterol varies with age. Even for the oldest age groups, however, most experts consider 240 to be the highest acceptable level. Those having higher levels are considered at high risk of heart disease.

L. M. Dalderup, M.D., of the Netherlands Institute of Nutrition, has studied the possible effects of vitamin D on blood cholesterol. In farmers aged 35 to 55, he found that those taking supplemental vitamin D in doses estimated at 700 to 2,500 I.U. daily averaged cholesterol levels of 268 mg. (per 100 ml. of blood). Those not taking vitamin D averaged cholesterol levels of 248 mg.— substantially less and more healthful. But, there hasn't been any follow-up work to confirm or refute Dr. Dalderup's study.

However, infants who develop the high blood calcium syndrome discussed earlier often have abnormally high blood cholesterol as well. So, I think there might be something here. Determining where the danger zone starts, though, is difficult based on just one study in adults.

HEART HEALTH: PART TWO

Blood cholesterol levels (along with high blood pressure and cigarette smoking) only increase the chances that an individual will develop heart disease. The second issue involving vitamin D, however, concerns those who've already had heart attacks.

Victor Linden, M.D., a researcher at the Institute for Community Medicine at the University of Tromso in Norway, has investigated vitamin D intake among confirmed victims of heart disease. His subjects were those who had qualified for a disability pension due to heart attack, angina pectoris, and degenerative diseases. Total vitamin D intake (past and present, if possible) was calculated for each participant. Both food and supplements were included.

The bottom line was this: Those who had suffered heart attacks had higher vitamin D intakes than those who had not. In fact, the vitamin D intake was about 50 percent higher in the heart attack group. According to Dr. Linden, the danger zone seemed to begin at a vitamin D intake of about 1,200 I.U. daily.

Critics protested that perhaps something other than the vitamin D in the fish liver or fish liver oil commonly used in vitamin D supplements might have led to the heart attacks. A valid argument for the fish liver, I think, because liver is high in the cholesterol that promotes heart disease. On the other hand, fish oil is rich in polyunsaturates that lower blood cholesterol, thereby helping to reduce risk of heart disease. Moreover, fatty fish usually contains the special agent EPA that has been linked to better heart health. When, despite this, the heart attack group consumed more fish fat and fish oil, I take seriously the possibility that vitamin D may have ill effects on the heart.

Research in animals does show that high intakes of vitamin D are hazardous to the arteries. C. Bruce Taylor, M.D., of the Veterans Hospital at Birmingham, Alabama, and his colleagues, summarized their concerns about these leads on vitamin D and heart health with the following comment in the *Annals of Clinical Laboratory Science*:

> The tragic "operation over-kill" of adding vitamin D to almost everything excepting cigars may well be one of the most important . . . factors in human atherosclerosis [hardening of the arteries]. People in the United States may well be the victims of Madison Avenue advertising tycoons, food manufacturers, unsuspecting dieticians and indifferent physicians who have probably all played a role in adding excessive amounts of vitamin D to foods.

Many years have passed since these words were written. Physicians' groups did call for a halt to the addition of vitamin D to food except milk. Prodded by doctors and the Food and Drug Administration (FDA), food manufacturers have cut back, either eliminating vitamin D or adding only small amounts of it to food.

But what better time to ask yourself: How much vitamin D are you consuming? You cannot make a sound decision about supplementation without knowing the answer.

D IN YOUR DIET

In amassing nutrition information from more than 100 major food companies, I usually found only cereal and milk to be fortified with vitamin D. In many cereals, though not all, the amount of

Vitamin D and Daily Intake

Since our major source of vitamin D comes from sunshine and not from the foods we eat, we'll forgo the quiz used in previous chapters to evaluate your daily intake. Besides, few foods other than liver and fatty fish are natural sources of the vitamin (cereals and milk are fortified sources).

Below I've listed the foods most likely to contribute to the vitamin D intake in the daily diet. From it you can get an idea of your dietary intake of the vitamin.

Food	I.U.
Cereals, most types,* 1 ounce dry	40
Cereals, superfortified, 1 ounce dry	100
Egg, one (or one yolk)	35
Herring, kippers, 4 ounces	994
Liver, 4 ounces	34
Mackerel, 4 ounces	300 (minimum)
Milk,† 1 cup	100

D added was small. Moreover, new FDA regulations limit the amount of vitamin D that can be added to cereals, grain products, milk, and milk products.

However, health food companies may generously fortify foods not covered by the new regulations with vitamin D. Some may be fortified the full allowance for vitamin D in a single serving. If you use such products frequently, you will want to consider their vitamin D content in addition to the foods listed below.

Liver and fatty fish are our natural sources of vitamin D. All values are but estimates, as the nutritional value can vary markedly from one piece of liver to the next. This simply means that your estimate will be a rough one if your diet typically includes these foods.

Food	I.U.
Milk shake, fast-food (estimate)	40
Salmon, canned, 4 ounces	565
Sardines, canned, 4 ounces	339
Tuna, canned, 4 ounces	271

*Quaker brand cereals are not fortified with vitamin D, except for King Vitaman.

†About 2 percent of the milk sold in the United States may not be fortified. To be sure, just check the front label of the milk you commonly buy. It should say "vitamin D fortified." It probably will.

Don't be alarmed if your diet does not contain the RDA for vitamin D. Remember, sunlight contributes, too. If you do make a level of 400 I.U. or more, however, read the section on "How Much Is Too Much" before deciding to take a supplement.

As for fatty fish not listed, chances are good that their vitamin D content is substantial—at least as high as tuna.

THE STAR SYSTEM SHINES ON VITAMIN D

Before setting some guidelines for safe use of vitamin D, let's sum up its record and look at some new facts, mostly about its interaction with certain drugs.

Side effects—Oddly enough, I found no side effects caused by vitamin D in the absence of a toxic reaction or an underlying condition such as disturbed kidneys or parathyroid function.

Acute ailments—Without question, excessive D can cause a toxic reaction within a short time. However, most cases have required at least a few weeks to develop, and some would argue that these are long-term problems. Certainly, as compared to the reactions to certain vitamins that occur within a half hour or a few days, the incubation period for vitamin D toxicity seems longer. To me this is an academic point, because the symptoms are the same in both acute and long-term reactions.

Long-term problems—Nausea, vomiting, loss of appetite, headache, dry mouth, abdominal or bone pain or distress, dizziness—these are the classic symptoms of vitamin D toxicity. As the condition progresses, signs of impaired kidney function, such as excessive urination, may arise. Itching, calcification of organs and blood vessels, osteoporosis, and seizures are still other signs that develop at the later stages. Intakes of 40,000 I.U. or more are often involved in adults, but the unusually sensitive have developed high blood calcium on as little as 2,000 I.U.

Aside from the toxicity syndrome are concerns that even moderate intakes of vitamin D might raise blood cholesterol, increase risk of heart disease, and contribute to kidney stones.

Conflicting combinations—Vitamin D is not known to prevent any drugs from doing their job. That does not mean that precautions are not in order. Adverse reactions can occur when vitamin D is taken along with two types of drugs.

First, the drug Crystodigin (brand name for digotoxin or digitalis glycoside). There is a risk of abnormal heart rhythm when it is combined with vitamin D. A second alert pertains to diuretics ("water pills") belonging to the thiazide class of drugs. There have been some reports of high blood calcium when these are combined with substantial doses of vitamin D. A list of common brand name drugs that fall under this category appears on page 77.

The following drugs can increase the need for vitamin D or adversely affect the body's use of it:

• Barbiturates such as Seconal, Amytal, Butisol, Nembutal, and phenobarbital and the sleeping pill, Doriden (glutethimide)
• Certain anticonvulsants
• Cholesterol-lowering drugs such as cholestyramine and colestipol
• Cortisone drugs
• Laxatives such as mineral oil and phenolphthalein

Hidden consequences—I found only one report of vitamin D interfering with laboratory tests. Vitamin D reportedly can cause a falsely high blood cholesterol reading by interfering with what is called the Zlatkis-Zak reaction. However, as best as I can determine, this method of measuring blood cholesterol is not in wide use.

HOW MUCH IS TOO MUCH

We have taken a long, hard look at the levels of vitamin D supplementation that have caused serious toxicity. But safe use means more than avoiding high blood calcium and the toxicity syndrome it brings. It also means minimizing the risk of kidney stones and harm to the heart.

You might say that an intake of 1,000 I.U. can be considered relatively untainted by current knowledge. The critical level for increased risk of heart attack, for instance, seemed to be 1,200 I.U. In the study of kidney stones, the average intake was 1,254 I.U. among those with no condition predisposing to stones. So an intake of up to 1,000 I.U. might seem like a safe bet. In fact, supplements containing 1,000 I.U. can be found easily.

Count me out as one who will endorse this level of supplementation as a general measure. It lacks something that I spoke of only a chapter ago—a margin of safety.

I also feel that too many questions remain unanswered about vitamin D to think in terms of a lowest dose known to be harmful. Rather, I think you should ensure that your needs for the vitamin are met and forgo additional amounts. I have not taken this approach for other vitamins, but for vitamin D, it is the only one that feels right.

I think of 400 to 600 I.U. as a safe range. This is two to three times the recommended allowance for adults and more than enough to reduce the risk of colon cancer. In a key study, men in the lowest risk group had vitamin D intakes of 100 to 300 I.U. daily. That's no megadose.

There are three exceptions to the range I recommend. First, pregnant and nursing women who are age 22 or younger have an RDA above 400 I.U. Second, the elderly. A distinguished group of bone health experts has argued convincingly that vitamin D requirements increase in the elderly, suggesting a range of 600 to 800 I.U. I can't oppose them, especially for those elderly at risk of osteoporosis. Finally, if your doctor prescribes a higher intake, that too is an exception.

The most recent expert opinion on vitamin D safety comes from an expert panel on osteoporosis of the National Institutes of Health. In 1984, they concluded, "No one should consume more than 600 to 800 I.U. daily . . . without a doctor's recommendation."

If you take both a calcium supplement and a multiple vitamin, be sure that the combination is not giving you more vitamin D than you realize. Some calcium supplements contain added vitamin D. If you take in 400 I.U. from a multiple vitamin and another 400 I.U. from a calcium supplement, you are taking in 800 I.U. in addition to the amount your diet provides.

CHECKING FOR SAFETY

If, for any reason, you choose or are instructed by your doctor to take a high dose of vitamin D, the safety of your regimen can be monitored by simple blood and urine tests. In fact, some physicians require these tests for all patients for whom large doses of vitamin D are prescribed. This makes it possible to catch any potential problems early.

Similarly, if you are concerned about whether your vitamin D intake (from food, sunlight, or supplements) is meeting your needs, your doctor can order a test of blood vitamin D that will give the answer.

C O O K I N G
for Vitamin D

SALMON IN A PACKET

(Makes 4 servings)

Vitamin D: 580 I.U. per serving
Calories: 250 per serving

1 shallot, minced	1 teaspoon minced orange rind
1 small carrot, cut into julienne strips	4 6-ounce salmon steaks
1 small stalk celery, cut into julienne strips	¾ cup orange juice
1 teaspoon minced fresh ginger	4 thin slices fresh ginger

Preheat oven to 450°F.

Set a piece of 30 × 18-inch aluminum foil shiny side down and fold up 2 inches of each long side and 8 inches of each short side, to form a box. Scatter the shallot, carrot, celery, minced ginger, and orange rind on the bottom of foil. Arrange the salmon steaks on top of the vegetables. Pour the orange juice over the salmon. Place a slice of ginger on top of each salmon steak. Bring the short sides of the foil up to the center to enclose the salmon. Seal tightly. Place on a baking sheet and bake for 15 to 20 minutes. Remove from foil and serve.

(continued)

C O O K I N G

for Vitamin D—continued

SARDINE GRINDER

(Makes 8 servings)

Vitamin D: 60 I.U. per serving
Calories: 195 per serving

Sandwich:

1 loaf French or Italian
    bread, halved
    lengthwise
2 red bell peppers,
    roasted* and
    chopped
1 green bell pepper,
    roasted* and
    chopped
4 scallions, minced
1 pint cherry tomatoes,
    chopped
4 sardines, drained and
    chopped

⅓ cup minced fresh
    parsley
⅔ cup packed watercress
    leaves

Dressing:

1 cup fresh parsley leaves
⅓ cup packed watercress
    leaves
1 clove garlic, chopped
3 tablespoons lemon juice
4 sardines, drained
2 tablespoons olive oil

To make the sandwich, remove the inside of bread from the loaf, leaving a ½-inch shell. Crumble the bread with your hands and reserve 1 cup.

In a medium-size bowl, combine the peppers, scallions, tomatoes, sardines, parsley, and watercress.

To prepare the dressing, combine the parsley, watercress, and garlic in a food processor or blender. Process until finely minced. Add the lemon juice, sardines, and reserved bread and process until thoroughly combined. With the motor running, slowly add the oil.

To assemble, stir ⅔ of dressing into the sandwich mixture. Spread the remaining dressing over the inside of the

C O O K I N G
for Vitamin D—*continued*

bread. Pack the filling into one of the bread shells. Put the remaining shell on top. Wrap the sandwich in aluminum foil. Place a 2-pound weight on top of the sandwich. Chill 4 hours or overnight. With a serrated knife, cut the sandwich into 2-inch slices.

*To roast peppers, place them whole on a broiler rack and broil, turning often, until skins are blistered and black. Remove from oven and place them in a paper bag. Cool. Remove skins, tops, and seeds and rinse with cold water. Drain the peppers on paper towels.

BAKED FONDUTA

(Makes 4 servings)

Vitamin D: 38 I.U. per serving
Calories: 295 per serving

8	slices French bread (½-inch slices)	1½ cups skim milk / pinch of dry mustard
½	cup grated Swiss cheese	1 tablespoon minced fresh parsley
½	cup grated Fontina cheese	pinch of freshly grated nutmeg
4	medium-size eggs	

Preheat oven to 350°F.

Spray an 8 × 8-inch glass baking dish with no-stick spray. Cube the bread and arrange in the baking dish. Combine the cheeses and toss them on top of the bread.

In a medium-size bowl, whisk together the eggs, milk, mustard, parsley, and nutmeg and pour the mixture evenly over the cheese. Bake for about 25 to 30 minutes, or until the fonduta is set. Serve warm for breakfast or lunch.

Vitamin D Content
of Selected Supplements

Dosage is one tablet or capsule unless otherwise indicated.

Supplement	Manufacturer	I.U.
Abdec Baby Drops (per 0.6 ml.)	Parke-Davis	400
Abdec Kapseal	Parke-Davis	400
Abdol with Minerals	Parke-Davis	400
Abron	O'Neal, Jones & Feldman	400
Bugs Bunny	Miles	400
Bugs Bunny Plus Iron	Miles	400
Bugs Bunny with Extra C	Miles	400
Calcium, Phosphate, and Vitamin D	Squibb	180
Cal-M	Anabolic	400
Cal-Prenal	North American	400
Centrum	Lederle	400
Chew-Vite	North American	400
Cluvisol 130	Ayerst	400
Cluvisol Syrup (per tsp.)	Ayerst	400
Cod Liver Oil Concentrate Capsules	Schering	400
Cod Liver Oil Concentrate Tablets	Schering	200
Cod Liver Oil Tablets with Vitamin A	Schering	200
Dayalets	Abbott	400
Dayalets plus Iron	Abbott	400
De-Cal	North American	125
Di-Calcium Phosphate Tablets	North American	333
Di-Cal D Capsules	Abbott	133
Di-Cal D Wafers	Abbott	133
Di-Cal D with Vitamin C Capsules	Abbott	133
Drisdol Drops	Winthrop	200
Engram-HP	Squibb	400
Feminins	Mead Johnson	400
Femiron with Vitamins	J.B. Williams	400
Filibon Tablets	Lederle	400
Flintstones	Miles	400
Flintstones Plus Iron	Miles	400

Supplements—continued

Supplement	Manufacturer	I.U.
Flintstones with Extra C	Miles	400
Ganatrex (per 0.6 ml.)	Merrell Dow	400
Gerilets	Abbott	400
Geritinic	Geriatric Pharm.	400
Geritol Junior Liquid (per tsp.)	J.B. Williams	400
Geritol Junior Tablets	J.B. Williams	100
Gest	O'Neal, Jones & Feldman	200
Gevral Protein	Lederle	217
Gevral T Capsules	Lederle	400
Multicebrin	Lilly	400
Multiple Vitamins	North American	400
Multiple Vitamins with Iron	North American	400
Multivitamins	Rowell	400
Myadec	Parke-Davis	400
Natabec	Parke-Davis	400
Natalins Tablets	Mead Johnson	400
Norlac	Rowell	400
Nutra-Cal	Anabolic	100
Obron-6	Pfipharmecs	400
One-A-Day	Miles	400
One-A-Day Core C 500	Miles	400
One-A-Day Plus Iron	Miles	400
One-A-Day Vitamins Plus Minerals	Miles	400
Optilets-500	Abbott	400
Optilets-M-500	Abbott	400
Os-Cal	Marion	125
Os-Cal 500	Marion	125
Os-Cal Forte	Marion	125
Os-Cal Plus	Marion	125
Paladec (per tsp.)	Parke-Davis	400
Paladec with Minerals	Parke-Davis	400
Panuitex	O'Neal, Jones & Feldman	400
Poly-Vi-Sol Chewable	Mead Johnson	400
Poly-Vi-Sol Drops (per 0.6 ml.)	Mead Johnson	400
Poly-Vi-Sol with Iron Chewable	Mead Johnson	400
Poly-Vi-Sol with Iron Drops (per 0.6 ml.)	Mead Johnson	400
Stuart Formula	Stuart	400
Stuart Prenatal	Stuart	400

(continued)

Supplements—continued

Supplement	Manufacturer	I.U.
Sugar Calcicaps	Nion	133
Super D Cod Liver Oil (per tsp.)	Upjohn	400
Super D Perles (per tsp.)	Upjohn	400
Super Plenamins	Rexall	400
Theragran	Squibb	400
Theragran Liquid (per tsp.)	Squibb	400
Theragran-M	Squibb	400
Theragran-Z	Squibb	400
Therapeutic Vitamins	North American	400
Thera-Spancap	North American	400
Tri-Vi-Sol Chewable	Mead Johnson	400
Tri-Vi-Sol Drops (per 1 ml.)	Mead Johnson	400
Tri-Vi-Sol with Iron Drops (per 1 ml.)	Mead Johnson	400
Unicap	Upjohn	400
Unicap Chewable	Upjohn	400
Unicap T	Upjohn	400
Vi-Aqua	USV	400
Vigran	Squibb	400
Vigran Chewable	Squibb	400
Vigran plus Iron	Squibb	400
Vio-Geric	Rowell	400
Vi-Penta Infant Drops (per 0.6 ml.)	Roche	400
Vi-Penta Multivitamin Drops (per 0.6 ml.)	Roche	400
Vitagett	North American	400
Vita-Kaps-M Tablets	Abbott	400
Vita-Kaps Tablets	Abbott	400
Vitamin-Mineral Capsules	North American	400
Viterra	Pfipharmecs	400
Viterra High Potency	Pfipharmecs	400
Zymacap Capsules	Upjohn	400
Zymasyrup (per tsp.)	Upjohn	400

Source: Adapted from the American Pharmaceutical Association, *Handbook of Nonprescription Drugs*, 7th ed. (1982), 240–57.

Note: This chart is intended only as a guide. Vitamin formulations change periodically; always read product labels for accurate and up-to-date information on their nutrient levels.

13
Vitamin E

After enduring 30 years of insults (and occasional accolades), vitamin E is coming into its own. Doctors and nutritionists who once regarded it as useless now take it very seriously. They have seen the research that presents vitamin E as a promising substance in the prevention of cancer and in the treatment of premenstrual syndrome.

The new research provides more than a testing ground for the benefits of vitamin E. It also offers information about the vitamin's safety, collected under the kind of controlled research that meets today's exacting scientific standards.

In my experience, no vitamin has been subject to the kind of claims and counterclaims that have been the hallmark of the vitamin E debate. One doctor, for instance, reports that vitamin E helps prevent blood clots. Another insists that it contributes to clots. One camp believes that high doses of E cause fatigue. Another says, to the contrary, E is energizing. Sorting out the conflicting comments has been an education in itself.

I'd like nothing better than to share the facts with you. I find them rather reassuring.

The Vitamin E Popularity Poll

When a supplement's popularity rises and falls within a few years' time, you have witnessed a fad. But when it stays on the scene for decades, with countless users coming back for more, you are seeing something that people believe in—often despite what their doctors or what scientists have to say.

Vitamin E seems to have a mystique of sorts . . . it's something that certain people will try on instinct or intuition. Of course, some users *are* following doctor's orders. And still others are acting on the latest scientific findings. So if you ask people why they take vitamin E, you'll get a list of reasons so long and varied that, well, it will probably look something like this:

To Combat:
- Arthritis
- Athlete's foot
- Blood fat disorders
- Dry skin
- Leg cramps
- Pain left by herpes infections
- Rare skin disorders
- Sunburn
- Tendency to abnormal "overclotting" of blood
- Wounds and skin irritation

To Prevent:
- Aging
- Cancer
- Decline of the immune system
- Deterioration of eyesight
- Hazards of pollution
- Heart attacks and strokes

E'S UNIQUE JOB

Vitamin E doesn't have much in the way of a classic role in human nutrition. There is no vitamin E deficiency disease that is the counterpart of scurvy (vitamin C deficiency) or rickets (vitamin D deficiency). So nothing truly dramatic happens when intake is low. But this doesn't mean vitamin E isn't important.

The vitamin plays a role in the metabolism of polyunsaturated fats, the kind that help lower blood cholesterol and keep heart disease at bay. Diets high in polyunsaturated fats take care of their vitamin E needs automatically. These fats are the best food source of vitamin E, so they naturally provide the vitamin E needed to use them well.

Vitamin E is best known, however, as an antioxidant—a substance that helps to prevent oxidation. Oxidation is not only a process that allows food to turn rancid, but also one that allows certain harmless chemicals in the body to become harmful ones. This has become an important issue in cancer research. Cancer scientists believe that an antioxidant might prevent a benign substance from being oxidized into a harmful one that contributes to the cancer process. There is little research on vitamin E's direct effects here—that is, how its antioxidant ability affects the cancer process. However, the value of another antioxidant in cancer prevention—vitamin C—has been well documented by cancer researchers. This is reason enough for me to accept vitamin E's antioxidant ability as a good bet for cancer prevention.

While many foods, from meat to cereals, provide some vitamin E, the amounts are small in relation to levels in common vitamin E supplements. Even for those on a good diet, total vitamin E intake from food is unlikely to exceed 20 International Units (I.U.) per day. That more than meets the Recommended Dietary Allowance (RDA) for all age groups, but is far from the three- and sometimes four-digit levels that many people take in supplement form. Which brings us to the very important question: Is vitamin E safe at such large doses?

TESTIMONIES OF SAFETY

I have watched the vitamin E debate for many years and feel confident in saying that detractors and unanswered questions notwithstanding, it has earned a reputation as a generally safe substance. Even those who oppose its use as unnecessary have been known to acknowledge that it has yet to show much toxic potential.

Here's some sample commentary from doctors who have conducted studies of vitamin E or prescribed it for patients:

No side effects were noted by any patient in this study [of 58 women taking 150–600 I.U. vitamin E daily for premenstrual syndrome.]

Robert London, M.D., and colleagues
Sinai Hospital of Baltimore, Baltimore, Maryland

In a series of well over 1,000 patients who have been treated with an average of 2,000 I.U. of synthetic vitamin E daily for more than two years, neither my associate nor I have noted any of the dangerous disease entities [that critics attribute to vitamin E].

James L. Baker, M.D.
Winter Park, Florida

We have had no complications after the use of vitamin E [1,600 I.U. daily in 22 men].

W. M. Toone, M.D.
Veterans' Hospital, Victoria, British Columbia

On the basis of 20 laboratory screening tests per individual, designed to test a wide range of organ functions, it must be concluded that no signs of toxicity were uncovered in this investigation [of 28 adults who had been taking 100 to 800 I.U. vitamin E daily for an average of three years].

Philip M. Farrell, M.D., Ph.D.
John G. Bieri, Ph.D.
National Institutes of Health (NIH), Bethesda, Maryland

THE FATIGUE FACTOR

To say the least, not everyone agrees with the rosy assessment. In 1973, Harold Cohen, M.D., of Sylmar, California, sent a letter about vitamin E that was published in several medical journals. As far as I can see, it was a letter that made history.

Dr. Cohen related how he had decided to test vitamin E himself after finding too much inconclusive information in medical journals. He included himself, his partner, and a number of patients in his study; all started on doses of at least 800 I.U. daily. Of the experience, he wrote:

After about one week on the medication, I began to feel an amazing weakness and fatigue as if suffering from a severe influenzal syndrome. The symptoms stopped after withdrawal of the vitamin E. Still thinking that I had likely suffered a viral illness, I resumed the vitamin E, and the symptoms returned. I did not relate this to my partner who was taking the vitamin in the same dosage. When he left the office early two days in a row because he felt very tired and "sick," I related to him my experiences. He stopped the vitamin E and his symptoms disappeared the following day. By this time, virtually all of the patients and colleagues to whom I was giving the therapy were calling me and relating the same thing, and had to stop their vitamin E. Some, I among them, were able to tolerate the vitamin at 400 I.U. daily, with only minimal fatigue.

After this experience, Dr. Cohen said, he examined numerous vitamin users who complained of severe fatigue. He noted that their physicals and laboratory tests were almost always normal, and that withdrawal of vitamin E was all that was needed to end the symptoms. In fact, he reported, vitamin E was second only to depression as the cause of fatigue in his young patients.

THE CONTROVERSY CONTINUES

Dr. Cohen's letter was read far and wide, and response was dramatic. As best as I can tell, the reaction was evenly divided between those who agreed and those who did not.

After running an antivitamin E editorial, the *Journal of the American Medical Association* reported that letters to the editor supporting the editorial mentioned fatigue prominently as a problem with the vitamin.

Michael Briggs, M.D., took the issue a step further by directly measuring body reaction to high doses of vitamin E. Dr. Briggs enlisted eight healthy young men who took 800 I.U. of vitamin E daily. After three weeks, two of the eight complained of severe fatigue and weakness. They asked to stop participating in the study.

In these two men, laboratory tests showed abnormally high

The RDA and Vitamin E: Clearing the Confusion

If you are taking vitamin E supplements, you are familiar with the term "International Unit" or I.U. as a measure of supplement potency. I think of vitamin E in those terms, too.

But the official RDA for vitamin E are issued in a different language. Rather than use the familiar I.U., the scientists in charge use mg. The reasoning is complex.

Even more complex, though, is converting mg. of vitamin E to I.U. That's because vitamin E comes in many forms that can differ in the amount of I.U. per mg. More complications.

If you think of vitamin E in terms of one common form found in supplements, d l-alpha-tocopherol acetate, your worries are over. A mg. of vitamin E is basically equivalent to an I.U. of that, so you can simply think of the numbers below in I.U. instead of mg.

For the trivia seeker, here is how some other common forms of vitamin E translate from mg. to I.U.:

• Synthetic free d l-alpha-tocopherol (not acetate) has 1.1 I.U. per mg.

• Naturally occurring alpha-tocopherol and d-alpha-tocopherol have 1.49 I.U. per mg.

levels of a substance called creatine kinase in the blood. They also had excessive levels of creatinine in the urine. Creatinine, which is made from creatine, is an end product of muscle metabolism. Coupled with the complaints of fatigue and weakness, Dr. Briggs suspected his findings meant the beginning of "some degree of damage to skeletal muscles." Fortunately, these laboratory tests returned to normal within a week after stopping supplemental vitamin E.

Six of Dr. Briggs's participants, however, remained normal throughout the study. They had no complaints while on vitamin E and a wide range of laboratory tests yielded normal readings for them. One can only conclude that sensitivity to vitamin E varies.

• Alpha-tocopherol acetate or d-alpha-tocopherol acetate have 1.36 I.U. per mg.

Now for those RDAs. As you can see, they pale in comparison to the vitamin E supplements we commonly take. And of course, the role of vitamin E in cancer prevention was not considered in formulating the allowances in 1980.

Group/Age	Mg.
Infants 0–6 mon.	3
Infants 6–12 mon.	4
Children 1–3 yr.	5
Children 4–6 yr.	6
Children 7–10 yr.	7
Males 11–14 yr.	8
Males 15+ yr.	10
Females 11+ yr.	8
Pregnant women	10
Nursing women	11

Note: The U.S. RDA for vitamin E is 30 I.U.

NO FATIGUE HERE

You have heard the advocates of the fatigue theory. Now let's give two of the skeptics a turn.

Samuel Ayres, Jr., M.D., and his partner Richard Mihan, M.D., who have pioneered the successful use of vitamin E in troublesome skin disorders, replied, "We have administered therapeutic doses of vitamin E in the range of 400 to 1,600 I.U. daily to hundreds of patients, including ourselves and several members of our office staff, without observing a single case of muscular weakness or fatigue."

W. M. Toone, M.D., of Victoria's Veterans' Hospital, who also had treated patients with 1,600 I.U. of vitamin E, countered the fatigue claim as well. None of his 22 patients complained of muscle weakness or fatigue. "On the contrary," he said, "there has been a sense of well-being in taking vitamin E."

My own feeling after reading all of this? There are too many conflicting claims on this subject and not enough formal research work to conclude that high doses of vitamin E cause fatigue. Certainly this possibility seems to exist in doses of 800 I.U. or so.

But, after all, fatigue is not the black plague. Anyone who develops fatigue or weakness after taking vitamin E can simply stop or lower the dosage. By all accounts, the condition clears up promptly. So I don't see this as reason to preach with a fervor against vitamin E.

E AND EMOTIONS

Taking the fatigue theory one step further is Albert Kligman, M.D., Ph.D., a prominent skin care specialist and dermatologist at the Hospital of the University of Pennsylvania in Philadelphia. Dr Kligman believes he has seen in his patients an "unusually high prevalence of emotional disorders with dosages of 800 I.U./day" of vitamin E. He cites such symptoms as depression, withdrawal, tiredness, mood swings, and loss of confidence as typical symptoms.

Dr. Kligman admits that such symptoms may have existed before vitamin E supplementation was started. But he concludes, "It is a near certainty that vitamin E does not relieve these feelings, and probably aggravates them."

No one else has reported these findings, so at this time, I consider this to be conjecture.

SOME SERIOUS CHARGES

Now it's time to consider the most serious charges ever leveled against vitamin E. In fact, until Hyman Roberts, M.D., brought them to the fore in 1978, vitamin E was considered generally nontoxic by proponents and opponents alike.

Times changed in 1978 when *Lancet*, a popular British medical journal, published a letter by Dr. Roberts proposing an association between vitamin E and thrombophlebitis. That's a tongue twister referring to inflammation of a vein brought on by a blood clot. For simplicity, I'll use the term phlebitis for the rest of this discussion.

Dr. Roberts also proposed a link between vitamin E and some other disorders, most notably breast enlargement in both men and women, and breast tumors. A few years later, he published an editorial in the *Journal of the American Medical Association* in which the charges were repeated. With coverage in two of the most widely read medical journals, these claims of adverse effects received a great deal of publicity.

After printing Dr. Roberts's editorial, the *Journal of the American Medical Association* received a large amount of correspondence. Some letter writers agreed that E is potentially harmful, while others contested the idea. According to the editor, the proposed link between vitamin E and phlebitis was "prominently challenged." Instead of printing the letters, the editor referred readers to the organization's reference book, *AMA Drug Evaluations*. It did not list phlebitis as an adverse effect of E.

I write this eight years since Dr. Roberts first made his charges. No confirming reports of phlebitis or breast enlargement have been reported since. Interestingly enough, vitamin E is now under study as a cure for breast lumps and premenstrual syndrome.

Because no confirmation has been made, I feel that these theories have not stood up well. Until shown otherwise, I consider it unwarranted to claim that vitamin E contributes to phlebitis, sore breasts, or breast enlargement.

TO CLOT OR NOT

After hearing one scientist charge that vitamin E might play a role in a condition marked by inflammation due to a blood clot, how odd to read that vitamin E can prolong the clotting of the blood under certain conditions.

Five of the factors that help blood to clot are related to vitamin K. In a select group of patients who are already short on vitamin K, vitamin E appears to make matters worse. What happens is that vitamin E prolongs the amount of time required for necessary clotting of blood. The result can be internal bleeding.

In one victim, for instance, the adverse effects were marked by discolored skin. The cause of the discolorations was blood that had leached into the tissues below the skin. These discolored areas are called ecchymoses. The patient had been taking up to 1,200 I.U. of vitamin E daily, and his symptoms were duplicated with 800 I.U. daily.

It is critical to understand two things: First, the potential seriousness of this condition, and second, the limited circumstances under which it is known to occur. The conditions involved are those where people might be short on vitamin K. These include:

- Biliary tract obstruction
- Liver disease
- Malabsorption syndromes such as sprue and celiac disease
- Use of coumarin-type drugs, such as warfarin (Coumadin)

The patient mentioned above had been taking warfarin and vitamin E. Apparently, it wasn't a good combination. However, for healthy individuals, no problems of this nature have been reported, with one somewhat related exception. One of the 28 vitamin E users studied by Drs. Farrell and Bieri at the NIH did show a prolonged clotting time on a test of 8 of 12 factors involved in the clotting process. However, no signs of abnormal bleeding were reported.

OTHER SPECIAL CONDITIONS

Even some of vitamin E's most ardent advocates admit that it should be used cautiously, if at all, in certain other conditions.

Dr. Toone, who reported positive findings mentioned earlier, nonetheless warns that patients with congestive heart failure should have only "small, guarded doses" under the monitoring of a physician.

Drs. Ayres and Mihan, two more advocates of vitamin E's therapeutic effects and relative safety, comment that, "We would strongly endorse the proposal that the administration of large doses of vitamin E should be under medical supervision, especially in patients with damaged hearts and hypertension, in whom an initial large dose, by improving the tone of the heart muscle, could further increase the blood pressure."

On another matter related to heart health, consider the results of a study at the University of Michigan. Researchers found that women—but not men—taking 600 I.U. of vitamin E daily for four weeks—showed a significant increase in their blood triglyceride levels. Triglycerides have long been considered by some experts to be a risk factor for heart disease. While the higher triglycerides of these women remained well within the normal range, those who already have high triglycerides should take note. Ditto for those with thyroid conditions, as the women in this study also had a significant reduction of blood thyroid hormones while taking the 600 I.U. daily of vitamin E.

Finally, I have read concerns that E might aggravate diabetes, particularly for those taking insulin. As a matter of principle, I feel that all diabetics should have their supplement program approved by their doctors.

E AND ALLERGY

Probably no vitamin is applied to skin as often as vitamin E. It has become a popular skin remedy and a widely used ingredient in cosmetics.

A rare user may react unfavorably to the vitamin E in skin preparations. There have been cases of itching, skin inflammation, and patches of redness from deodorants, creams, and oils containing vitamin E. Testing revealed victims to be specifically allergic to the vitamin E that these products contained. In two of the cases, the reactions occurred when vitamin E was applied to scar tissue.

Tabulating the results, I have read a total of only nine cases. That's enough to establish that reactions can occur. But it's also enough to demonstrate how safe these products are. So few reactions to the large volume of vitamin E preparations that have been sold annually speaks well for their safety.

THE STAR SYSTEM SHINES ON VITAMIN E

To me, vitamin E is pretty safe stuff when taken at reasonable doses. But safety cannot be guaranteed for all. Accordingly, I am summarizing below the adverse effects that have been reported. The list does include some effects that are rare or not well established.

Side effects—High doses of vitamin E can cause nausea, gastric distress, diarrhea, chapping of the lips, hives, or giddiness. All of these are rare, but when side effects do occur, the gastrointestinal symptoms seem most common.

Acute ailments or long-term problems—I feel that there are too few cases of vitamin E toxicity to draw a distinction between acute and long-term problems. Accordingly, I have combined these two categories for vitamin E. Factors attributed to vitamin E toxicity include: blurred vision, change in blood coagulation factors, fatigue and weakness, gonadal dysfunction or hormonal changes, decreases in blood thyroid factors, lowered response to iron therapy, or worsening of heart risk factors (such as blood pressure). In addition, allergic skin reactions have occurred from the vitamin E in products applied to skin. These reactions have been rare.

Conflicting combinations—High doses of vitamin E may interfere with the effect of iron therapy in anemic children. How iron and vitamin E interact in healthy adults has not been studied well, but one medical handbook notes that vitamin E requirements may increase in those taking large amounts of iron. On the other hand, substantial intakes of vitamin E reportedly lower vitamin A requirements. However, I would not lower vitamin A intake below the recommended allowance on this basis.

Vitamin E should be used only under the supervision of a physician if you take an anticlotting drug such as warfarin. If you have any other condition that can contribute to vitamin K deficiency (liver disease, biliary tract obstruction, or a malabsorption syndrome), you should also take vitamin E only under medical supervision.

Finally, frequent use of mineral oil may increase the need for vitamin E.

Hidden consequences—Vitamin E is not known to cause false readings in any laboratory tests, nor to interfere with the diagnosis of any diseases.

HOW MUCH IS TOO MUCH

Vitamin E has been reported harmless in such doses as 600, 800, and 1,200 I.U. daily. Its most ardent proponents insist that even doses of 2,000 I.U. can be tolerated safely.

Even opponents of vitamin E use concede that it is generally safe in reasonable doses. The Food and Nutrition Board of the National Academy of Sciences, for instance, issued a statement opposing supplemental vitamin E for most people. Still, its book on Recommended Dietary Allowances concedes that there is little evidence of harm at doses less than 1,000 I.U. Says its Committee on Dietary Allowances, "isolated but inconsistent reports have appeared of adverse effects from large intakes (400–1,000 I.U.) ...but most adults appear to tolerate these doses." A group of scientists charged with evaluating vitamin E safety for the Food and Drug Administration reached similar conclusions.

All things considered, including a margin of safety, I would say that 400 I.U. daily is a good safe dose. At 400 I.U., adverse effects would be very unlikely to occur. Many people, of course, can tolerate more. This is always the case when defining the lowest dose known to cause side effects.

Despite its relatively clean reputation, do keep in mind that vitamin E is far from an inert substance. It is an active agent, affecting hormones and possibly blood fats in ways that remain to be understood. Research on how vitamin E affects individual blood fats is just beginning, as is concerted study of its hormonal effects. Whether its antioxidant properties are all to the good, one can only guess. In this context, it is hard to consider vitamin E a completely benign substance. That's a good reason to reserve judgment on very high doses until we get to know it better.

C O O K I N G
for Vitamin E

ALMOND ANGELS

(Makes 12 pastries)

Vitamin E: 8 I.U. per pastry
Calories: 199 per pastry

½	cup blanched, slivered almonds	¼	teaspoon grated orange rind
1	tablespoon wheat germ	1½	tablespoons honey
¼	teaspoon ground cinnamon	12	sheets of phyllo
	dash of freshly grated nutmeg	⅓	cup safflower oil (or less)
		½	cup wheat germ

In a small bowl, combine the almonds, wheat germ, cinnamon, nutmeg, orange rind, and honey and set aside.

Lay the phyllo on a dry counter under a slightly damp cotton towel. To assemble an angel, remove a sheet of phyllo from the pile and cut it into 3 strips vertically. Brush 1 strip with oil and sprinkle a scant teaspoon of wheat germ over the oil. Lay the second strip over it, brush with oil, and sprinkle again with wheat germ. Do the same with the third strip.

Place a well-rounded teaspoon of filling at the bottom left-hand corner of the stack of strips and fold 1 corner over it, to make a triangle. Continue folding the strips tightly in triangles (like you would fold a flag), until there's no more to fold. Brush with oil and repeat with remaining phyllo and filling.

Bake at 350°F on a baking sheet sprayed with no-stick spray for about 20 minutes, and serve with Honey Orange Sauce (recipe follows).

C O O K I N G
for Vitamin E—*continued*

HONEY ORANGE SAUCE

½ cup orange juice
1 tablespoon honey

Combine the orange juice and honey in a small saucepan and heat until the honey has dissolved. Drizzle sauce over warm pastries.

FRAGRANTLY MARINATED MACKEREL

(Makes 4 servings)

Vitamin E: 3 I.U. per serving
Calories: 253 per serving

1 tablespoon safflower or
   soybean oil
3 tablespoons lime juice
½ teaspoon mustard seed,
   crushed
3 allspice berries,
   crushed
½ teaspoon coriander
   seed, crushed
1 pound mackerel fillets
   lime slices, for garnish

In a flat glass baking dish, combine the oil, lime juice, mustard, allspice, and coriander. Place the mackerel skin-side up in the dish, so that the exposed flesh will soak in the marinade. Let the fish marinate at room temperature for 30 minutes, then broil, skin-side up, for about 7 to 9 minutes. Garnish with lime slices and serve. Lift the cooked meat from the skin as you eat it.

(continued)

C O O K I N G
for Vitamin E—*continued*

AVOCADO SALSA

(Makes approximately 2½ cups)

Vitamin E: 3 I.U. per ½ cup
Calories: 124 per ½ cup

Serve over eggs for breakfast or over poached fish. This sauce can also be served with corn chips for a snack.

1 tablespoon safflower or soybean oil	½ teaspoon cumin seed, crushed
1 small bell pepper, seeded and chopped	½ teaspoon dried oregano pinch of cinnamon
1 medium-size onion, chopped	1 avocado, peeled and chopped
1 clove garlic, minced	5 medium-size tomatoes, peeled and seeded
½ teaspoon chili powder	

In a medium-size sauté pan, warm the oil and sauté the pepper, onion, and garlic for about 2 minutes. Add the chili powder, cumin, oregano, and cinnamon and sauté 2 minutes more. Remove from heat.

In a medium-size nonmetallic bowl, combine the avocado, tomatoes, and pepper mixture. Cover and refrigerate for at least 4 hours (overnight is best) to blend the flavors.

Vitamin E Content
of Selected Supplements

Dosage is one tablet or capsule unless otherwise indicated.

Supplement	Manufacturer	I.U.
Abdec Kapseal	Parke-Davis	5
Allbee C-800	Robins	45
Allbee C-800 plus Iron	Robins	45
Aquasol E Capsules (100)	USV	100
Aquasol E Capsules (400)	USV	400
Aquasol E Drops	USV	50
Bugs Bunny	Miles	15
Bugs Bunny Plus Iron	Miles	15
Bugs Bunny with Extra C	Miles	15
Calciwafers	Nion	67
Centrum	Lederle	30
Chew-E	North American	200
Cluvisol 130	Ayerst	1
Dayalets	Abbott	30
Dayalets plus Iron	Abbott	30
E-Ferol Succinate (200)	O'Neal, Jones & Feldman	200
Engram-HP	Squibb	30
Epsilan-M	Warren-Teed	100
Feminins	Mead Johnson	10
Filibon Tablets	Lederle	30
Flintstones	Miles	15
Flintstones Plus Iron	Miles	15
Flintstones with Extra C	Miles	15
Ganatrex (per 0.6 ml.)	Merrell Dow	30
Gerilets	Abbott	45
Geriplex	Parke-Davis	5
Geriplex-FS Kapseals	Parke-Davis	5
Gevral	Lederle	30
Gevral Protein	Lederle	4
Gevral T Capsules	Lederle	45
Lufa Capsules	USV	4
Multicebrin	Lilly	7
Multivitamins	Rowell	10
Myadec	Parke-Davis	30
Natalins Tablets	Mead Johnson	30

(continued)

Supplements—*continued*

Supplement	Manufacturer	I.U.
Norlac	Rowell	30
Nutra-Cal	Anabolic	3
One-A-Day	Miles	15
One-A-Day Core C 500	Miles	15
One-A-Day Plus Iron	Miles	15
One-A-Day Vitamins Plus Minerals	Miles	15
Optilets-500	Abbott	30
Optilets-M-500	Abbott	30
Os-Cal Forte	Marion	1
Paladec with Minerals	Parke-Davis	10
Poly-Vi-Sol Chewable	Mead Johnson	15
Poly-Vi-Sol Drops (per 0.6 ml.)	Mead Johnson	5
Poly-Vi-Sol with Iron Chewable	Mead Johnson	15
Poly-Vi-Sol with Iron Drops (per 0.6 ml.)	Mead Johnson	5
Selenace	Anabolic	200
Stresstabs 600	Lederle	30
Stresstabs 600 with Iron	Lederle	30
Stresstabs 600 with Zinc	Lederle	45
Stuart Formula	Stuart	15
Stuart Prenatal	Stuart	30
Super Plenamins	Rexall	2
Surbex 750 with Iron	Abbott	30
Surbex 750 with Zinc	Abbott	30
Tega-E Caps (400)	Ortega	400
Tega-E Caps (1000)	Ortega	1,000
Theragran	Squibb	15
Theragran-M	Squibb	15
Theragran-Z	Squibb	15
Therapeutic Vitamins	North American	15
Unicap	Upjohn	15
Unicap Chewable	Upjohn	15
Unicap T	Upjohn	15
Vi-Aqua	USV	1
Vicon Iron	Glaxo	30
Vicon Plus	Glaxo	50
Vigran	Squibb	30
Vigran Chewable	Squibb	10

Supplements—*continued*

Supplement	Manufacturer	I.U.
Vigran plus Iron	Squibb	30
Vio-Geric	Rowell	30
Vi-Penta Infant Drops (per 0.6 ml.)	Roche	2
Vi-Penta Multivitamin Drops (per 0.6 ml.)	Roche	2
Vitagett	North American	3
Viterra	Pfipharmecs	4
Viterra High Potency	Pfipharmecs	5
Vi-Zac	Glaxo	50
Z-Bec	Robins	45
Zymacap Capsules	Upjohn	15

Source: Adapted from the American Pharmaceutical Association, *Handbook of Nonprescription Drugs*, 7th ed. (1982), 240–57.

Note: This chart is intended only as a guide. Vitamin formulations change periodically; always read product labels for accurate and up-to-date information on their nutrient levels.

Part 3: Minerals

14

Magnesium

Conventional wisdom in nutrition holds that minerals are more toxic than vitamins. Conventional wisdom is right.

But at least one mineral has a safety record—as an oral supplement, that is—rivaling that of untainted vitamins like thiamine and riboflavin. Magnesium is the one.

This mild-mannered mineral has all sorts of traditional roles in nutrition. Physicians also use drugs containing magnesium to treat certain conditions. Meanwhile, the debate continues as to whether magnesium is another weapon in the war on heart disease. Let's start with magnesium's role in good health.

THE OLD AND NEW

The importance of magnesium is beyond debate. It is a component of every body cell. It allows for smooth functioning of the nervous system, helping in the task of transmitting nerve impulses. Numerous enzyme systems in the body also depend on magnesium.

These are the long-known facts about magnesium. Recently,

though, it has won the attention of heart scientists, for new reasons. First, some studies have shown heart disease to be less common where drinking water contains higher levels of magnesium. Second, autopsies of heart attack victims have repeatedly found them to have had lower than expected levels of magnesium.

This is another chicken-or-egg issue, of course; did the magnesium level fall because of the heart attack, or did the heart attack come because of a low magnesium level? Even with the question unanswered, the link between magnesium and heart disease is under serious investigation.

Also at issue is the role magnesium might play in preventing osteoporosis. About half of the body's magnesium is stored in the bone. When the bone loses calcium to the process called osteoporosis, some of this magnesium must be lost also. That makes one wonder if magnesium, not just calcium, plays a role in combating osteoporosis.

No one has conducted research that answers this question to my satisfaction. I wish I knew the answer, but frankly I don't.

Among the minerals necessary for health, magnesium is classified as a "major" one. Major minerals are those the body needs in substantial amounts. Trace minerals, also known as trace elements, are needed only in tiny quantities. The designation of major or trace refers only to these required amounts. It in no way reflects a judgment on the mineral's importance to good health, though in the case of magnesium, its importance goes without saying.

THE MAGNESIUM MONITOR

Magnesium overdose from supplements? It's almost impossible to imagine in a healthy adult taking even a sizable dose.

This mineral owes its safety to what I call the Magnesium Monitor. You know the monitor already as the kidneys. Healthy ones can and will go to great lengths to keep too much magnesium from accumulating in the body, specifically in the blood.

Too much magnesium in the blood goes by the name hypermagnesemia. Depending on how much excess magnesium is involved, the condition can be mild to life threatening. We'll talk shortly about the signs of this disorder and the circumstances that favor its development.

Many doctors have long believed that hypermagnesemia cannot occur in healthy people having normal kidney function. However, I would like to share with you a case that made me suspect that even healthy kidneys can be overwhelmed if assaulted with too much magnesium.

MORE THAN THE MONITOR COULD TAKE

This is a story about a middle-aged man named George who proved once again that if some is good, more isn't necessarily better.

George had long-standing gastritis—an inflammation of the stomach lining. For several years, he had been taking a common over-the-counter antacid to relieve his symptoms. Few would expect that such medication would land him in the emergency room, but it did. I'll let Carol Millet and Gary Snodgrass, the pharmacists who managed his case and reported it in the *American Journal of Hospital Pharmacy*, explain more:

> A 51-year-old Caucasian man came to the emergency room with a chief complaint of "total body swelling," feeling bloated, and vomiting for the past two days.
>
> Two weeks before admission, the patient developed anorexia [loss of appetite], malaise, and diarrhea ... During the week before admission, the patient noted a dull, diffuse abdominal pain, difficulty in [urinating], and a "puffy appearance" of his face.
>
> The patient had a long history of esophagitis and hiatal hernia. He also had a history of mental depression ... He denied any previous renal problems.

Doctors in the emergency room diagnosed George's problem as acute kidney failure. For four days, he underwent dialysis. In the process he lost more than 30 pounds, no doubt because he had retained an enormous amount of water during his period of kidney failure.

(continued on page 268)

The Diet Detective Searches for Magnesium

More and more, nutritionists are wondering if magnesium intake in the United States has been another casualty of the flour mill. During the refining of wheat, much of its magnesium is removed, leaving reduced amounts in the resulting white flour.

The average magnesium intake of Americans has been estimated at about 300 mg., a level that meets or comes close to the RDA for most adults. But with magnesium remaining a possible contender for promoting heart health, some nutritionists wonder if intake should be boosted. As you test your diet for magnesium, you'll see that a diet rich in whole grain foods, nuts, and beans is one way to do it.

The rules for the quiz are the same as for past quizzes. Just tally up the points assigned to any of the foods you ate yesterday.

1 point

3 raw apricots
1 cup canned apricots
1 cup apple juice
1 cup canned asparagus
1 cup canned green beans
4 ounces beef
1 slice rye bread
1 slice whole wheat bread
1 cup raw cabbage
1 ounce cheddar cheese
1 cup cottage cheese
1 ounce Swiss cheese
1 medium raw fig
1 cup vanilla ice cream
4 ounces lamb
4 ounces beef liver
1 orange
1 cup strawberries
1 ripe tomato
1 tablespoon toasted wheat germ
1 tablespoon brewer's yeast

2 points

1 cup frozen green beans
1 cup canned beets
1 cup raw or frozen broccoli
1 cup frozen brussels sprouts
1 cup raw carrots
1 cup raw or frozen cauliflower
1 cup chopped celery

1 cup canned, drained
  cherries
1 cup canned or frozen
  corn
1 cup frozen peas
1 medium baked potato
1 cup canned tomato
1 cup crab
4 ounces flounder
4 ounces chicken
4 ounces turkey
4 ounces canned herring
4 ounces canned salmon
½ grapefruit
1 cup canned grapefruit
  juice
1 cup orange juice from
  concentrate
1 cup milk
1 tablespoon peanut butter
⅓ cup pecans
10 frozen French fries
  (4 inches long)
1 slice pumpernickel bread
½ cup Wheatena
1 cup chicken noodle soup
¼ cup barbecue sauce

3 points
1 medium banana
1 cup blackberries
½ cup chopped dates
1 cup raw spinach
⅔ cup oatmeal

4 points
⅓ cup roasted peanuts
1 cup raw or canned
  oysters
⅓ cup bran
½ cup dry lentils

5 points
1 cup frozen lima beans
1 cup kidney beans
1 cup canned pork and
  beans

6 points
⅓ cup Brazil nuts
1 cup black-eyed peas

7 points
1 avocado
⅓ cup almonds
⅓ cup cashews

14 points
½ cup dry soybeans

Scoring

Add up your total number of points. Multiply that total by 5. The result is an estimate of the percentage of the U.S. RDA for magnesium in your diet for the day tested. If you scored 10 points, for instance, multiply 10 by 5 for a score of
(continued)

The Diet Detective—
Magnesium (continued)

50 percent of the U.S. RDA.

One note of caution in interpreting your results. Information on the magnesium content of foods is somewhat sparse, and for some foods, only facts for its raw state are available even though it is cooked before eating.

There is no foolproof way to account for these shortcomings, but I do recommend viewing your results flexibly. Assume that your magnesium intake is probably higher than your score indicates. If your score is only 40 or 50 percent of the allowance, however, even the magnesium that the quiz misses isn't likely to bring it up to 100 percent.

Tests also showed that George had multiple kidney stones; these were removed. Analysis of the stones revealed a high magnesium content, a fairly uncommon finding. His blood magnesium level was also abnormally high.

During his hospital stay, George was questioned further about his customary medications. He had told the staff on arrival at the hospital that he had been taking Gelusil, a popular antacid. Later, he told them *how much* he had been taking: an astonishing 25 to 30 tablets a day, for a weekly total of about 200 tablets. That's overuse, or abuse, by any standard.

Before leaving the hospital, George was educated about appropriate use of antacids. Four months later, follow-up testing showed no remaining damage to his once-failing kidneys.

THE UNDERLYING PROBLEM

As you have probably guessed, George's problem was an excessive magnesium intake due to abuse of antacids. Many, though certainly not all, antacids contain magnesium; as the chart on pages 270 to 271 shows, the amount varies from one product to another. Some laxatives also contain magnesium. Milk of magnesia, for example, is used as both an antacid and laxative. As the name implies, it is magnesium rich.

As I mentioned earlier, it's been long believed that healthy kidneys can handle the magnesium from these antacids, even when used regularly. George's case suggests otherwise, since his kidneys appeared healthy until he suddenly fell ill.

Of course, George was not just using, or even mildly overusing antacids, he was greatly overusing them. But would reasonable use of magnesium-containing antacids, laxatives, or supplements cause excessive magnesium to accumulate in individuals with healthy kidneys?

That's a judgment call. But I think George's doctors would agree that he might have never suffered his episode of kidney failure if he had been using antacids within reason. His magnesium intake from the antacid alone was 1,710 to 2,052 milligrams (mg.) daily.

Though antacids provided the excess magnesium in George's case, his experience tells us much about taking magnesium supplements safely. Both antacids and supplements are taken orally. So the amount of magnesium from antacids that can be taken safely is probably a good barometer of the amount from supplements that can likewise be consumed safely.

Of course, the analogy isn't perfect. That's because the magnesium in antacids and laxatives derives from different magnesium compounds than the magnesium contained in magnesium supplements. The magnesium compounds in the antacids, for instance, could have effects that the type in supplements don't.

THE EXCESSIVE
MAGNESIUM SYNDROME

George's experience tells only part of the story. His case centers on kidney failure, but there are other aspects of magnesium overload. In fact, when we talk about hypermagnesemia, we are really talking about a complex of symptoms that result when there is too much magnesium in the blood.

Hypermagnesemia refers to a blood magnesium level in excess of 2.5, generally considered the maximum normal reading. (The reading measures the amount of magnesium in milliequivalents per liter, a term that will probably interest you only if you like the technicalities of medicine.)

Symptoms of hypermagnesemia are typically related to the

Magnesium Content of Some Antacids

Brand Name	Mg.*
Aludrox Suspension	43
Aludrox Tablets	35
Camalox Suspension	83
Camalox Tablets	83
Delcid Suspension	302
Di-Gel Liquid	36
Di-Gel Tablets	50
Gelusil Liquid	82
Gelusil-M Liquid	82
Gelusil II Liquid	164
Kolantyl Liquid	63
Kolantyl Tablets	112
Kolantyl Wafers	71
Maalox No. 1 Tablets	84
Maalox No. 2 Tablets	167
Maalox Plus Suspension	84
Maalox Plus Tablets	84
Maalox Suspension	84
Milk of magnesia (1 tbsp.)	500

severity of overdose. The following is a list of its symptoms and signs in order of their severity.

- Low blood pressure
- Drowsiness, lethargy, weakness
- Slight slurring of speech
- Unsteadiness
- Changes in mental status
- Nausea and vomiting
- Flushing of the skin
- Retaining of urine
- Changes on the ECG test of heart function
- Decrease in (or absence of) deep tendon reflexes

Brand Name	Mg.*
Mylanta Liquid	84
Mylanta Tablets	84
Mylanta II Liquid	167
Mylanta II Tablets	167
Riopan Plus Chew Tablets	103
Riopan Plus Suspension	103
Riopan Suspension	93
Riopan Tablets	93
Silain-Gel Liquid	119
Simeco Suspension	125
WinGel Liquid	66
WinGel Tablets	66

Source: Adapted from Richard Ratzan et al., *Geriatrics* (September 1980): 77 and information provided by manufacturers.

Note: The magnesium levels listed are subjected to change due to product reformulations.

*Milligrams of magnesium per tablet or teaspoon unless otherwise noted.

- Respiratory depression
- Coma
- Cardiac arrest

TREATMENT AND RECOVERY

Effective treatment is available for the high blood magnesium syndrome. If the condition is mild, withholding the source of the magnesium will often do the trick. By the way, this offending source of magnesium is never food. Only pills, as well as injected sources of magnesium used by doctors, can be responsible.

When high blood magnesium is more severe, there are two tried-and-true remedies. The first of the classic approaches is to give calcium intravenously; the second, preferred when the kidneys are not fully functioning, is dialysis. Recovery is often complete, and sometimes surprisingly fast.

In fact, high blood magnesium normally can't continue very long after the offending high-magnesium substance is withdrawn. The healthy kidneys simply won't tolerate it. Without new doses of the magnesium-rich substance coming in, the kidneys work on the excess magnesium in the blood, excreting it rapidly.

You noted, I am sure, my use here of the word "normally." When kidney function is not normal, high blood magnesium can continue and become more severe—even life threatening. If we could identify everyone who falls under this category, we could prevent high blood magnesium through careful use of the antacids, drugs, and supplements that contain magnesium.

Total kidney failure, of course, is obvious and easily diagnosed by experts. But a mild and undetected decline in the kidneys' functioning, such as occurs with age, may make one vulnerable to high blood magnesium if magnesium-rich antacids, laxatives, or supplements are overused. Specialists in this area urge using these compounds sparingly if declining kidney function may exist. Laboratory tests can check for this possibility.

Generally speaking, then, those with healthy kidneys should not be at risk from magnesium supplements unless the dose is extremely high. We'll talk more about a sensible dose later, under "How Much Is Too Much."

THE DOLOMITE DEBATE

Magnesium safety is more than a matter of how much can be taken without harm. Also at issue is whether one source of magnesium—the ever-popular dolomite supplement—is safe.

A 1979 study by the Food and Drug Administration (FDA) revealed unexpected contamination of dolomite with toxic metals such as lead. But the question turned to controversy in 1983, when Hyman Roberts, M.D., reported that several dolomite users in his practice had a variety of health problems. Writing in *Southern Medical Journal*, Dr. Roberts told of:

• A 68-year-old diabetes sufferer who had severe nerve-damage syndrome similar to that seen in vitamin B_6 overdose. The man had been taking large amounts of dolomite for several years.

• A 23-year-old seizure sufferer who experienced new seizures on three occasions a few days after taking dolomite. Just one tablet was enough to cause a metallic taste, as well as excessive salivation and jitteriness that preceded the actual seizures.

• A retired engineer, also a seizure sufferer, who had ten times the normal amount of arsenic and 50 percent more than the normal mercury count in his hair. He had been taking four to six tablets of dolomite daily.

Dr. Roberts arranged for a medical laboratory to test samples of dolomite. Sure enough, the analysis revealed a variety of toxic metals, in concentrations he found of great concern. Among the list were aluminum, antimony, arsenic, barium, cadmium, cobalt, and of course the best-known metal—lead. Needless to say, the amount of these metals varied greatly from one brand tested to another.

It's no surprise that dolomite—a mineral deposit—would have trace amounts of toxic metals. There are two issues here: First, are the levels unsafe, and second, are the alternative sources of magnesium known to be purer?

On the first count, I would have to say that there is too little evidence to conclude that dolomite is a clear hazard or that the problems of Dr. Roberts's patients must have been the result of dolomite. No similar cases have been reported by any other physicians. Moreover, the degree of danger would be expected to vary with the dosage of dolomite one takes and the relative purity of the specific brand.

Nonetheless, I would like to share with you the FDA's advice to doctors in light of both their own laboratory findings and those of Dr. Roberts. An excerpt of the FDA announcement follows. (We'll talk about the bonemeal issue separately, in the next chapter, Calcium.)

> Due to the unknown but often substantial lead content of individual samples of bonemeal and dolomite, [the] FDA advises practitioners that these substances should be used as little as possible in infants, young children, and pregnant or lactating women.
>
> Although levels are usually lower, FDA scientists

have found some samples of bonemeal containing lead at concentrations as high as 17 to 20 parts per million (ppm). Comparably high levels of lead have also been detected in some samples of dolomite.

Individuals at special risk of lead toxicity from the consumption of bonemeal or dolomite include infants, children, women of childbearing age, and possibly the elderly. Others who ingest bonemeal at the recommended doses (usually not more than 5 to 10 grams) [5000 to 10,000 mg daily] would not ordinarily exceed the ... guideline for a tolerable daily adult intake of 430 micrograms of lead.

Pregnant or lactating women taking bonemeal or dolomite ... may have sufficient increased lead intake and absorption to present a health hazard to the developing fetus, via placental transfer of lead, or to the nursing infant from the mother's milk.

The message here is clear: red light for infants, children, mothers-to-be, potential mothers-to-be, nursing mothers, and possibly for the elderly. But as for the rest of the population, only a plea to use moderation in doses.

I have to admit that I was initially alarmed by these reports and remain concerned. But I also have become aware that dolomite and bonemeal are hardly the only items we ingest that may be contaminated with toxic metals. Common foods such as milk can be unanticipated sources as well.

That brings me to the second issue I mentioned above. Is dolomite known to be a more contaminated source of magnesium than other supplements? Unfortunately, there is no basis for comparison; that is, no information on metal contamination in supplements such as magnesium gluconate and magnesium-amino acid chelates is available.

The bottom line is this: There might be a problem with dolomite. I cannot assure you that similar contamination doesn't exist in other magnesium supplements. I would venture a guess that alternative sources that are not drawn from mineral deposits, as dolomite is, would probably be less tainted. And so I would have to recommend such an alternative source of magnesium for anyone concerned about metal contamination.

Perhaps intense consumer concern about this matter will lead to research that will settle the unanswered questions shortly once and for all.

THE STAR SYSTEM SHINES ON MAGNESIUM

Magnesium has a safety record that is hard for other supplemental minerals to beat. But it is not without its special considerations. I'll tell you about them next, as we run through the five points of the star system.

Side effects—I have found no reports of side effects from magnesium supplements. Side effects from antacids containing magnesium, of course, are another matter. However, the magnesium in supplements is not supplied by the same compounds as the magnesium in antacids.

Acute ailments—I have also found no reports of acute ailments traced to magnesium supplements. Certain magnesium-rich prescription drugs have produced the high blood magnesium syndrome shortly after administration. Such drugs are usually injected, increasing the chances of both effectiveness and adverse reactions. And their magnesium content is enormous when compared to that found in typical supplements.

Long-term problems—The high blood magnesium syndrome is the key long-term problem related to magnesium ingestion. So far, I have not found one case due to supplemental magnesium; magnesium-containing antacids, laxatives, and prescription drugs have been the guilty parties. As we already have discussed the symptoms in detail, I won't repeat them here.

The possibility of metal toxicity from dolomite might also be considered here. Any toxicity, however, stems from the contaminants, such as lead, and not from the magnesium itself. That means that magnesium remains an unlikely cause of long-term problems in healthy people.

Conflicting combinations—You already know that high doses of magnesium and impaired kidneys don't go together. A second conflict relates to two types of prescription drugs.

The most commonly used of the two are tetracycline antibiotics. Magnesium, as well as minerals discussed in later chapters, reduces your body's ability to absorb these antibiotics. But the solution is simple: Take the drug 2 to 3 hours before eating foods rich in magnesium. If you are taking these drugs for a short period of time, it might be best not to take magnesium supplements until you finish the drug. Alternatively, follow the same advice as for food; refrain from taking the supplement for 2 to 3 hours after you take the drug.

The other drug of concern is lithium, a psychoactive drug. Lithium can raise the blood magnesium level—the very basis for magnesium toxicity. Even though the magnesium toxicity syndrome is exceedingly rare in those without kidney problems, I think that lithium users should take magnesium supplements only under a doctor's supervision.

As is so often the case, more drugs interfere with nutrients than vice versa. Drugs that can cause the body to excrete more magnesium or to lose it from the blood include some of the antibiotics, anticonvulsants, and diuretics ("water pills"). The antigout drug probenecid and the heart drug digitalis can have these effects also, and the possibility of increased magnesium needs should be considered.

Needless to say, alcohol can also interfere with magnesium nutrition.

Hidden consequences—Magnesium might be an impostor in the laboratory. Excessive amounts of magnesium in the blood or urine may be taken for calcium instead, falsely increasing the reading. Results of a urine test for lead may be lowered by the presence of magnesium.

I have not found any reports of serious consequences related to the effect of magnesium on these tests.

HOW MUCH IS TOO MUCH

In setting a safe dose for magnesium supplementation, a few facts bear repeating. First, experience shows that magnesium generally is a safe mineral as long as the kidneys are working up to par. That is reassuring indeed. On the other hand, the effectiveness of these organs can decline with age, without our realizing it. This makes me wary of putting the stamp of approval on unlimited doses of magnesium.

Second, as best as I can determine, there are no cases on record of magnesium toxicity caused by a supplement. That makes it almost impossible to set an upper limit for safety, for it would not derive from any experience with magnesium supplements. The only facts to go on come from the antacids containing magnesium, and even here there is far too little experience for sound judgment. The lowest level on record as causing harm in an individual with presumably healthy kidneys amounted to about 1,700 mg. daily of extra magnesium. Of course, George's case may have been a fluke. He may have had some hidden kidney problems after all. However, those who use magnesium-containing

Recommended Dietary Allowances for Magnesium

Group/Age	Mg.
Infants 0–6 mon.	50
Infants 6–12 mon.	70
Children 1–3 yr.	150
Children 4–6 yr.	200
Children 7–10 yr.	250
Males 11–14 yr.	350
Males 15–18 yr.	400
Males 19+ yr.	350
Females 11+ yr.	300
Pregnant and nursing women	450

Note: The U.S. RDA for magnesium is 400 mg.

antacids regularly should consider this before deciding to take a supplement.

As for those with any degree of kidney impairment, a doctor's advice is a must. The picture changes dramatically here, with caution often advised at intakes of 600 mg. daily.

Those who want to take large doses of magnesium probably should use a source other than dolomite until the questions about its safety are resolved. This is especially true for children, pregnant and nursing women, and possibly the elderly. It's possible that for these people even a standard dose may be "too much" because of the contaminants. There are more than enough alternatives available.

These facts aside, I would say that a combined intake of less than 1,000 mg. from diet and supplements should have a high degree of safety in the absence of kidney impairment. No doubt, higher doses—even much higher doses—can often be taken safely, but I have my reasons for not approving of them as a general measure. I wonder, for instance, about the combined effects of high-dose magnesium plus large doses of other minerals. Each mineral may be safe by itself, but are the combined effects safe, too? We need to know more here.

One thing I do know is that magnesium users often take other minerals, especially calcium. We'll look at calcium's safety in the next chapter.

C O O K I N G

for Magnesium

CAJUN CAKES

(Makes 10 cakes)

Magnesium: 133 mg. per 2 cakes
Calories: 68 per 2 cakes

A tasty blend of mashed black-eyed peas, vegetables, and herbs. Serve as an accompaniment to meats, poultry, and fish.

1½ cups cooked black-eyed peas	generous dash of freshly ground pepper
3 tablespoons minced fresh parsley	¼ teaspoon dried thyme
2 tablespoons minced bell pepper	1 teaspoon olive oil, optional
2 tablespoons minced onion	2 tablespoons plain low-fat yogurt
	2 tablespoons tomato sauce

Puree the peas in a food processor, then transfer them to a medium-size mixing bowl or place them in a medium-size mixing bowl and use a potato masher. Add the parsley, bell pepper, onions, ground pepper, and thyme and mix by hand until well combined.

Place a large no-stick skillet over low to medium heat and brush with olive oil, if desired. Then form the pea mixture into 10 well-rounded tablespoon-size balls. Flatten the balls between your hands and set 4 or 5 in the skillet. When brown, flip them gently and brown the other side. Repeat with remaining cakes.

Combine the yogurt and tomato sauce and serve with warm cakes.

(continued)

C O O K I N G

for Magnesium—*continued*

AVOCADO AND SCALLOP SALAD

(Makes 3 servings)

Magnesium: 183 mg. per serving
Calories: 360 per serving

½ pound bay scallops	½ teaspoon corn oil
10 small cherry tomatoes (about ⅔ cup)	2 avocados, peeled and chopped into chunks
2 tablespoons minced scallions	juice of 1 lime
1 tablespoon minced fresh coriander	freshly ground black pepper

In a large no-stick skillet, sauté the scallops, tomatoes, scallions, and coriander in the oil until the scallops are opaque, about 3 minutes.

Scoop the scallop mixture into a serving bowl and mix in the avocados and lime juice. Sprinkle with pepper and serve immediately in lettuce cups as a first course or salad.

TOASTED NUT APRICOT GRANOLA

(Makes 7 cups)

Magnesium: 68 mg. per ½ cup
Calories: 365 per ½ cup

1 cup cashews, coarsely chopped	¼ cup vegetable oil
1 cup Brazil nuts, coarsely chopped	¼ cup almond butter
1 cup slivered almonds, coarsely chopped	⅓ cup honey
3 cups rolled oats	¼ teaspoon ground cinnamon
	1 cup chopped dried apricots

```
C    O    O    K    I    N    G
```
for Magnesium—*continued*

Preheat oven to 300°F.

In a large bowl, combine the cashews, Brazil nuts, almonds, and oats and set aside.

In a small skillet, combine the oil, almond butter, honey, and cinnamon and heat, stirring frequently until warm, liquid, and well combined.

Pour the warm liquid into the nut mixture and toss until all of the ingredients are coated. Pour into a large (or 2 small) jelly roll pan and bake for 25 to 30 minutes, stirring about every 10 minutes.

Allow the granola to cool slightly, then toss with apricots.

Cool completely before storing in tightly covered jars.

Magnesium Content
of Selected Supplements

Dosage is one tablet or capsule unless otherwise indicated.

Supplement	Manufacturer	Mg.
Abdol with Minerals	Parke-Davis	20.0
Abron	O'Neal, Jones & Feldman	20.0
B6-Plus	Anabolic	20.0
Centrum	Lederle	20.0
Cluvisol 130	Ayerst	50.0
Engram-HP	Squibb	20.0
Filibon Tablets	Lederle	20.0
Geralix Liquid (per tbsp.)	North American	0.0
Gerizyme (per tbsp.)	Upjohn	33.3
Gevrabon (per 2 tbsp.)	Lederle	50.0
Gevral	Lederle	20.0
Gevral Protein	Lederle	6.5
Gevral T Capsules	Lederle	30.0

(continued)

Supplements—*continued*

Supplement	Manufacturer	Mg.
Hi-Bee Plus	North American	100.0
Myadec	Parke-Davis	100.0
Natalins Tablets	Mead Johnson	20.0
Norlac	Rowell	20.0
Nutra-Cal	Anabolic	62.0
Obron-6	Pfipharmecs	20.0
One-A-Day Vitamins Plus Minerals	Miles	20.0
Optilets-M-500	Abbott	100.0
Os-Cal Forte	Marion	15.0
Paladec with Minerals	Parke-Davis	20.0
Stuart Formula	Stuart	20.0
Stuart Prenatal	Stuart	20.0
Theragran-M	Squibb	100.0
Vicon-C	Glaxo	100.0
Vicon Iron	Glaxo	20.0
Vicon Plus	Glaxo	25.0
Vio-Geric	Rowell	20.0
Vitagett	North American	20.0
Vitamin-Mineral Capsules	North American	20.0
Viterra	Pfipharmecs	25.0
Viterra High Potency	Pfipharmecs	100.0

Source: Adapted from the American Pharmaceutical Association, *Handbook of Nonprescription Drugs*, 7th ed. (1982), 240–57.

Note: This chart is intended only as a guide. Vitamin formulations change periodically; always read product labels for accurate and up-to-date information on their nutrient levels.

15
Calcium

When it rains, it pours, says the old saying, and for the mineral calcium, the words ring so true. In just the last five years there has been an outpouring of new findings about the health-promoting benefits of this very important mineral. In fact, calcium now appears capable of protecting health in ways never before imagined.

First came the headlines about calcium's ability to prevent and slow osteoporosis, the brittle bone disease affecting one out of four American women. The ink had hardly dried on these reports when calcium made the news again, this time for an apparent role in controlling high blood pressure. And on the heels of that finding came still another piece of good news, this one linking a healthy calcium intake to lowered chances of developing colon cancer.

Naturally, people wanted to reap these benefits, and sales of calcium supplements skyrocketed. From 1984 to 1985 alone, sales jumped by an estimated 40 percent, and one distributor of vitamins and minerals reported that calcium supplements had become its top-selling product. That's quite a feat, for it requires outperforming the long-time favorite—the multiple vitamin.

Still, much confusion and concern remains. There are now so many types of calcium supplements that some consumers are bewildered about which one is best. At the same time, others are aware of the long-standing concerns of developing kidney stones from taking too much. Health professionals also worry that an occasional consumer might become so enthused about calcium supplementation that he'll take far more than is beneficial.

But before looking at calcium's safety record, I think you might want to know more about the wonderful benefits calcium can have on your health.

THE CARE AND FEEDING OF BONES

One could write a book on this subject (as I have done) because bone health and nutrition are closely intertwined.

To some extent, bone thinning is a natural part of aging. But mild bone loss does not qualify as osteoporosis; loss of about 30 percent or more of one's original bone mass does. Yet, until the last few years, the importance of calcium for preventing abnormal bone loss has too long been underestimated. Here are a few highlights from new findings that convinced me of the oversight:

The bones' need for calcium is lifelong and just as critical in later years as in early life. For decades, nutritionists thought calcium most important for children, because their bones are still growing. It was all but assumed that the strong bones would become solid, unchanging pillars that would last for decades.

In fact, an adult's bones are not pillars at all. They are changing every day in a process called remodeling. Without a good calcium intake, remodeling can result in bones that grow progressively thinner. That's why calcium is as important for adults as it is for children.

Osteoporosis may be a factor in loss of bone from the jaw, leading to loss of teeth. Preliminary evidence hints strongly that loss of bone from the jaw is an early warning sign of osteoporosis. Research has found that loss of bone from the jaw often occurs in the same individuals suffering from osteoporosis in the bones of the spinal column. That tells us that both conditions may have the same underlying cause or causes.

Calcium requirements for adults are such that the 800 milligram (mg.) Recommended Dietary Allowance (RDA) set in 1980 is too low. The recommended allowance is not a minimum requirement, but rather a level that is supposedly set high enough to meet the needs of 98 percent of the population. In both its 1974 and 1980 reports, the Committee on Dietary Allowances deemed 800 mg. daily as sufficient to meet the needs of all adult men and women— pregnant and nursing women excepted.

New research, however, shows that for women, the RDA should not be the same throughout adulthood. On the contrary, when women reach menopause, their need for calcium rises dramatically. The sharp drop in a woman's own estrogen production that comes with menopause is responsible, for estrogen is a bone-protecting factor with enormous influence. To make up for her sharp decline in estrogen production at menopause, a woman needs one of two things: a major increase in calcium intake or estrogen drugs that replace her body's diminished supply.

The calcium RDA for premenopausal women also has been challenged as too low. Newer studies, as well as criticism of past research, suggest that an allowance of 1,000 mg. daily—not 800 mg.—is required to insure that the needs of almost all younger women will be met.

The key numbers now are no longer the RDA last published in 1980. Much better advice about calcium comes from a special Consensus Panel on Osteoporosis convened by the National Institutes of Health (NIH) in 1984. Here are their recommendations, which, as far as I can see, are supported by almost all bone health experts:

• Premenopausal women: 1,000 mg. calcium daily
• Postmenopausal women not taking estrogen replacement: 1,500 mg. calcium daily
• Postmenopausal women taking estrogen: 1,000 mg. calcium daily

Some bone health experts suggest increasing calcium intake slightly, from 1,000 to about 1,200 mg., during the decade before menopause. The reason is that some bone loss does occur before menopause, perhaps most of this loss taking place as a woman approaches her menopause. The degree of bone loss involved is not as great as after menopause, but it is still significant.

Calcium intakes among many American adults have been far below recommended amounts, but little attention was paid to the problem until recently. Surveys dating back to 1955 show that calcium was among the nutrients most likely to be consumed in amounts below the recommended allowances. More recent studies have found that about two-thirds of young American women (aged 18 to 35) have calcium intakes below the RDA. Among women over 35, an even larger number—75 percent—are not meeting the RDA. And these surveys base their findings on the recommended allowance of 800 mg. daily. Had the current NIH recommendations of 1,000 to 1,500 mg. daily been used, even fewer women would have had calcium intakes meeting the recommended levels.

Too little calcium, however, isn't the only thing contributing to osteoporosis. Individual characteristics and personal habits also play a role. They are:

• Childlessness
• Frequent use of aluminum-containing antacids
• High alcohol intake
• Removal of ovaries (without estrogen replacement)
• Sedentary lifestyle
• Small build
• Smoking
• Stress
• Thinness (10 percent or more below desirable weight)

In addition, white women are more frequently affected than black women.

The more risk factors you have, the more you need to insure that your calcium intake is in line with the latest advice.

If you are male, your chances of developing osteoporosis are smaller, but it can happen. Of men living to age 90, 17 percent suffer a hip fracture, and osteoporosis is the most frequent cause. But there are more compelling reasons for men to consider their calcium intake. We'll look at them next.

BETTER BLOOD PRESSURE

Women are more likely to develop osteoporosis, but among whites, men are more likely to develop high blood pressure. Along with smoking and high blood cholesterol, high blood pressure is one of the major risk factors for heart disease. High blood pressure is the greatest risk factor for strokes.

Of course, high blood pressure is not a new issue to nutritionists. Authorities have long recognized excesses of two nutritional factors—sodium and calories—as culprits contributing to the condition. Losing excess weight and cutting back on sodium does help reduce blood pressure in some, though not all, of those afflicted. Lowering the sodium content of the American food supply has been a major goal of those seeking ways to prevent—not just treat—the problem.

Now it's clear that a third food factor—calcium—is joining the ranks of nutritional strategies against high blood pressure. Some highlights of recent findings show why:

• A 1,000 mg. calcium supplement taken daily for 22 weeks significantly lowered (diastolic) blood pressure in young men (by 9 percent) and in young women (by 6 percent).
• In another study, subjects with normal blood pressure reported a calcium intake averaging 200 mg. higher than those with high blood pressure.
• A California-based survey reported that both a rough estimate of daily milk consumption and a one-day diet analysis found that high blood pressure in men was associated with low calcium intake from dairy products. Since dairy products supply about three-fourths of the calcium in the average American diet, use of dairy products is probably a fairly good index of total dietary calcium.

Most authorities on the subject of high blood pressure probably consider these findings preliminary. Regardless, they look very promising, and I grow more convinced with each study that is published.

Based on results so far, it is likely that calcium will influence blood pressure for some of us, but not all. I am sure that researchers would like nothing better than to devise a simple, inexpensive

(continued on page 290)

Recommended Dietary Allowances for Calcium: A Hot Dispute

In 1984, the NIH, concerned over the prevalence of osteoporosis in American women, appointed a special panel to look into the causes and treatments of the disease. The panel held a conference where experts in the field made presentations on the many factors affecting bone health.

After considering the knowledge at hand, the panel wrote a consensus statement summarizing its findings and conclusions. Among them was a frank statement that the RDA for calcium—the mineral which defends the body against this crippling disease—is too low. The panel recommended that women in their postmenopausal years, the time when bone depletion is most rapid, should have calcium intakes almost twice the RDA set in 1980, unless taking estrogen replacement therapy. In addition, the panel felt that the RDA for both premenopausal women and postmenopausal women taking estrogen was, likewise, too low. They recommended a 20 percent increase in the allowance for these women.

Naturally these recommendations did not go unnoticed by the National Research Council's Food and Nutrition Board (FNB), the body responsible for the RDA. In 1985, the FNB's Committee on Dietary Allowances was scheduled to release a new report, updating the RDA last set in 1980. All concerned expected that the criticisms of the NIH panel would be reflected in a new, higher RDA for calcium. But the president of the National Academy of Sciences—National Research Council, refused to release the new report. According to press reports, an impasse arose because committee members wanted to lower the allowances for quite a few nutrients, including vitamins A, C, and B_6. Experts reviewing drafts of the report protested that the reductions were unjustified, and inconsistent with a 1983 report by the National Research Council's Committee on Diet, Nutrition and Cancer. That report urged Americans to increase their intakes of fruits and vegetables rich in vitamins A and C. With the 1985 edition halted, the 1980 RDA for all nutrients, including calcium, remain in force.

As a result, we now have two sets of standards for calcium—the official RDA and the unofficial NIH recommendation. Which one should you use?

The answer comes easily to me. Without a doubt the NIH panel's recommendation is much sounder, especially if prevention of the disease is the goal.

Although the NIH panel recommended increases only for women, I think men should also strive for the 1,000 mg. level advised for premenopausal women and postmenopausal women taking estrogen.

Just for the record here are the 1980 RDA for calcium:

Group/Age	Mg.
Infants 0–6 mon.	360
Infants 6–12 mon.	540
Children 1–10 yr.	800
Males 11–18 yr.	1,200
Males 19+ yr.	800
Females 11–18 yr.	1,200
Females 19+ yr.	800
Pregnant or nursing women	
18 yr. or less	1,600
19+ yr.	1,200

Note: The U.S. RDA for calcium, designed solely for nutrition labeling purposes, is 1,000 mg.

Also for the record are the NIH recommendations:

Group	Mg.
Premenopausal women and postmenopausal women taking estrogen replacement therapy	1,000
Postmenopausal women not taking estrogen replacement therapy	1,500

test that will pinpoint who will respond and who will not. But if you have high blood pressure, you should not try to find out for yourself if calcium will help reduce it. It is important that you test the effect of calcium on your blood pressure only under medical supervision. Above all, let your doctor be the judge regarding any changes in your current medication.

Similarly, if you are on a sodium-restricted diet, stick with it (unless your doctor decides it is not helping you). The newly discovered link between calcium and blood pressure in no way undermines the much better established relationship of high salt intake to high blood pressure.

CALCIUM AGAINST CANCER

In my last book, *The Calcium Bible*, I wrote of calcium's role in bone health and its emerging role in blood pressure. Unfortunately, I didn't have the chance to share new findings linking calcium to cancer prevention. The landmark study on the subject was published in the medical journal *Lancet* ten days after the typeset manuscript was handed over to the printer! Just one of those things in an author's life.

Now I would like to make up for the lost opportunity by telling you about this exciting new research. The landmark study I refer to compared calcium intake to risk of colorectal (colon or rectal) cancer among almost 2,000 male employees of the Western Electric Company in Chicago. The project, known among researchers as the Western Electric Health Study, began in the late 1950s. Over the course of two decades, it provided some of our finest knowledge about how nutrition and other factors influence heart health. I have always held it in great esteem.

Naturally, when a study I admired so much turned its attention to calcium and cancer rates, I took notice. And I was impressed by the findings. The men were divided into four groups, based on their daily calcium intake (per 1,000 calories). The men with the highest calcium intake had only one-third the risk of colorectal cancer as the men with the lowest intake.

I decided to see if I could find anything more to support these results. I succeeded. I found research from Scandinavian countries linking intake of milk—one of the best sources of calcium—with reduced risk of colon cancer. I found studies in animal research, too, that found both a protective effect of calcium and a possible explanation for it. The research hints that calcium binds up harmful substances in the digestive tract, preventing them from exerting any effects that might enhance the cancer process.

As with the link between calcium and blood pressure, many authorities will call these findings just the first few steps in what will be a long process of confirming or refuting calcium's effect on cancer risk. Be that as it may, I am extremely impressed with the information available. It has helped me solve a puzzle that has been on my mind for almost a decade.

For years, I had been baffled that colon cancer rates in Florida were significantly lower than in northeastern states such as New York. How can this be, I would wonder, since many Florida residents were lifelong New Yorkers until retiring to the sunny state late in life.

Now I am no longer bewildered. Instead, I am betting that thanks to their sunnier skies, Florida residents make more vitamin D. That vitamin, in turn, enhances calcium absorption in the digestive tract where it can exert cancer-preventing effects.

Fortunately, nothing that has turned up so far shows that calcium intakes have to be unusually high to reduce cancer risk. The desirable range looks no greater than the new intakes recommended by the osteoporosis panel for preserving bone health. So there is no need for excessive amounts of calcium. From here on, we'll focus on the toxic effects of such excess as well as possible side effects.

WHICH SUPPLEMENT IS BEST?

Judging from the mail I have received since publication of The Calcium Bible, the question of "which supplement is best" remains on the minds of many. One bone health expert queried by a major newspaper responded to this four-word question with a four-word answer. "They're all the same."

In a very general sense, his words are true. For many people, any of the countless brands of calcium supplements on the market today will provide calcium in a form as usable as any other. For these lucky people, there is no "right" source of supplemental calcium; only a right dose to take. The quiz on page 292 will help you figure out what this amount should be for you.

(continued on page 294)

The Diet Detective Searches for Calcium

Millions of Americans take calcium supplements, and considering the potential benefits, that's no surprise. But along with concerns that too many Americans take in far too little calcium are concerns that some people get too much.

The easiest way to overdo things and perhaps the most likely way is through supplements. But even modest supplement use added to a diet naturally high in calcium can also mean exceeding a sensible intake—accidentally, of course. For example, the NIH panel on osteoporosis recommends 1,500 mg. daily for a woman who has passed menopause and is not taking estrogen replacement. If such a woman takes 1,500 mg. of supplemental calcium daily and eats a diet high in calcium-rich foods, she might exceed recommended limits on calcium intake.

As you'll read in this chapter, the recommended maximum varies from one authority to another. Nonetheless, I think all would agree that you should consider the calcium content of your diet before deciding how much supplemental calcium to take.

This quiz will help you estimate the calcium content of your usual diet. On a day that you are eating as you normally do, check off any of the following foods that you consumed. Then see the scoring section to determine how much, if any, additional calcium is advisable for you.

1 point

1 cup carrots
1 cup brussels sprouts
1 cup squash
1 sweet potato
1 cup turnips
1 cup sliced zucchini
1 cup mashed potatoes
   from mix
1 cup green beans
1 cup wax beans
1 cup mixed vegetables
1 cup green cabbage
1 cup Boston lettuce
1 cup sauerkraut
1 cup canned clams
1 cup crabmeat
1 cup lobster
1 cup uncreamed cottage
   cheese

1 tablespoon nonfat dry
milk
1 tablespoon Parmesan
cheese

2 points
⅓ cup almonds
1 small can (8 ounces)
baked beans
1 bean burrito
1 serving cocoa from mix
1 Fudgsicle
½ cup oysters
1 cup broccoli
1 cup okra

3 points
1 cup creamed cottage
cheese
1 ounce (2 tablespoons
crumbled) blue cheese
1 slice processed cheese
(American, Velveeta)
3 pancakes made with
milk
4 ounces shrimp (about 1
small can)
4 ounces scallops
1 cup ice cream
1 cup soybeans
4 ounces (¼ of a 1-pound
package) tofu
1 slice Hollywood special
formula bread
1 cup beet greens
1 ounce cheese spread

1 wedge Camembert
cheese
1 cup kale
1 cup mustard greens

4 points
½ frozen medium pizza
1 cup vegetable in cheese
sauce
1 serving any entrée with
cheese
1 cup ice milk or frozen
yogurt
1 ounce (¼ cup shredded
or 1½-inch cube) any
hard cheese except
Swiss
1 long slice (8 by 4 inches)
Swiss cheese
1 cup turnip greens

5 points
1 cup bok choy
⅔ cup pink salmon with
bones
1 ounce Swiss cheese
(1½-inch cube)
1 fast-food milk shake
½ cup ricotta cheese
1 cup plain whole milk
yogurt

6 points
1 cup fruit yogurt
1 cup milk
½ cup mackerel
1 tin herring steaks

(continued)

The Diet Detective—
Calcium (continued)

7 points
1 cup collard greens
⅔ cup red salmon with
    bones

8 points
1 tin sardines with bones
1 cup plain low-fat yogurt

10 points
1 cup Calcimilk

14 points
1 ounce Dairy Crisp cereal

Scoring

Add your total number of points, and multiply by 5. If you collected 15 points, for instance, multiply 15 by 5 for a final score of 75. This means your diet contains about 75 percent of the intake level now advised for premenopausal women. If you had 20 points, multiplying by 5 yields a final score of 100. In this case, your diet already supplies 100 percent of the latest recommended intake.

Remember, however, if you are a woman who has passed menopause and are not taking estrogen replacement therapy, the NIH panel advises a total calcium intake that is 50 percent greater than that recommended for premeno-

But for some people, the type of calcium in supplements does matter. Why? Because certain medical conditions make some forms of calcium preferable to others. And because some people experience side effects from one form of calcium that others do not.

To make understanding supplements as simple as possible, I will discuss the various types of calcium supplements along with their pluses and minuses. But first I'll explain one of the key characteristics that some have and some don't.

THE ACID TEST

Each substance in nature has a chemical personality of its own, and calcium supplements are no exception. A key charac-

pausal women or women on estrogen therapy. To be meeting the higher allowance by diet alone, your final score would have to be 150. Chances of a score this high are slim. In fact, the average American woman would have a final score of only 50 to 55 on this quiz.

The goal now is to find your calcium gap. To do so, you need to turn your final score (e.g., 50 percent of the recommendation) into milligrams. It's easy. Simply attach a zero to your score. For instance, if you scored 75, attach a zero for a calcium intake of 750 mg. on the day tested.

Now subtract this amount from the NIH recommendation for your age group—1,000 mg. if you have not reached menopause or are taking estrogen therapy. (I also recommend the 1,000 mg. level if you are male.) If you are postmenopausal and not on estrogen, subtract your intake in milligrams from 1,500 mg.

The remainder is your calcium gap—the amount you need to add each day. You can close the gap with dietary changes or with supplements. The choice is entirely up to you.

teristic of any substance is its solubility—that is, the conditions under which it can be dissolved. A substance may be soluble in water, alcohol, or both; others may be soluble in neither, but easily dissolved in an acid. Solubility matters in calcium nutrition, because the body absorbs calcium only in soluble form.

Certain forms of calcium supplements are naturally soluble in something our body has plenty of—water. As a result, they need no assistance to be absorbed. But supplements that won't dissolve in water—known as insoluble calcium supplements—must first be combined with something in which they are soluble.

In the case of insoluble calcium supplements, the problem-solver is acid. For many of us, this is no problem; we have acid in our stomachs that does the job nicely, allowing us to absorb calcium from insoluble supplements just as well as from soluble ones.

But some people—most commonly the elderly—do not secrete normal amounts of stomach acid. They have conditions called hypochlorhydria or achlorhydria. In the former, the stomach secretes lower than normal amounts of acid. In the latter and more severe condition, the necessary acid is absent.

Precise statistics on how many Americans are afflicted with one of these two disorders are not available, since this is not the kind of condition reported to disease registries. Most often the problem is simply said to be common among the elderly. One gastroenterologist I questioned, however, estimated that about 10 percent of people over age 60 secrete below normal amounts of acid, with the rate climbing to about 30 percent among those age 70 and older. Fortunately, however, the condition is not common around the time of menopause, when some women first begin to use calcium supplements.

There are a few other situations where the amount of acid in the stomach can fall below normal levels. Treatment of ulcers often includes drugs that reduce acid secretion. The reduction here usually brings the acid down to below normal levels. In patients with pernicious anemia, acid secretion is absent. Finally, patients with stomach cancer may also secrete reduced amounts of acid. (Regardless, stomach cancer patients should not take calcium supplements except as prescribed by their doctors.)

THE ABSORPTION PROBLEM

Authorities on calcium nutrition have always believed that those with these low-acid problems can't convert enough (or in some cases, any) of the insoluble forms of calcium into the soluble form that the body requires. In an often-cited study, for instance, absorption of an insoluble calcium supplement was tested in five normal subjects and five who secreted no acid. The latter group absorbed only 0 to 2 percent of the supplemental calcium, while the normal subjects absorbed much more: 9 to 16 percent. (Don't be surprised by the results among the normal patients; the body normally absorbs only a fraction of the calcium contained in food or supplements.)

Results such as these led the medical world to conclude that patients with low-acid or no-acid conditions should use only soluble forms of calcium. This notion prevailed for many years, only to be challenged recently when Robert Recker, M.D., measured absorption of calcium in nonacid secreters under both fasting and nonfasting conditions.

Sure enough, his achlorhydric volunteers absorbed very little of the insoluble calcium supplement when taken on an empty stomach. But when the same insoluble calcium was given with a breakfast meal containing an egg, toast, juice, and coffee, the subjects absorbed the calcium normally. The most likely explanation is that food—or more specifically, something in one or more of these foods—provided enough acid to permit normal calcium absorption.

Of course, it will take a bit more investigation to determine if certain conditions do allow those with impaired acid secretion to absorb insoluble forms of calcium. Until the matter is settled, though, I feel that those with impaired acid secretion should choose naturally soluble forms of calcium.

That's all for my preamble. Now for the characteristics of the various supplements.

THE COMMON CARBONATES

As I said before, calcium supplements are proliferating. And if you're a label reader, you already know that the form of calcium in the vast majority of them is calcium carbonate. Whether from oyster shell, eggshell, or other source, this form of calcium is Number One.

But calcium carbonate isn't packaged just as a dietary supplement. In fact, decades before calcium supplementation became commonplace, drug companies were marketing calcium carbonate for a different purpose: as an antacid. If you have certain antacids in your medicine chest—such as Tums, Titralac, Chooz, or Alka 2—you already have a calcium supplement that is inexpensive and easy to take. USA Today found this information so newsworthy that it ran a page-one story proclaiming "TUMS spells relief for brittle bones."

Unbelievable as it may seem, the only important differences between the calcium carbonate antacids and the calcium carbonate products sold as supplements is that the supplements tend to contain more calcium per tablet or capsule. In addition, the antacids may contain some amount of sodium, so check the label if you are a sodium-watcher.

Naturally, calcium carbonate didn't get to be number one without good reason. Its strong points are that it is:

• The most concentrated source of supplemental calcium, containing 40 percent calcium by weight
• The least expensive choice in many cases
• A form available in a wide range of dosages, from 140 to 600 mg. per tablet or capsule
• The supplement packaged for an array of palates: as capsules, chewable tablets (flavored or unflavored), coated tablets, and even gum; powder is also available, with both pluses and minuses that I'll discuss shortly

Not a bad track record, to be sure. However this supplement that enjoys the largest share of the market also has some side effects that other (but often less convenient) forms do not: nausea, gas, and constipation. The nausea can often be alleviated by taking the supplement with meals. If that doesn't work, or the other side effects of gas and constipation persist, you have plenty of other supplements to choose from.

A bit more troublesome can be a problem called "acid rebound." This term refers to the ironic ability of calcium carbonate to neutralize excess stomach acid, then later do an about-face, causing the stomach to secrete more acid. Naturally, the symptoms of sour stomach again return. Once more, however, taking your supplement with meals may do away with the problem.

How common is "acid rebound"? I would love to know. One classic pharmacy textbook says that as little as 500 mg. of calcium carbonate (supplying 200 mg. of calcium) has been reported to produce the problem. Nonetheless, it is my impression that few individuals experience acid rebound on such a low dose. As far as I can tell, most cases develop at much higher doses.

Of the many people I know who take calcium carbonate supplements daily, not one has complained of acid rebound. Nor have I read that this was a complaint among women taking calcium carbonate in research studies of osteoporosis. Sales of calcium carbonate antacids, such as Tums, have skyrocketed so much during the past year that it is difficult to believe that acid rebound occurs with much frequency at the dosages commonly taken to provide supplemental calcium.

The main drawback of calcium carbonate? It's insoluble and needs acid in order to be made soluble.

THE PHOSPHATE FAMILY

The high concentration of calcium in calcium carbonate is probably the best explanation for its success. The next most concentrated calcium compounds are various forms of calcium phosphate. These provide the mineral phosphorus as well as calcium.

There are three forms of calcium phosphate: monophosphate, diphosphate, and triphosphate. Only the first, calcium monophosphate, offers any significant degree of solubility. It is partially soluble. It is also, as far as I can determine, not a form of calcium that any manufacturer is using in supplements.

The supplements from this family that I have found are dibasic or tribasic calcium phosphate. Both are practically insoluble in water, requiring acid for solubility. But they have their pluses, including:

• A respectable concentration of calcium. The dibasic form is about 23 percent calcium, and the tribasic form, containing about 39 percent calcium, rivals calcium carbonate as a concentrated source of this mineral.
• Reported absence of the gas distress sometimes experienced with calcium carbonate. (According to Ayerst Laboratories, manufacturer of a tribasic calcium phosphate supplement called Posture, this form produces no gas.)
• Chemical characteristics well suited to the purpose of adding calcium to food. Calcium-fortified products, such as Dairy Crisp cereal, often contain this tribasic form.
• A calcium-to-phosphorus ratio that is favorable, supplying about 30 percent more calcium than phosphorus.

I would like to explain a little more about the calcium-phosphorus ratio. One theory claims that the high rate of osteoporosis in the United States has to do with the balance between calcium and phosphorus. Because phosphorus-containing compounds are added to many processed foods (such as colas) and because the American diet is meat-heavy, the average American takes in much more phosphorus than calcium. I have calculated that some women may easily consume four times more phosphorus than calcium.

There is some evidence that, after infancy, calcium and phosphorus intakes should be about equal for best health, or at least not so different that phosphorus intake is more than double calcium intake. Thus, a supplement with more calcium than phosphorus is a step in the right direction of bringing the calcium-to-phosphorus ratio into better balance.

As for side effects, there is not much to say. Until very recently, calcium phosphate supplements were not widely used, so there may be too little experience with them to know much about potential side effects. I did find one study, though, where 20 women took dicalcium phosphate supplements providing 350 mg. calcium daily for six months. The authors did not mention any complaints from the treatment. None of the women dropped out of the study—a good sign that the treatment was well tolerated at the dose studied.

Both dicalcium and tricalcium phosphates reportedly have some antacid activity. But as yet, I have not found any reports of acid rebound as a possible side effect of calcium carbonate.

Should you have any side effects, of course, you can turn to other supplements.

CHELATES AND CHLORIDES

Chelates are one of the most expensive forms of calcium. They are basically supplements in which the calcium is bound to an amino acid—the building block of proteins—rather than to substances such as carbonate or phosphate. Manufacturers often claim that chelated calcium is better absorbed, but I have found no published evidence to support the claim. Appealing to manufacturers for evidence also brought none.

However, if for some reason you prefer chelated calcium, you will want to know two facts:

• The solubility of chelated calcium varies among brands, depending on manufacturing techniques. Ron Martin of the Thompson Vitamin Company advised me that "partially soluble" would be an appropriate description for most brands. This raises concern for those with impaired acid secretion.

• The precise concentration of calcium may vary among products, but the one brand (Arco) for which I have full information contains 20 percent calcium.

I have not found any information on side effects from chelated calcium.

For calcium chloride, the story changes. This form of calcium is used to pickle foods, but is not recommended as a calcium supplement because it can irritate the stomach—sometimes severely. However, it is highly soluble.

Calcium chloride is available in granulated form for use as a salt replacement by those who must avoid the most common salt substitute—potassium chloride. Even these individuals, however, are advised to use it sparingly. I do not know of any calcium tablets or capsules that contain this form of calcium. If I did, I would not recommend them.

LACTATE, GLUCONATE, AND COMPANY

If you suffer adverse effects from calcium carbonate or calcium phosphate, or if you want a supplement that is unquestionably soluble because you have an acid secretion problem, calcium lactate and calcium gluconate are good choices for you. Both are nonconstipating, soluble in water, and well tolerated.

According to my trusted pharmacy text, these two forms of calcium do not irritate the gastrointestinal tract. I have found only one report to the contrary, a set of studies dating back more than a half century. In this research, extremely large doses of calcium gluconate (10,000 mg., about 900 mg. of which is calcium) caused a tendency toward diarrhea if taken by fasting subjects. But the same amount taken after a meal apparently produced no side effects.

The same researcher also found that the identical dose of calcium lactate (10,000 mg. providing about 1,300 mg. of calcium) caused severe vomiting, diarrhea, and abdominal distress if taken all at once. When the dose was halved—to the equivalent of about 650 mg. of calcium—the severe reaction did not occur.

Given that no one else has reported this type of reaction to these forms of calcium, I can't help but wonder if the calcium lactate and calcium gluconate we have today is better in quality than what was available in the 1930s. So, I remain optimistic that these two forms of calcium are, in fact, well tolerated.

There is, however, one drawback with the lactate and gluconate forms—it is their low calcium concentration. Only 13 percent of the material in the lactate form is calcium, with the concentration falling to 9 percent calcium for the gluconate form. This means, as the chart of calcium supplements on pages 304 to 307 shows, that getting a substantial dose of calcium from these supplements requires taking numerous tablets per day. Most contain less than 100 mg. of calcium per tablet.

CALCIUM POWDERS: PRO AND CON

Some have suggested that one way to eliminate the problem and cost of taking numerous calcium lactate or calcium gluconate tablets per day is to take it in powdered form. You can order these powders over the counter in any pharmacy, usually in 1-pound containers. Some of the more concentrated sources of calcium, such as calcium carbonate and phosphate are also available in powdered form.

I have very mixed feelings about using these powders. On the one hand, their ease of use and often substantial cost savings are attractive. But getting the dose you want can be a problem when using a powder.

Tablets or capsules will almost certainly contain the amount of calcium stated on the label. With powders, however, the calcium content per measure—per teaspoon, for instance—will vary. Factors such as the fineness of the powder or crystals and how tightly you or the manufacturer pack it into a spoon or container will affect the calcium content in any given amount. So you can't be sure that you are getting the dosage of calcium you want if you take this route.

If the manufacturer states the calcium content per teaspoon, you have a chance of coming within striking range of your desired dose. In my experience, however, the label rarely provides this information.

I have been able to obtain the calcium content for one powdered product. It is intended as a substitute for baking soda, but it is nonetheless pure calcium carbonate. Called Ener-G Baking Soda, it is available in many health food stores or from the manufacturer, Ener-G Foods, P.O. Box 24723, Seattle, Washington, 98124. Unlike the 1-pound size of calcium powders available through drug stores, this product is packaged in smaller ¼- to ⅓-pound packages.

A single teaspoon of this product (measure carefully) contains a full 800 mg. of calcium. If you want 600 mg. of supplemental calcium—the amount in many popular tablets—you would use ¾ teaspoon. Purchased in a store, free of shipping charges, the cost is very low as compared to most tablets or capsules. To preserve the low cost when ordering by mail, where shipping charges are made, buy several bottles at a time. Remember, however, that you should not assume that other brands of calcium carbonate powder contain the same amount of calcium per teaspoon as this product does, for the reasons discussed above.

LIQUID CALCIUM, ANYONE?

Also available is a special liquid similar to calcium gluconate. It is a good alternative for those who need a soluble form of calcium but have difficulty swallowing multiple tablets or capsules daily. Marketed under the brand name Neo Calglucon, it is available at any pharmacy without a prescription.

It takes almost 2 tablespoons to equal the 600 mg. of calcium in some of the leading tablets, but if the cost and dosage don't bother you, it is a fine option. Controlling dosage is much easier with this product than with powdered forms of calcium.

THE "OTHER" CALCIUMS: BONEMEAL AND DOLOMITE

Both bonemeal and dolomite have become popular as calcium supplements. From what I have seen, the concentration of calcium in these two sources is respectable—on the order of 20 percent for dolomite and roughly 30 percent for bonemeal, although the calcium content of bonemeal is bound to vary from one sample to another due to the complex makeup of bone.

But those who are cautious about what goes into their bodies may want to avoid bonemeal and dolomite. As mentioned in
(continued on page 306)

The Many Faces of Calcium

There is so much to say about calcium supplements. But one thing you can't say is that manufacturers are giving us too few of them. There are literally hundreds to choose from: carbonates, gluconates, and phosphates, just to name a few.

After reading this chapter, you will have a good idea of the dose and type that's best for you. The following chart should help you pinpoint some of the products that most closely match your needs. The calcium values, of course, are for one tablet or capsule, unless otherwise noted. Within each category, products are arranged in order of calcium content, starting with the product containing the most calcium. If you are looking for only a modest amount of extra calcium, in the range of 250 mg. or less, you may be able to find it in a standard multiple vitamin/mineral supplement. The calcium content of a number of multiples is listed on pages 328 to 329.

In this chart, an asterisk (*) indicates a product marketed as an antacid rather than as a calcium supplement. Two asterisks (**) indicate a product containing more than one type of calcium, such as calcium gluconate plus calcium lactate. Often these products combine an insoluble form of calcium with a soluble form, meaning those with low stomach acid should probably look for a different form of calcium supplement.

Bonemeal (insoluble)	
Bone Meal Powder (GNC), ½ tsp.	500
Natural Bonemeal (Arco)	220

Calcium Carbonate (insoluble)	**Mg.**
Calciday-667 (Nature's Bounty)	667
Calcitab (American Pharmaceutical)	600
Calcium-600 mg (CVS)	600
Calcium-600 mg (Nature Food Centers)	600
Caltrate 600 (Lederle)	600
Potent Calcium-600 mg (GNC)	600

Suplical (Warner-Lanbert)	600
New Biocal-500 mg. (Miles)	500
Os-Cal Chewable (Marion)	500
Os-Cal 500 (Marion)	500
Oyster Shell Calcium-500 mg (Your Life)	500
Calcium Complete (GNC)	400
New Potent Calcium Plus (Advantage)	400
Oyster-Cal (Nature Food Centers)	375
Oyster Calcium (Nature's Bounty 375)	375
Alka-2 Mints* (Miles)	340
Calcium Junior-Chewable (GNC)	300
Tums-Ex* (Norcliff-Thayer)	300
Generic Calcium Carbonate (Lilly)	260
Chewable Biocal-250 mg (Miles)	250
Os-Cal 250 (Marion)	250
Oyster Shell Calcium (Rexall)	250
Alka-2* (Miles)	200
Calcium Carbonate-500 mg (GNC)	200
Chooz* (Plough)	200
Tums-Regular* (Norcliff-Thayer)	200
Titralac* (Riker)	168
Calcium with vitamin D (GNC)	140

Calcium Gluconate (soluble)

Calcium Gluconate (Thompson)	63

Calcium Lactate (soluble)

Calcium Lactate (Schiff)	100
Calcium Lactate-0.65 mg. (Rexall)	85
Calcium Lactate (GNC)	84
Calcium Lactate (Gray)	84
Calcium Lactate-10 grains (CVS)	84
Calcium Lactate (Nature Food Centers)	83
Calcium Lactate (Plus)	83
Calcium Lactate (Thompson)	83

(continued)

The Many Faces of Calcium—continued

Calcium Phosphates: Dibasic and Tribasic (insoluble)

Posture: high-potency (Ayerst)	600
Posture: moderate potency (Ayerst)	300
Di-Cal D wafers (Abbott)	232
Di-Cal D capsules (Abbott)	117
Dicalcium Phosphate (Gray)	112
Dicalcium Phosphate (North American)	89

Chelated Calcium (partially soluble, varying among brands)

Chelated Calcium (Thompson)	200
Chelated Calcium (Arco)	150
Chelated Calcium (Schiff)	130

Dolomite (insoluble)

Dolomite Mint Wafers (GNC)	158
Natural and Organic Dolomite 600 mg. (Arco)	130

chapter 14, work at both the Food and Drug Administration (FDA) and a private laboratory in Florida have found worrisome metals, such as lead, in some samples of both of these calcium sources.

If you are pregnant, contemplating pregnancy, elderly, or have been advised to consider calcium supplementation for an infant or child, you will want to reread the text of the FDA's statement, printed in full on pages 273 to 274. In short, it advises that "these substances should be used as little as possible in infants, young children, and pregnant or lactating women." The FDA also notes that the elderly are possibly at risk from the metal levels found in some samples of bonemeal and dolomite.

Miscellaneous	
FEMCAL Powder (Retech), 1 tsp.	317
Ca-Plus (Miller)	280
Calciwafers** (Nion)	165
Calcet** (Mission)	153
Calcicaps Tablets** (Nion)	130
Neo-Calglucon Syrup (Dorsey), 1 tsp.	115
Calcium Orotate (Sturdee)	50

Sources: Adapted from *Facts and Comparisons; The Calcium Bible,* (New York: Rawson Associates, 1985), 91–102; *Physicians Desk Reference,* (1986); *Tufts Diet and Nutrition Newsletter,* (July 1984): 6; and information provided by manufacturers.

Note: Supplement formulations can and do change—in both the amount of calcium per pill and the type(s) of calcium used. Therefore, use this chart only as a guide. Always check the label of a product for the most up-to-date and accurate information of its contents.

BETTER ALTERNATIVES?

As I said when I discussed the contamination problem in chapter 14, I have to wonder whether alternative sources of calcium are known to be any purer than bonemeal or dolomite. One scientist, for instance, challenged the basis for advising against bonemeal and dolomite for this very reason.

In a letter to *Southern Medical Journal,* where Hyman Roberts, M.D., first published his findings of metal contamination and bizarre symptoms in several patients using these supplements (described in detail on pages 272 to 273), Richard B. Holtzman,

Ph.D., of Argonne National Laboratory argued that "the information is not presented in a form that allows the medical profession or the user to judge the conclusions effectively."

Dr. Holtzman pointed out that the amount of lead in alternative sources of calcium must also be considered, for as experts such as he are well aware, even common foods are contaminated with the metal. Dr. Holtzman chose milk as his point of comparison. He first calculated that most of the bonemeal and dolomite samples tested by Dr. Roberts would supply less than 10 micrograms (mcg.) of lead per 1,000 mg. of calcium, with the most contaminated samples providing up to about 50 mcg. of lead. He then computed the amount of milk needed to supply 1,000 mg. of calcium and reported that the milk would contain no less lead than many (though not all) of the bonemeal and dolomite samples tested. According to his calculations, the milk "would have at least several hundred calories, would cost about five times as much, and would contain at least 10 to 20 mcg. of lead."

Dr. Holtzman makes a good case here when comparing bonemeal and dolomite to dairy sources of calcium. What remains to be published, however, is an analysis of how contaminant levels between bonemeal and dolomite compare to those found in other commonly used supplements.

My curiosity has been provoked further on coming across a chemical company's specifications for its calcium carbonate and gluconate powders. These powders are sold to drug and vitamin manufacturers, who convert them into tablets and capsules. These information sheets simply state that the powders contain less than 10 parts per million (ppm.) of lead. How much less is not said, but many of the bonemeal and dolomite samples that have been tested also contained less than 10 ppm. of lead. Some, however, contained almost twice this maximum.

DECISIONS, DECISIONS

For the sake of argument, let's assume that you want 500 mg. of supplemental calcium. Let's also assume that, contrary to all the fuss, the calcium carbonate, bonemeal, and dolomite that you are considering as sources actually contain the same percentage of lead. (The measurement that scientists use—parts per million—is a concept we think of as a percent level.)

Because the calcium carbonate is more concentrated (about twice as concentrated as the dolomite, for instance), you would need less of it to provide that 500 mg. of calcium than you would need for bonemeal or dolomite. As a result, the lead content per 500 mg. of calcium would be lower in calcium carbonate.

Until more precise information about metal contaminants in each alternative form of calcium is available, the possibility remains that these other types also contain their share of lead— maybe even amounts similar to that of bonemeal and dolomite. That, of course, addresses only the question of lead. Other unwanted minerals have also turned up in bonemeal and dolomite.

Because of the popularity of bonemeal and dolomite, I have given much thought to this matter. For now, I have concluded that the risk always exists that a particular brand or batch has an unusually elevated level of metal contamination. And scientists have barely scratched the surface regarding the significance of the toxic metals other than lead found in bonemeal and dolomite. How the levels of these compare to other forms of calcium remains unknown.

In light of these uncertainties, I do think it wiser to use other sources of calcium, particularly if you are in one of the high-risk groups cited by the FDA or if your need for supplemental calcium is high. Should the day come when all batches of bonemeal and dolomite are tested for metal contamination and certified to be within the same limits as other sources, I would be much happier.

By the way, neither bonemeal nor dolomite offer any particular advantage to those with impaired acid secretion. Both are insoluble. Dolomite does offer a dose of magnesium with its calcium, while bonemeal provides extra phosphorus in a favorable balance with calcium. Other types of calcium supplements offering these extra minerals, however, are readily available.

Because bonemeal and dolomite are rarely, if ever, used as calcium sources in scientific research, there is precious little information as to their side effects. Dolomite, however, is officially known to scientists as magnesium calcium carbonate. Because of its similarity to calcium carbonate, I have to wonder if it can produce any of the side effects associated with calcium carbonate—nausea and constipation, for instance. The same strategies for avoiding side effects described under calcium carbonate would be worth a try in this event for those who, for whatever reason, choose to forgo the warnings and use dolomite as a calcium supplement.

TIMING SUPPLEMENTS
FOR BEST EFFECT

A question I am often asked is, "When is the best time to take my calcium supplement?" Actually, there are several options. You can decide which is best for you based on your needs, habits, any side effects you experience, and your ability to remember to take pills.

One theory holds that bedtime is the best time to take at least some of your calcium supplement. We know from experience with bedridden patients that inactivity promotes bone loss. Since sleep is the most inactive part of the day for most of us, some have proposed that calcium supplementation should be taken as we settle into bed.

I have to say, however, that no one has actually produced evidence of better results with this method. Until researchers actually compare calcium absorption from supplements taken at different times of day, I can't tell you with certainty that when you take your supplement will affect your calcium nutrition.

Nonetheless, I think it's fine to take your calcium supplement at night (I do so myself). However, most of us go to bed on an empty, or relatively empty stomach. If taking your supplement without food causes nausea, this may not appeal to you. Also, in the event that you have impaired acid secretion, any calcium supplement that you take at night, without a meal, definitely should be a soluble one, such as calcium lactate or calcium gluconate.

For obvious reasons, a once-a-day schedule for supplementation is easiest—whether morning, noon, or night. But some argue that calcium is best absorbed when taken in divided doses. Nutritionists have long held this to be true, but, in my opinion, it has not been proven with certainty. In light of this belief, however, some advocate that calcium supplements be taken in divided doses, perhaps three times a day.

I have no objection to timing supplements in this way, but am concerned that remembering to take all of the doses may be a real problem for some. When you are sick, your discomfort provides a good reminder to take your medicine as many times a day as prescribed. But when you are simply trying to stay healthy, I think that remembering to take multiple doses is much more difficult.

I also feel that most of us are already getting some of our calcium spread throughout the day—in the form of the calcium-containing foods that we eat at mealtimes. So I remain a little skeptical that divided doses are really necessary for most users. However, when the amount of supplemental calcium is substantial (on the order of more than 600 mg. per day), or if recommended by a doctor, I would definitely divide the doses and spread them throughout the day.

Of course, anyone taking lower doses who prefers this method—or wants to use it in hopes of better absorption—should feel free to do so. As noted earlier, this does help minimize side effects in some people.

Now let's look beyond the minor side effects to the issue of serious toxicity.

FACT VERSUS FEAR

Of all supplements, fear of overdosing seems to be greatest about calcium. I imagine that the fears originate from hearing that many kidney stones contain calcium, or from knowing that hardened arteries contain calcium, or from having friends who talk of calcium deposits in their necks or joints. But after an exhaustive search of medical journals, I can tell you that the fears about calcium overdose are not backed by a long list of victims.

With all the talk of overdosing, I assumed I would find an abundance of case histories in the medical literature. To the contrary, I was shocked to find far fewer reports of adverse reactions than I had expected. Nonetheless, if they do occur, these reactions can be serious ones.

HOW CALCIUM CAN HURT

Might you overdose on calcium? Of course. But, as I have just noted, not as easily as you may think.

Problems from excessive calcium intake result only if the body actually absorbs too much of what is taken in. Depending on the size of the dose, the body has the option of simply letting the excess calcium pass through the digestive tract, unabsorbed. Research has turned up no reason to worry about this unabsorbed calcium.

If the body does absorb too much, the possible consequences can be serious: too much calcium in the blood (hypercalcemia); too much calcium in the urine, which increases the risk of kidney stones; calcification of various body tissues, especially in the kidneys; and excessively dense bones (osteosclerosis). Should the excessive absorption result from heavy use of both dairy products and certain antacids, a rare but serious disease known as the milk-alkali syndrome can occur.

To be sure, none of these conditions can be taken lightly. But the odds of developing them, in the absence of certain special conditions, is far lower than I ever imagined. Those of us with normal calcium metabolism seem to have a "calcium thermostat" that regulates our absorption of this all-important mineral. Unless overwhelmed with excessively high doses, the thermostat does a surprisingly good job of preventing the body from absorbing too much calcium.

Let's take a closer look at how typical levels of calcium supplementation affect the two most crucial issues: blood and urine calcium levels.

BLOOD: A CALCIUM LEACH

The importance of normal blood calcium cannot be overestimated. In fact, the body places a higher priority on maintaining enough calcium in the blood than in the bones. Should the blood calcium fall lower than necessary to maintain normal functioning of the muscles and heart, the body helps itself to the calcium in bone. That avoids an acute crisis from low blood calcium, but allows the bones to deteriorate, slowly and silently, to the point of weakness and fractures.

With overuse of calcium supplements, however, the concern is not of too little, but rather of too much calcium in the blood. We have already discussed the problem of high blood calcium in relation to overdoses of vitamin D in chapter 12. The case described on page 224 of Jon and his mother, who had been drinking an extremely concentrated vitamin D formula, illustrates some of the classic symptoms of high blood calcium.

The list of symptoms associated with high blood calcium is long: nausea, vomiting, loss of appetite, diarrhea, constipation, abdominal pain, depression, fatigue, dry mouth, thirst, excessive urination, high blood pressure, and muscle wasting have all been reported as symptoms. Unbeknownst to the patient, the excess calcium also can be deposited in body organs and walls of the arteries. If left untreated, the blood calcium level can rise so high as to cause stupor, coma, and even death. But the earlier symptoms are unpleasant enough that few would delay medical treatment long enough for the worst to happen.

Now for the happy news. Writing in the medical journal *Postgraduate Medicine*, Dan Keyer and Charles Peterson, both Doctors of Pharmacy, state that "hypercalcemia rarely develops as a result of calcium administration alone." At least at the dosages now used to prevent and treat osteoporosis—in the latter case, as much as 2,000 mg. daily—calcium supplementation is quite unlikely to cause high blood calcium.

I have not heard any concern that intakes such as these will cause high blood calcium levels among those with normal calcium metabolism. In fact, an FDA panel evaluated this matter in 1979 and concluded that "calcium intakes ranging from 1,000 to 2,500 mg. daily do not result in hypercalcemia in normal individuals." Those of us with normal calcium metabolism apparently are blessed with a line of defense mechanisms—ranging from hormones to kidney activity—that help resist high blood calcium even at moderately high intakes.

Odd as it may seem, oversupplementation with vitamin D is probably more likely to cause high blood calcium in a normal individual than is a high intake of calcium itself.

THE KIDNEY CONNECTION

The NIH panel on osteoporosis did express concern that too much calcium could cause kidney stones in "susceptible people." Those affected often overabsorb calcium; then, having no use for the excess, send it to the kidneys for excretion. In the process, the calcium content of the urine increases, setting the stage for kidney stones.

Doctors often refer to this condition as "idiopathic hypercalciuria." That simply means you have excessive amounts of calcium in your urine without any underlying condition to account for it. By all indications, this is a metabolic disorder in which the intestine does not adequately regulate its absorption of calcium. Many of those afflicted know who they are, for they already have had kidney stones. Some of these individuals seem to develop stones regardless of how much or how little calcium they consume.

But for those with normal calcium metabolism and no signs of this disorder, experts say that there is little evidence of kidney stones developing at the higher calcium intakes now recommended to improve bone health. According to Robert Heaney, M.D., a leading authority on osteoporosis, "development of [kidney stones] in connection with high calcium intakes is rare."

Dr. Heaney, professor of medicine at Creighton University in Omaha, Nebraska, explains that adding an extra 1,000 mg. of calcium daily increases the calcium content of the urine by an average of 50 to 70 mg. per day in middle-aged and elderly people. That is not an enormous amount. Moreover, the average premenopausal women or postmenopausal women taking estrogen should be adding only about 500 mg. of additional calcium to meet the recommended intakes set by the osteoporosis panel. Presumably their urinary calcium would increase somewhat less at this lower level of supplementation.

SECOND OPINIONS

Despite assurances such as Dr. Heaney's, I hear almost constant concern about calcium supplementation and kidney stones. As a result, I have researched the issue in depth and sought other expert opinions on the question. Based on what I have found published so far, I see little, if any, reason to suspect that a calcium intake of 2,000 mg. per day or less would have much effect on the risk of kidney stones among those with normal calcium metabolism. In fact, I have not found even one report of a woman with normal calcium metabolism who developed kidney stones as a result of calcium supplementation for osteoporosis.

I feel the same way about calcium and kidney stones as I do about high blood calcium. In both cases, I have a hunch that overdoing vitamin D is more likely than a high calcium intake to set the stage for trouble.

THE EXPERTS SPEAK

In addition to my own opinion, I would like to share with you the voices of others who have carefully considered the effect of calcium intake on urinary calcium levels and the risk of kidney stones.

> Calcium overload is rare in patients with postmeno-pausal osteoporosis. [High blood calcium, abnormal urine calcium levels, and kidney stones] are more likely in the following circumstances: immobilizations, very high doses of calcium (much more than 2,000 mg/day) ... [and] disorders associated with increased intestinal absorption of calcium.
>
> The Medical Letter on Drugs
> and Therapeutics

> Urinary calcium excretion varies widely among in-dividuals, but under most conditions appears to be rela-tively constant for any given individual. Major changes in calcium intake produce only slight shifts in the quan-tity of urine calcium.
>
> Committee on Dietary Allowances
> Food and Nutrition Board
> National Academy of Sciences

> Wide variations in [calcium] intake are accompa-nied by parallel, but only slight alterations in excretion. The urinary excretion of calcium is determined more by the absorption of calcium from the intestine than by dietary intake.
>
> Louis V. Avioli, M.D.
> Washington University
> School of Medicine

> While it is true that a very high consumption of calcium can increase your risk of kidney stones, quanti-ties under 2,000 mg daily constitute a very small risk. On the other hand, if you have a history of kidney stones, it is

necessary to consult your physician before taking large amounts of calcium.

Morris Notelovitz, M.D., Ph.D.
Director, Center for Climacteric Studies
University of Florida
and coauthor of *Stand Tall! The Informed Woman's Guide
to Preventing Osteoporosis*

As Dr. Notelovitz and others have pointed out, those who do have a history of kidney stones or have abnormally high levels of calcium in the urine should always consult a doctor about calcium intake. In fact, calcium is often not the only dietary factor of concern here—all the more reason to seek expert professional advice.

Several people who never have had kidney stones have asked me if they might be excreting too much calcium without knowing it. The only honest answer is that in medicine, virtually anything is possible. If this worries you, you can ask your doctor for a urinary calcium test, which I hope will settle the matter for you. The test is fairly inexpensive and painless, though it does require you to collect your urine for 24 hours. Some doctors use the test at regular intervals to monitor patients on very high doses of calcium.

THE MILK-ALKALI SYNDROME

Put together everything that can go wrong when the body absorbs too much calcium—high blood calcium and the discomfort it brings; kidney stones; impairment or failure of kidney function; deposits of calcium in tissues of the kidney and eye; abnormal readings in a variety of laboratory tests—and you have the once-mysterious illness that afflicted an unknown number of (mostly) ulcer patients for about four decades.

This constellation of symptoms was first reported in 1923, but it wasn't until 1949 that Charles Burnett, M.D., showed that the condition could be reversed by decreasing the intake of milk and absorbable antacids. Because these antacids are called "alkali" in the medical jargon, the term milk-alkali syndrome became the official name for the disease. Some, however, refer to it as Burnett's Syndrome in honor of Dr. Burnett's contribution to our understanding of its cause and treatment.

Today, the milk-alkali syndrome is mostly history. Long gone are the days when ulcer patients were encouraged to take large amounts of both milk and absorbable antacids, such as calcium carbonate or baking soda (sodium bicarbonate). These antacids were replaced by newer, nonabsorbable antacids that were considered more effective and without risk of milk-alkali syndrome. Prescription drugs for ulcer treatment appeared on the scene. The effectiveness of enormous milk consumption was challenged. Sodium bicarbonate, one of the guilty antacids in milk-alkali, fell into great disfavor as the antisodium message grew louder.

But the milk-alkali syndrome, though almost nonexistent today, has not been forgotten. Critics of calcium supplementation charge that medical history may repeat itself now that calcium carbonate is coming back, this time as a calcium supplement.

Is milk-alkali syndrome about to make a comeback? Hardly a likely happening. The calcium intakes now advocated for better bone health are a far cry from those taken in by victims of the milk-alkali syndrome.

The calcium intake of milk-alkali patients dwarf today's recommended intake of 1,000 to 1,500 mg. daily. Between the 1 to 5 quarts of milk and dozens of calcium carbonate tablets they took daily, milk-alkali victims easily consumed 4,000 mg. of calcium a day. I found one case where calcium intake was estimated at almost 10,000 mg. daily. I wouldn't be surprised if some patients had even higher intakes.

My favorite pharmacy textbook says that milk-alkali syndrome can be avoided if calcium carbonate intake is limited to 8,000 mg. a day—the equivalent of 3,200 mg. of calcium. You don't have to make a trip to the medical library to confirm this; just read the label of a Tums package. "Warning: Do not take more than 16 tablets in a 24-hour period." Sixteen Tums tablets yield exactly 8,000 mg. of calcium carbonate, of which 3,200 mg. are calcium.

There are even those who doubt that this level of calcium carbonate alone could produce milk-alkali syndrome. Dr. Heaney, for instance, estimates that without use of baking soda as an antacid—which was clearly a major factor in many cases—calcium carbonate intakes would have to be much higher than the level quoted above to create a risk of milk-alkali. Why might there be such a difference? Though both sodium bicarbonate (baking soda) and calcium carbonate are absorbable antacids, the baking soda is absorbed better—in fact, it's almost fully absorbed. As a result, the body conditions that invite milk-alkali may be more likely to appear, another reason why use of baking soda as an antacid is not recommended.

But whether it's a calcium carbonate intake of 8,000 mg. (3,200 mg. calcium) or 24,000 mg. (9,600 mg. calcium) that brings on the risk of milk-alkali in the absence of baking soda seems almost academic to me. We're talking about recommended calcium intakes of 1,000 to 2,000 mg., of which calcium carbonate would contribute but a part. And some supplement users don't take any calcium carbonate. Unless they regularly take baking soda as an antacid along with a high calcium intake from food or noncarbonate supplements, they have no known risk of milk-alkali syndrome.

Just for the record, I have yet to find a published report of milk-alkali syndrome in a patient taking calcium carbonate for osteoporosis. And I don't expect to as long as we use some common sense about dosage—and don't use baking soda as an antacid.

WHO CALCIUM CAN HURT

Throughout the sections above, I have referred to the relative safety of calcium supplements for normal individuals. For these purposes, normal means those who do not have any of the conditions associated with abnormal calcium metabolism, calcium overload, or the need for a doctor to monitor calcium requirements.

Those who fall into one or more of the latter categories should, of course, seek and follow a doctor's advice about calcium intake. The conditions involved here include:

- Cancer of any type
- Cushing's Syndrome
- Fanconi's Syndrome
- Gout
- Heart disease
- High blood calcium from any cause
- Hyperparathyroidism
- Hyperthyroidism
- Hypothyroidism
- Immobilization due to illness or injury

- Kidney conditions, including kidney stones, kidney failure, as well as a successful kidney transplant
- Metabolic acidosis
- Sarcoidosis
- Vitamin D overdose

Your physician's advice is just as important if you take any of the following medications:

- Cortisone drugs, on a regular basis
- Digitalis glycoside therapy
- High-dose vitamin D therapy
- Thiazide diuretics (see list of brand names on page 321)

Though uncommon, high blood calcium sometimes develops in Addison's disease. Though the odds are not high, those afflicted would do best to consult their physicians about calcium intake.

Keep in mind that vitamin D and calcium interact closely. Ask your doctor for advice on your calcium intake if you have any conditions related to vitamin D nutrition, including use of drugs, such as certain anticonvulsants, that can cause vitamin D deficiency. See chapter 12 for a refresher on the conditions and drugs that affect vitamin D nutrition.

THE STAR SYSTEM SHINES ON CALCIUM

Side effects—Gastrointestinal complaints such as nausea, gas, and constipation, can occur, and most commonly are associated with calcium carbonate. In my experience, such side effects are fairly infrequent. Strategies for alleviating these are dividing doses and taking them with meals; or, if necessary, switching to a different form of calcium.

Acute ailments—The early signs of high blood calcium—vomiting, nausea, loss of appetite, etc.—can occur among individuals with normal calcium metabolism who have taken or been given enormous doses—far more than recommended for preserving bone health. However, the high blood calcium generally does not last very long; sometimes only a few hours, provided that calcium treatment is discontinued or the dosage greatly reduced.

Naturally, when special conditions or drug treatments that alter the blood calcium level are present, supplement use poses more risk. Under these circumstances, high blood calcium is more likely to develop and less likely to clear up as quickly. Whether a single or a few large doses of calcium would cause long-lasting damage in affected individuals is debatable.

Long-term problems—Here is where too much calcium can have truly serious effects. With long-term use, a number of problems can occur. Those afflicted are most likely to have an underlying abnormality of calcium metabolism. Such a disorder increases their risk of high blood or urine calcium levels and the events, such as kidney stones, that can follow.

When an absorbable antacid—calcium carbonate or sodium bicarbonate—contributes to, or is taken with a high calcium intake, the milk-alkali syndrome may occur. In severe cases, some of its damage may be irreversible. Avoiding use of sodium bicarbonate as an antacid and keeping calcium carbonate intake at reasonable levels should keep this condition at bay.

Without an abnormality of calcium metabolism, toxic effects are unlikely at levels currently advocated. But at doses above 2,500 mg. daily, healthy individuals can succumb to high blood calcium. Unless taking an antacid such as sodium bicarbonate or calcium carbonate along with the high calcium intake, however, the troublesome milk-alkali syndrome is not among the ill effects. An exception to this rule might occur among individuals taking astronomical amounts of calcium carbonate alone—according to one estimate, on the order of 24,000 mg. daily, which yields 9,600 mg. of calcium.

The calcium intake needed to increase the risk of calcium-containing kidney stones in normal individuals is not easily defined. The level probably varies markedly from one person to the next and may depend on factors other than calcium intake alone. However, intakes of 2,000 mg. daily or less have not been shown to increase this risk when calcium metabolism is normal.

Conflicting combinations—The list of drugs that interact with calcium is long. However, far more drugs interfere with calcium than vice versa. In fact, the only drug that calcium is definitely known to meddle with is tetracycline, the familiar antibiotic. Calcium impairs its absorption, so always try to take the drug 2 to 3 hours apart from calcium supplements or calcium-rich foods.

Now for the drugs that have adverse effects on calcium balance in one way or another. Heading the list are thiazide diuretics, a widely prescribed type of "water pill," often used to treat high blood pressure. As noted earlier in the section about special conditions, you should consult a doctor about advisable calcium intake if you use any of these drugs. During long-term therapy, these drugs may cause the blood calcium level to rise and excretion of calcium to fall. Supplemental calcium may therefore pose an additional risk.

Doctors often favor thiazides over other diuretics, and they have no shortage of choices when doing so. The list of drugs that contain one of the various thiazides is long. Some of the best known brand names are: Aldactazide, Aldoril, Apresazide, Corzide, Diuril, Dyazide, Hydrodiuril, Hydropres, Naturetin, Rauzide, and Ser-Ap-Es. If your prescription bottle is labeled with only a generic term, and the last eight letters are thiazide, take the hint. Generic names such as chlorothiazide, cyclothiazide, and hydrochlorothiazide may look like Greek at first, but on second glance, the three final syllables they have in common identify the drug family from which they hail.

Diuretics other than thiazides can also increase calcium excretion. Sometimes these other varieties are combined with a thiazide, sometimes not. Again, ask your doctor how much calcium is right for you if you take any of the following brand name drugs (the nonthiazide generic ingredient of concern is listed in parentheses):

- Aldactazide or Aldactone (spironolactone)
- Diamox (acetazolamide)
- Dyrenium or Dyazide (triamterene)
- Edecrin (ethacrynic acid)
- Lasix (furosemide)

Drugs of many other classes can also affect calcium nutrition. Remember, of course, that the key concern is long-term use, and that not everyone will be adversely affected. Nonetheless, ask your doctor to advise you on calcium intake if you regularly take:

• The antibiotic neomycin (or viomycin, an antibiotic given by injection)
• The anticancer drug dactinomycin (Cosmegen), also given by injection
• The antigout drug probenecid (Benemid, ColBenemid)
• The antituberculosis drugs cycloserine (Seromycin) or capreo-mycin (Capastat)
• The cholesterol-lowering drug cholestyramine (Questran)
• Cortisone drugs, such as predisone, (Deltasone); dexametha-sone (Decadron), methylprednisolone (Medrol), to name just a few (long-term use of cortisone drugs is a well-established risk factor for osteoporosis)
• The laxatives mineral oil or phenolphthalein (the latter is found in a variety of popular over-the-counter antacids)
• Phenobarbital, an anticonvulsant that is also used as a sedative
• The psychoactive drug lithium

Finally, there are certain drugs that adversely affect bones in a variety of ways. Some encourage breakdown of bone; others interfere with the ever-important vitamin D nutrition. In this category are a number of anticonvulsant drugs, a sleeping pill called glutethimide (Doriden), and aluminum-containing antac-ids. The latter, bought easily over the counter, are a clear risk factor for osteoporosis when used regularly.

Ask your doctor about calcium intake if you are using any of these drugs regularly. If you are taking an aluminum-containing antacid frequently, ask if switching to another antacid might be possible.

Hidden consequences—I haven't found much evidence that calcium causes many false readings in laboratory tests. There is one report that it might increase the reading in a urine lead test. I have also noted a finding that readings for magnesium in the urine or blood may be falsely reduced by calcium if a certain test (called the titan-yellow method) is used.

HOW MUCH IS TOO MUCH

By now, you know that current recommendations for better bone health call for calcium intakes in the 1,000 to 1,500 mg. range.

As for calcium's contribution to better blood pressure and protection against colon cancer, findings so far lead me to believe that the desirable intake is the same for these conditions, too.

So much for the recommendations. The question that remains is how far beyond them can you go before risking your health in some way. Hardly a week goes by when someone doesn't pose this question to me.

One of the authorities that I trust most, Dr. Robert Heaney, writes that, "Calcium intakes up to 2.5 grams (2,500 mg.) [per] day do not result in hypercalcemia or other untoward effects in normal individuals." That is a full 1,000 mg. beyond the highest intake recommended by the NIH panel on bone health, though doctors do use doses this high sometimes in individual cases of osteoporosis.

Dr. Heaney isn't alone in his confidence. Others have "guesstimated" that the trouble range might begin around 3,000 mg. or so—the level warned against on the Tums label. And a 1967 editorial to doctors in the *Annals of Internal Medicine* warning of possible kidney damage from high doses of calcium drew a clear distinction between ulcer therapy and treatment of osteoporosis. "The doses of calcium salts used [for osteoporosis] are lower than those of calcium carbonate in peptic ulcer," noted the editorial. "[T]here is at present no conclusive evidence that [calcium-induced kidney damage] is a hazard at these dosage levels." During the 20 years since, I don't think evidence has come along that would cause the editorial writer to have a change of heart.

Oddly enough, however, the NIH panel that made headlines by declaring the need to increase calcium intake took an extremely conservative position on the matter of maximum intakes. In fact, the maximum level recommended by the panel is the most conservative I have found anywhere, excepting, of course, restrictions recommended for those with abnormal calcium metabolism.

A REALISTIC SAFE DOSE

The NIH panel on osteoporosis recommends a maximum calcium intake of 1,500 mg. for postmenopausal women not taking estrogen replacement therapy. I believe that the NIH panel could have safely extended its ceiling by about 20 percent, to a maximum recommended intake of 1,800 mg. This would not apply, of course, to those with special conditions cited throughout this chapter.

How about just a little more—say 2,000 mg.? The additional risk looks small to me. It does, however, rest mostly on the issue of kidney stones. Though very painful, kidney stones hardly rank as a major cause of death in the United States. Complications from osteoporosis do. Therefore, I think that minimizing the risk of osteoporosis is more important when setting a maximum recommended intake than is concern about the real, but less deadly, problem of kidney stones.

Another approach that appeals to me is an aged-linked safe dose. Since we absorb calcium better when we are young, I like the idea of setting a lower maximum for the earlier years of life. I think a good goal for premenopausal women and men under 60 is a maximum long-term intake of 1,500 mg. daily; for postmenopausal women and men over 60, again, 1,800 mg. seems quite safe to me.

These are still very cautious recommendations. No doubt there are tens of thousands of men (although few women) who habitually consume diets containing 1,500 to 2,000 mg. daily of calcium for many years, with no evidence of harm.

As for those whose doctors prescribe intakes as high as 2,500 mg., I feel you have little to worry about. Usually these doses are prescribed during the later decades of life—not as a lifelong measure. Moreover, when such doses are taken under medical supervision, doctors can monitor for and inquire after potential problems. So for those under regular care, I think there is little to fear.

I sincerely believe that most of us have a calcium thermostat operating with remarkable efficiency. But, without much research available on the long-term effects of intakes in the 1,800 to 2,500 mg. range, and because of unknown, but possible risk to some small number of people, I am most comfortable reserving these higher doses to those under regular medical care.

C O O K I N G
for Calcium

COLLARD PUREE IN ONION GLOBES

(Makes 4 servings)

Calcium: 507 mg. per serving
Calories: 218 per serving

4 large sweet onions (like
   Spanish or Vidalia),
   about 3 pounds total
½ cup beef stock
2 10-ounce packs collard
   greens, thawed and
   well drained
3 allspice berries,
   crushed

4 ounces cheddar cheese,
   cubed
2 tablespoons bread
   crumbs
   olive oil, for rubbing
   Parmesan cheese, for
   sprinkling

Preheat oven to 450°F.

Peel the onions and chop off a slice at the bottom so they
can sit without rolling. Then use a melon baller to scoop out
the insides of each onion, leaving about a ¼-inch-thick shell.

Chop the scooped-out parts and add them, with the beef
stock, to a large skillet. Simmer for about 5 minutes or until
the onions have wilted.

Scoop the mixture into a food processor and puree. Add
the collards, allspice, cheese, and the bread crumbs and
process until the mixture is smooth. Use a teaspoon to pack it
into the onion globes. Reserve any leftover puree.

Rub each onion with a bit of olive oil, sprinkle with
Parmesan, and set into a lightly oiled baking dish. Scoop
reserved puree into a small baking dish. Bake both dishes
uncovered for about 20 minutes. Serve immediately.

(continued)

C O O K I N G

for Calcium—continued

RICOTTA AND SALMON SAUCE

(Makes 1 cup)

Calcium: 81 mg. per ¼ cup
Calories: 55 per ¼ cup

Serve over pasta or steamed broccoli.

⅓ cup salmon with bones
    (3¾-ounce can)
⅓ cup part-skim ricotta
2 scallions, minced

½ teaspoon dried dillweed
¼ cup skim milk
½ teaspoon prepared
    white horseradish

Drain the salmon and scoop it into a food processor or blender. Add the ricotta, scallions, dill, milk, and horseradish and process until the sauce is thick and smooth.

VARIATION: Create a spread for sandwiches or a topping for baked potatoes by omitting the skim milk from the recipe.

PAPAYA AND MANGO BREAKFAST SOUP

(Makes 2 servings)

Calcium: 311 mg. per serving
Calories: 225 per serving

1 ripe papaya
1 ripe mango
  pinch of freshly grated
    lime rind

1 tablespoon freshly
    squeezed lime juice
1¼ cups plain low-fat
    yogurt

Cut the papaya in half the long way and scoop out the seeds with a spoon. Cut each half into manageable-size strips and

C O O K I N G
for Calcium—*continued*

peel off the skin with a sharp paring knife. Then drop the strips into a food processor fitted with the steel blade or blender.

Peel the mango. With the food processor running, hold the mango over the feed tube and slice the flesh right in. The mango will be slippery so grip it well. Keep slicing until there's no flesh left, then discard the mango's huge stone. Process the fruits until they're pureed. Add the lime rind, lime juice, and yogurt and process again, just until smooth.

Serve in chilled mugs with a twist of lime for garnish.

The Multiple Choice for Calcium Users

Multiple vitamin supplements are available in countless combinations. Most common, perhaps, is the long-standing multiple vitamin that contains only vitamins—no minerals. A second frequent form is the tablet containing vitamins and one mineral—iron.

Some multiples, namely those listed below, do contain calcium. As you can see, however, the calcium content is generally less than 300 mg., with the exception of supplements designed for pregnant women. There's no secret explanation for these low calcium levels; higher ones simply won't fit in the size of the supplement. A multiple containing a substantial dose of calcium would be larger than most of us would want to swallow.

For those who need only a modest amount of supplemental calcium because their diets provide the rest, one of the following multiples may do the trick—saving you the need to buy calcium supplements separately.

Dosage is one tablet or capsule unless otherwise indicated.

Supplement	Manufacturer	Mg.
Abdol with Minerals	Parke-Davis	44
Abron	O'Neal, Jones & Feldman	260
Beminal 500	Ayerst	20
Beminal Forte with Vitamin C	Ayerst	10
Cal-M	Anabolic	250
Cal-Prenal	North American	230
Centrum	Lederle	162
Cluvisol 130	Ayerst	120
De-Cal	North American	250
Di-Cal D with Vitamin C Capsules	Abbott	120

Supplements—*continued*

Supplement	Manufacturer	Mg.
Engram-HP	Squibb	650
Filibon Tablets	Lederle	125
Geralix Liquid (per tbsp.)	North American	33
Geriplex	Parke-Davis	59
Geriplex-FS Kapseals	Parke-Davis	59
Gerizyme (per tbsp.)	Upjohn	100
Gest	O'Neal, Jones & Feldman	130
Gevral	Lederle	162
Gevral Protein	Lederle	359
Gevral T Capsules	Lederle	162
Gevrite	Lederle	230
Livitamin Chewable	Beecham Labs	17
Natabec	Parke-Davis	600
Natalins Tablets	Mead Johnson	200
Norlac	Rowell	200
Nutra-Cal	Anabolic	185
Obron-6	Pfipharmecs	243
One-A-Day Vitamins Plus Minerals	Miles	100
Paladec with Minerals	Parke-Davis	23
Panuitex	O'Neal, Jones & Feldman	250
S.S.S. Tablets	S.S.S.	2
Stuart Formula	Stuart	160
Stuart Prenatal	Stuart	200
Vio-Geric	Rowell	220
Vitagett	North American	215
Vitamin-Mineral Capsules	North American	46
Viterra	Pfipharmecs	140
Viterra High Potency	Pfipharmecs	50
VM Preparation (per 2 tbsp.)	Roberts	94

Source: Adapted from the American Pharmaceutical Association, *Handbook of Nonprescription Drugs*, 7th ed. (1982), 240–57.

Note: This chart is intended only as a guide. Vitamin formulations change periodically; always read product labels for accurate and up-to-date information on their nutrient levels.

16
Potassium

Sodium—the mineral of the sea and shaker—is a familiar one to us all. But its metabolic coworker, potassium, had long been relatively anonymous.

All that changed about a decade ago, when potassium suddenly made the headlines. The occasion was the meteoric rise and crashing fall of the liquid protein diet. Dozens of its users—mostly young and female—had succumbed to fatal heart ailments rarely seen in women their age. Soon, reports began flowing into the Food and Drug Administration (FDA) noting that some of the victims had too little potassium in their blood. Though experts ultimately concluded that a general state of malnutrition, not the low blood potassium alone, likely had caused the deaths, potassium had been etched permanently in the minds of the nutrition conscious.

Today, attention is on potassium once again—a beneficial effect of the mineral on blood pressure is emerging. Although no Recommended Dietary Allowance (RDA) for potassium has been set, the Committee on Dietary Allowances has acknowledged its importance by offering a new "safe and adequate" range for daily intakes of the mineral.

THE SODIUM-POTASSIUM PARTNERSHIP

Naturally, a nutrient linked to blood pressure might be expected to interact with sodium, the mineral best known for its effect on blood pressure. And, as we mentioned before, that's exactly what potassium does. With sodium on the outside of body cells, and potassium on the inside, the two work together to maintain the body's water balance.

Some potassium does exist outside of body cells. Its purpose there is to allow normal functioning of nerves as well as muscles—particularly the heart. Potassium also assists in the body processes that synthesize protein and store carbohydrates.

With important roles such as these, it's no wonder that nature has given us so many ways to get potassium naturally. Often a nutrient will be present primarily in certain categories of food. Vitamin B_{12}, for instance, is found almost exclusively in animal foods. Fruits and vegetables are the domain for vitamin C. But potassium is different. Though plant sources tend to be richest in the mineral, a wide variety of other foods such as meat and dairy products also contain potassium. As a result, potassium deficiency is rarely seen.

THE POTASSIUM POOR

When potassium deficiency does occur, the cause often is not poor food choices, but rather specific medical conditions. In order to develop potassium deficiency, the body must lose more than it takes in. Typical conditions allowing this to happen include chronic diarrhea or vomiting, alcoholism, anorexia nervosa, and other illnesses causing severe loss of appetite.

Diabetics whose condition progresses to the state called ketoacidosis are at risk of potassium deficiency, as are those with Addison's disease or hyperaldosteronism, both disorders of the adrenal glands. Excessive loss of potassium in sweat, such as occurs in cystic fibrosis, can also deplete the body of potassium. And certain types of kidney impairment predispose to potassium deficiency.

Several kinds of drugs can also contribute to potassium deficiency. First, many—but not all—of the commonly prescribed diuretics ("water pills") can deplete body potassium in the process of routing out excess water. (I'll give you specifics later.)

(continued on page 334)

The "Safe and Adequate" Story

In 1980, the Committee on Dietary Allowances decided to give the public some guidelines on desirable potassium intakes. Count me among those who were gratified by the news.

The recommended intakes for potassium, however, differ from the usual RDA for common vitamins and minerals. Instead of a specific number, the recommended potassium intakes span a wide range. Rather than refer to this range as an RDA, the committee instead coined the term "safe and adequate" intake. The committee explained that a range, rather than a specific number, was set "because there is less information on which to base allowances" than is available for nutrients having a specific RDA.

It's not the decision to use a range that bothers me, but rather the term "safe and adequate" intake. Such a label implies that an intake exceeding the range given might be unsafe. The range for adults, for example, was set at 1,875 to 5,625 mg. daily. Someone unfamiliar with the committee's basis for its recommended range might get the impression that an intake of 6,000 mg. is considered unsafe.

Reading the fine print of the committee's report, however, reveals that the recommended range apparently did not evolve from a thorough study of potassium's safety. Rather, the range is a calculation derived from recommended sodium intakes.

In its 1980 report, the committee issued guidelines not only for potassium, but also for sodium. The latter long-awaited recommendations were based on an abundance of research showing that sodium limitation often helps reduce blood pressure. The committee set a recommended sodium range for adults at 1,100 to 3,300 mg. daily. This is a fine goal, but well below customary intakes in the United States.

From here, the committee reasoned—and I agree—that

a desirable diet would contain approximately equal amounts of sodium and potassium. They decided that this one-to-one balance would exist when the number of potassium and sodium molecules were the same. A molecule of potassium weighs 1.7 times as much as a molecule of sodium. Therefore, the "safe and adequate" potassium range of 1,875 to 5,625 mg. daily for adults is simply the recommended sodium range multiplied by 1.7.

Given this basis for the potassium recommendations, I feel one cannot conclude that intakes beyond the top of the range are unsafe. After all, the 5,625 mg. ceiling wasn't based on a study of potassium toxicity. It was more a matter of arithmetic. And in its prior report on dietary allowances—issued in 1974—the committee set no maximum nor minimum recommendations for potassium, simply acknowledging that our potassium thermostat allows for "a wide range of intakes."

Since the potassium range is actually a reflection of the sodium range, I am giving the committee's "safe and adequate" recommendations for both sodium and potassium in the chart below.

Group/Age	Sodium (mg.)	Potassium (mg.)
Infants 0–6 mon.	115–350	350–925
Infants 7–12 mon.	250–750	425–1,275
Children 1–3 yr.	325–975	550–1,650
Children 4–6 yr.	450–1,350	775–2,325
Children 7–10 yr.	600–1,800	1,000–3,000
Males 11–18 yr.	900–2,700	1,525–4,575
Males 19+ yr.	1,100–3,300	1,875–5,625
Females 11–18 yr.	900–2,700	1,525–4,575
Females 19+ yr.	1,100–3,300	1,875–5,625

Some doctors automatically prescribe potent potassium supplements when placing their patients on these drugs. Unquestioned for many years, this practice has become quite controversial. Opponents now argue that this routine practice is unnecessary for many patients. They believe that supplementation should be reserved for those who actually develop potassium deficiency while taking the diuretic in question. And as I will be telling you shortly, some diuretics actually keep potassium in the body, making supplementation a potentially dangerous practice.

In addition to long-term use of certain diuretics, excessive use of laxatives (especially if coupled with a food-restricted regimen) can also lead to potassium deficiency. The drug carbenicillin (an antibiotic given by injection), as well as use of high-dose penicillin has been associated with deficiency as well.

THE SIGNS OF DEFICIENCY

Symptoms of potassium deficiency include weakness, fatigue, abnormal heartbeat, and irregularities in the electrocardiogram (ECG), a test of heart function. If severe, the deficiency may be associated with muscle abnormalities such as twitches, muscle wasting, and hypoventilation. Kidney impairment may also occur.

A laboratory test showing a low blood potassium level, officially known as hypokalemia, will confirm a diagnosis of potassium deficiency. However, potassium depletion sometimes exists even when the blood level is normal. As a result, a normal blood potassium level of 4 to 5 or 5.5, does not always insure that potassium nutrition is adequate. In normal individuals, however, there is no reason to suspect that deficiency may exist despite a normal reading.

THE BLOOD PRESSURE CONNECTION

For most Americans, getting so little potassium as to cause the deficiency described above is not the problem. The question is: Is our intake near optimal?

As I have already mentioned, scientific signals now point to a possible beneficial effect of potassium on blood pressure. To reap the benefit, however, we may need to take in more potassium than we currently do, even though our current intake is adequate to prevent deficiency.

Here are some of the clues linking potassium to better blood pressure:

• In two Japanese villages where salt intakes (a known factor in high blood pressure) were similar, blood pressures differed greatly. A skilled researcher examined other aspects of the diets and found a higher potassium intake in the village with healthier blood pressures.

• A study of teenage girls showed that those with higher blood pressure had lower urine potassium levels.

• Research in animals, and one study in humans, has found that additional potassium can help reduce high blood pressure.

Even though the number of studies is small, the link looks promising. It makes sense, too, given the way that potassium and sodium work together so closely—sodium is pumped into cells, potassium is pumped out.

THE SALT ASSAULT

As impressed as I am with the possibility that potassium benefits blood pressure, I have to wonder what counts most: our potassium intake itself, or the *balance* between sodium and potassium.

In the twentieth century, the balance between these two minerals has shifted dramatically. Our ancestors, lacking salt-laden processed foods and easy access to the salt shaker, ate diets containing far less sodium than the meals we eat today. In some parts of the world, these low-sodium diets remain—accompanied by low rates of high blood pressure.

While we unwittingly have increased our sodium intake, we no doubt also have reduced potassium. Fats and sugars—two elements that contribute many calories but no potassium to the typical American diet—have replaced some of the potassium-rich plant foods of earlier centuries.

Food processing has also helped reduce our potassium intakes. Apparently, some potassium gets lost at the food factory. According to tables published by the U.S. Department of Agriculture, a cup of fresh cooked peas supplies 314 milligrams (mg.) of potassium. Put them in a can, however, and the potassium content drops to only 163 mg. per cup. Peas that come from the frozen food

(continued on page 340)

The Diet Detective Probes Potassium

Of all of the self-tests in this book, none was harder to design than this one. So many foods contain a significant amount of potassium that a complete list would go on for pages—not my idea of an easy way to test your potassium intake.

Another difficulty in composing the quiz is the absence of an RDA for the mineral. In quizzes for other nutrients, I often listed only those foods that contain 10 percent or more of the U.S. RDA. Recommended potassium intakes are in the form of a wide range: 1,875 to 5,625 mg. daily for adults. It isn't easy to decide what number along this range to take 10 percent of in order to find foods that qualify as significant sources.

I decided to adopt the middle point of the recommended range—3,750 mg.—as a starting point. Ten percent of that is 375 mg., so I initially planned to list only foods providing 375 mg. or more per serving. I noticed, however, that a number of foods considered good sources of potassium just missed meeting this 375 mg. minimum. Accordingly, I lowered the minimum to 300 mg. In the scoring section, I'll suggest a way to adjust your results to account for foods that contribute less than 300 mg. per serving.

To take the test, jot down the number of points associated with any of the foods that you ate yesterday. Remember to adjust the point value if you ate more than the serving size listed; for instance, two tomatoes would rate as 14 (2 × 7) points. Similarly, if you ate only half the serving size listed, halve the number of points.

Incidentally, it is not a mistake that the point system begins with 7 points, not 1 point. I intentionally allotted points this way to make scoring much easier.

7 points
1 cup turnips
1 cup grape juice

4 ounces ground beef
1 cup summer squash
5 prunes

1 medium tomato
1 boiled eggplant
3 apricots
⅓ cup Bran Buds
1 cup yellow corn
4 ounces broiled chicken
½ cup cashews
4 ounces water-packed
  tuna
1 veal chop
1 cup peach slices
1 cup mixed vegetables

8 points
½ cup chopped pecans
½ cup shelled chestnuts
½ cup dried apples
1 cup sliced beets
4 ounces lamb chop
4 ounces leg of lamb
1 cup bok choy
1 boiled sweet potato
4 ounces round roast beef
1 cup pineapple juice
1 cup cauliflower
4 ounces pork roast
1 cup apricot nectar
4 ounces pork chop
4 ounces round steak
1 pomegranate

9 points
4 ounces sirloin steak
1 nectarine
1 cup milk

4 ounces canned pink
  salmon
1 cup fruit cocktail
1 cup broccoli
1 cup grapefruit juice
1 cup brussels sprouts
1/16 watermelon
10 French fries
4 ounces beef liver
1 cup low-fat fruit yogurt
1 cup hash brown potatoes
1 medium banana
4 ounces roasted goose

10 points
½ cup peanuts
½ cup soybeans
4 ounces broiled cod
1 cup beet greens
1 cup lentils
1 cup collard greens

11 points
½ cup chopped almonds
1 cup orange juice
4 ounces broiled salmon
4 ounces calf liver
10 dates
1 cup canned tomatoes
½ cup tomato puree
1 cup plain low-fat yogurt
4 ounces steamed scallops
1 cup rhubarb, sweetened
1 cup mashed potatoes
  (made with milk)

(continued)

The Diet Detective—
Potassium (continued)

12 points
1 cup tomato juice
1 boiled potato
4 ounces untrimmed rump
  roast
1 cup black-eyed peas
1 cup spinach
1 cup parsnips
1 cup split peas

13 points
½ cup dried apricots
1 cup prune juice
1 cup apricots with syrup

14 points
½ cup sunflower seeds
½ cup pumpkin seeds
4 ounces baked flounder
4 ounces sardines

1 cup kidney beans
½ cantaloupe

15 points
½ cup dried peaches
1 cup Great Northern
  beans

16 points
1 cup navy beans

19 points
1 cup winter squash

21 points
1 plantain

24 points
1 cup lima beans

27 points
1 avocado

Scoring

Add up your total number of points. Multiply this total by 50. If you scored 60 points, for instance, multiply 60 times 50 for a final tally of 3,000. This number represents, in milligrams, a rough estimate of your potassium intake. Of course, the estimate is based only on foods included in the quiz.

Allowing for potassium contributed by foods with less than 300 mg. per serving is difficult, for this will vary greatly from one individual to another. I feel some adjustment is desirable, though, so I offer a suggestion based on the typical calorie count of your diet.

To your final tally in milligrams from above, add the adjustment below that most closely corresponds to your typical calorie intake.

Calorie Content of Diet	Potassium Adjustment
1,500	add 300 mg.
2,000	add 400 mg.
2,500	add 500 mg.
3,000	add 600 mg.

One last note about improving your estimate. If you use a salt substitute (including Lite Salt, which contains both table salt and potassium chloride), estimate your daily use—for instance, ¼ teaspoon. Consult the box "Sizing Up Salt Substitutes" on page 346 for the potassium content of your brand. Add the appropriate amount of potassium to your intake as estimated above.

All that remains now is rating your result. Although there is no RDA for potassium, you can compare your result to the RDA Committee's "safe and adequate" range of 1,875 to 5,625 mg. daily for adults. You can also weigh your result against the average adult intake of 2,300 mg. for women, 2,800 mg. for men.

My own inclination is to compare results to the recommendation of Herbert Langford, M.D., of the University of Mississippi. Dr. Langford, author of pioneering research on potassium and blood pressure, recommends a potassium intake of 4,000 mg. daily. This level is well within the "safe" range set by the RDA Committee, yet substantially above the average American intake. I agree with Dr. Langford that striving to do better than this average intake is a goal well worth the effort.

section fall in between, with 216 mg. per cup. Checking the numbers for corn and green beans, I found a similar pattern—more reason to suspect that modernization has taken some of the potassium from our food.

Today, the average dietary potassium intake among Americans stands at an estimated 2,800 mg. daily for men and 2,300 mg. for women. Sodium, by comparison, weighs in at about 4,000 to 6,000 mg. daily—in other words, two to three times typical potassium intakes. That's a dramatic shift from the old days when potassium intake probably dwarfed sodium. I wonder whether this lopsided balance between potassium and sodium isn't a major part of the blood pressure problem.

Should we cut back on salt? Of course. And increase potassium? Why not? To me, the big question is not *whether* we should look for more potassium, but *where* we should look. In other words, can we look to the supplements shelf for a safe source of additional potassium?

SUPPLEMENT OR DRUG?

Like calcium, potassium is available in numerous forms. Makers of potassium supplements have a selection of potassium-containing compounds from which to choose. But the average over-the-counter supplement buyer does not. Federal regulations have made some potassium compounds suitable mostly for supplements requiring a doctor's prescription. (I'll tell you why in a moment.)

Consumers looking for an over-the-counter supplement will quickly find that potassium gluconate dominates the market. Containing slightly less than 17 percent potassium by weight, this form of potassium supplement is clearly the favorite for over-the-counter use. Six of seven large mail-order companies that I surveyed offer potassium supplements composed exclusively of gluconate. The seventh marketed a chelated potassium supplement.

But regardless of the source, the potency of the supplements I checked was the same in almost every case. All but one contained 595 mg. of potassium gluconate, yielding 99 mg. of potassium. The chelated brand also yielded 99 mg. of potassium. One manufacturer parted company with the rest by offering potassium gluconate in two potencies—one with the same 99 mg. potassium as the others, and a lower-potency tablet yielding 83 mg. of potassium.

The almost universal potency of 99 mg. may seem quite a coincidence. But it isn't. Law, not coincidence, accounts for this standard. Federal regulations limit the amount of potassium in over-the-counter supplements because high doses of potassium in supplement form can have serious adverse effects in some people. The limit, as you can guess, is less than 100 mg. of potassium per pill.

For over-the-counter liquids (hard to find, in my experience), the FDA limits potassium content to 20 mg. per milliliter (ml.), which amounts to 100 mg. per teaspoon.

In addition to potassium gluconate, supplements also come in various forms of potassium citrate or potassium carbonate, although, for the most part, these are prescription-only items. However, they are not widely used and, therefore, I have little basis for comparing their safety to potassium gluconate. By far, the most popularly prescribed potassium compound is one you may be familiar with as a salt substitute—potassium chloride.

ENTER POTASSIUM CHLORIDE

Because it is highly concentrated, potassium chloride is the powerhouse of supplements. Containing 52 percent potassium by weight, this form has three times the potassium concentration of the gluconate form. An ounce of potassium chloride, for instance, has three times as much potassium as an ounce of potassium gluconate.

Thanks partly to its concentration, potassium chloride is widely used in high-potency potassium supplements. A glance at any drug manual shows that dozens of such potassium chloride supplements are available—by prescription, that is. Each year in the United States, doctors write hundreds of thousands of prescriptions for these products. I found no over-the-counter supplements containing potassium chloride as the sole source of the mineral.

These potassium chloride supplements come in a variety of forms: liquids, effervescent tablets to be dissolved in liquid, and two forms of tablets designed to be swallowed whole. The latter come in two notable forms. The first type is called "enteric-coated." Enteric coatings prevent medication from dissolving in the stomach and are widely used in drug manufacturing. The second—and also newer—type of potassium tablet comes in a waxed form designed to release its contents slowly. These tablets are called slow-release potassium; however, many people refer to them simply as "Slow-K," the brand name of one of the best known of these products.

THE EXPERT'S CHOICE

Of the four prescription potassium supplements discussed above, those taken in liquid form are considered the safest. According to experts, any potassium supplement may irritate the stomach, but those taken after meals as a diluted liquid are less likely to do so.

Both the enteric-coated and slow-release tablets have been associated with serious ulceration of the gastrointestinal tract, with the enteric-coated version more likely to cause such trouble. And the physicians newsletter *The Medical Letter* has recommended avoiding both, arguing that potassium supplements in liquid form or potassium-rich foods are better choices. This well-regarded publication for doctors has even advocated a ban on the enteric-coated form.

The FDA, however, has not banned enteric-coated potassium. The agency has acknowledged its "worst offender" status, though, by classifying all enteric-coated versions as prescription drugs, regardless of the potassium content. The FDA also requires that each brand of enteric-coated potassium be treated as a "new drug." This means that any new enteric-coated product must be approved by the FDA, even though other companies already market similar products. By requiring product-by-product approval, the FDA seeks to ensure that the quality of the enteric coating used is acceptable.

PRESCRIPTION STATUS IN PERSPECTIVE

With such strict FDA regulations on potassium, your impression may be that this mineral is a dangerous one. Actually, potassium itself is remarkably safe for most people because healthy kidneys maintain the body's potassium balance with extraordinary efficiency. This potassium thermostat is not easily deterred in healthy people. In addition, too much potassium will often induce vomiting—another defense against overdosing, because excess potassium is expelled.

Ironically, though, the safety profile of potassium packaged in certain ways—such as in these enteric-coated or slow-release forms—differs from that of the potassium dispersed throughout food or beverages. Supplements taken in tablet form can cause damage along the digestive tract. (Disturbing of the potassium thermostat, however, usually requires more than supplements alone, as we'll discuss shortly.)

Doctors usually are advised not to prescribe these concentrated potassium tablets to patients having conditions that delay passage of material through the digestive tract. An example would be a disorder of the esophagus in which "motility" or movement is impaired, causing food (or drugs) to remain in the esophagus longer than is normal. Liquid preparations are recommended instead in these cases. However, whether the 99 mg. of potassium in an over-the-counter product poses a risk to these individuals is unknown.

I don't want any of the information about prescription potassium supplements to discourage you from taking them if prescribed. Though the risk of digestive ulceration is undeniable, according to several reports, only one person among tens of thousands treated will develop this trouble.

USE VERSUS ABUSE

I included this information about prescription-strength supplements simply to show how over-the-counter potassium supplements might be abused. By abuse, I mean swallowing over-the-counter tablets in large numbers in order to reach the dosages that require a doctor's prescription.

Prescription tablets typically contain 300 to 1,000 mg. of potassium chloride, sometimes in the safer, slow-release form, sometimes not. Users of over-the-counter supplements should not take, all at once, enough 99 mg. tablets to reach these levels unless so instructed by a doctor. I am concerned that such a practice might irritate the gastrointestinal tract.

Granted, the potassium gluconate in most over-the-counter supplements probably has much less potential for producing ulcers and irritation than the potassium chloride in these high-potency prescription tablets. A classic study in animals supports this view. However, a few reports of ulceration from potassium gluconate solutions are on the record. I don't want you to take these reports so lightly as to dismiss them entirely, especially in light of the reassuring news I'm about to tell you next.

SO FAR, SO GOOD

I have not found any published reports of injury from potassium supplements sold over the counter. This means that over-the-counter potassium supplements actually have a clean bill of health in the medical literature. With 99 mg. per pill, I suppose that's not too surprising; a meal could easily supply ten times as much. Of course, as I have discussed, potassium packaged in tablets seems to have a different effect on the body than the potassium found in food and drink. Nonetheless, with no published cases of harm from over-the-counter supplements, I'm not losing any sleep over it.

What then, you must be wondering, are the tragedies from nonprescription potassium supplements that I mentioned only a few paragraphs ago? These were poisonings caused by potassium-rich products not labeled or intended as supplements. You can buy these products in the drugstore. You can also find them at the supermarket. Just look right next to the salt.

THE SAGA OF THE SALT SUBSTITUTE

As long as there have been salt-restricted diets, so has there been a demand for a seasoning that tastes like table salt, but lacks its sodium. I don't have to tell you that sodium contributes to high blood pressure in some people.

A stand-in for the trouble-making table salt proved to be its sodium-free cousin, potassium chloride. For years, it has been marketed under familiar names: Morton's Salt Substitute, Adolph's Salt Substitute, and more recently, as a new product simply called NoSalt. (NoSodium would actually be a more accurate name, for chemically speaking, potassium chloride is a type of salt.)

At any rate, potassium chloride marketed as a salt substitute is not subject to the FDA regulations that apply when the same substance is marketed as a potassium supplement. To make a long story short, salt substitutes are not classified as supplements. Because these products are intended as flavoring agents, the FDA considers them similar to food additives, not supplements. And potassium chloride is an approved food additive. As a result, consumers can buy it freely when packaged as a salt substitute, but not when packaged as a supplement.

GENERALLY RECOGNIZED AS SAFE

In addition, potassium chloride sold as a flavoring agent has "GRAS status." GRAS is shorthand for Generally Recognized As Safe, and the FDA monitors GRAS substances less stringently than food additives. As a result, few rules apply to potassium chloride in salt substitute form.

Were the label of a salt substitute to claim, however, that the product is designed for a specific medical condition, the FDA could require special labeling or warning statements. Even though their salt substitutes carry no such claims, some manufacturers nonetheless include warning statements directed at those with heart or kidney disease, diabetes, and people taking certain medications.

Contradictory as it may seem, no compelling reason exists for the FDA to bring salt substitutes under the strict regulations that apply to potassium chloride supplements. Used to flavor food in reasonable amounts, these products are better for many of us than table salt. That's because they are almost sodium-free (or sodium-reduced) and also provide potassium that can benefit our health. I have not bought a single box of table salt since sodium-reduced salt became available.

So if you are using salt substitutes, chances are that you should continue. Used as intended to replace table salt, these products haven't hurt healthy people—to the contrary. But in the wrong hands, wrong amounts, or taken with the wrong drugs, there has been big trouble.

THE SADDEST STORY
IN SUPPLEMENT HISTORY

Deaths from supplement abuse are rare, but unfortunately, have occurred. Of all cases in which supplement abuse (or misuse)

(continued on page 348)

Sizing Up Salt Substitutes

Even if their use posed widespread safety problems (hardly the case), it's unlikely that potassium chloride salt substitutes would ever become a widespread health hazard. The reason? Many—if not most—people simply don't like their taste.

Granted, these substitutes taste enough like table salt to some people (I even met a person who claimed to prefer them to table salt!), but countless people find potassium chloride to be a bitter, unacceptable stand-in for salt. In fact, doctors believe that many patients defy their instructions to use these salt substitutes for this reason.

A compromise between table salt and the standard salt substitute has been on the market for some time now. This new blend is part potassium chloride, part table salt. It tastes much more like table salt than potassium chloride alone does. I have yet to meet anyone who objects to its flavor or claims it's unsuitable for any type of cooking. In my opinion, this blend represents a major advance in the war against high sodium intakes because it may gain the widespread acceptance that potassium chloride alone has not.

One such blended product—Morton's Lite Salt—contains 1,100 mg. of sodium per teaspoon, about half that of table salt. I would say that is quite an improvement, wouldn't you? Unfortunately, though, some sodium-restricted diets cannot even accommodate these blended salt substitutes because the sodium content is still not low enough.

For those not on strict low-sodium diets, however, a blended salt substitute can help lower sodium intake without changing the taste of food. In the process, the balance between sodium and potassium will improve. This better balance is something that I like to see.

Needless to say, such blends should be used only with a doctor's approval if you have a medical condition requiring restriction of sodium or potassium intake. Similarly, if you have any of the medical conditions or take any drug that can interfere with potassium balance, consult your doctor before using a salt substitute containing only potassium chloride.

Finally, do not combine both a salt substitute and a potassium supplement. Cases of potassium overload have resulted from using salt substitutes and prescription-strength supplements together. Whether users of lower-strength over-the-counter supplements might develop such a problem is unknown. However, no problems from using both an over-the-counter supplement and a salt substitute have been reported so far.

Despite these cautionary notes, I feel that one comment bears repeating. For healthy adults not on a salt-restricted regimen, salt substitutes are at least as safe as table salt when used in similar amounts. For many of us, they are much safer, if not desirable. Just to play it safe, however, I wouldn't use more than a teaspoon daily.

Here is the approximate potassium content (in milligrams per teaspoon) of some common salt substitutes, based on information published in the April 1985 issue of the *Journal of the American Dietetic Association*.

Morton's Regular Salt Substitute	2,730
NoSalt	2,652
Adolph's Salt Substitute	2,535
Featherweight K Salt Substitute	1,911
Morton's Lite Salt	1,560
Adolph's Seasoned Salt Substitute	1,287

was a contributing or direct factor, I know of none sadder than the following tale.

The tragic episode involved a mother, her two-month-old infant, and a well-meaning but misinformed author. The author, in a popular health book, had offered the following advice for alleviating a baby's colic: "1. Offer to the infant, after nursing, a supplement made with ¼–½ teaspoonful Morton's Salt Substitute and ½ teaspoonful lactobacillus acidophilus culture to each 4 oz [ounces] water bottle. 2. The mother should use Morton's Salt Substitute in her diet."

Good intentions notwithstanding, this was *extremely danger-ous* advice. Unfortunately, it went unchallenged until the worst occurred. Charles Welti, M.D., and Joseph Davis, M.D., of the University of Miami and Dade County, Florida Medical Examin-er's office, reported the upsetting outcome in a letter to the editor of the *Journal of the American Medical Association*. An excerpt from their letter follows:

> A 2-month-old 4.8 kg [11 pound] boy had "colic." The mother, following directions in a popular health book, mixed 3,000 mg. potassium chloride [just under a half teaspoon] with her breast milk and administered it to the baby in two divided doses. The symptoms were re-lieved but recurred the next morning. In the same man-ner, 1,500 mg. of potassium chloride [almost ¼ of a teaspoon] was fed to the child. A few hours later the baby became listless and cyanotic [having bluish-purple skin], stopped breathing, and was rushed to a hospital. The initial serum potassium level was 10.1 . . . [about twice normal levels] and remained elevated until he died 28 hours later despite intensive treatment.

There was virtually no doubt that the infant had died from the overload of potassium provided by the salt substitute. Infants can't handle the same amount of potassium chloride as healthy adults, as this tragic case illustrates all too well.

I would love to tell you that no one else fell victim to this terribly hazardous advice, but six years later a similar incident occurred. The baby boy was barely a month old; his mother, too, read and followed these instructions to feed a salt substitute to remedy colic. After keeping her baby on this regimen for four days, his appetite lessened, and he became irritable and tired. Finally, his skin turned blue, his breathing suspended, and he became limp. His parents tried mouth-to-mouth resuscitation and took him to a hospital emergency room.

Tests at the hospital revealed abnormal heart rhythm and an extremely high blood potassium level. Thanks to immediate treatment, to which the boy responded well, he recovered after three days.

There are more stories of accidental poisonings—not based on this dangerous advice for treating colic—but from neglecting to keep potassium out of children's reach. The moral of them all is the same: infants and children should never be given large amounts of potassium chloride. And to prevent accidental ingestion of large amounts, salt substitutes and potassium supplements should be inaccessible to them.

RISKY BUSINESS

As is so often the case in medicine, what is safe—or even potentially beneficial—for healthy people can be hazardous to those with special conditions. Potassium is a perfect example of this basic truth.

Most people regulate potassium with extraordinary accuracy, excreting any unnecessary or potentially harmful amounts. However, certain conditions and drugs can affect the body's ability to keep potassium in balance. In these instances, supplemental potassium—whether from salt substitutes or products sold as supplements—can be risky business.

The potential problem is accumulation of too much potassium in the blood. This condition, called hyperkalemia, was responsible for the tragic death of the infant boy described earlier. Obviously, the condition is potentially fatal; it can seriously disrupt the heart rhythm. As far as I can see, however, more cases than not are brought to medical attention before such an extreme outcome. These episodes often end with successful treatment.

Initially, high blood potassium generally produces few—if any—symptoms. Loss of muscle tone and diminished tendon reflexes sometimes signal development of the problem. Unfortunately, in other cases, no symptoms occur until toxic effects on the heart become evident. These changes can be seen on the electro-

cardiogram. Routine measurement of blood potassium also un-
covers some cases.

Regardless, high blood potassium is a toxicity syndrome distinct from the supplement-induced gastrointestinal problems discussed earlier. Each can exist independently—and to the extent
that they occur—often do.

Healthy adults almost never develop high blood potassium
simply from taking large amounts of the mineral orally. No doubt,
a high enough dose might cause an exception to the rule. Owing to
the potassium thermostat, however, such an occurrence is rarer
than rare.

On the other hand, supplementation should be used only as
directed by a doctor if a condition exists that can interfere with the
potassium thermostat. Here are some of the conditions that can
predispose to high blood potassium, setting the stage for it to
develop or worsen if already present:

- Addison's disease, untreated stage
- Certain ECG abnormalities and heart conditions
- Dehydration
- Heat cramps
- High blood potassium, from any cause
- Impaired kidney function
- Use of potassium-sparing diuretics ("water pills") or the digitalis
heart drugs

DETAILS ON THE DRUGS

At the beginning of this chapter, I recited a list of the "Potassium Poor"—people at risk of potassium deficiency. Prominent on
that list were users of many diuretics ("water pills"), such as the
common thiazides. These drugs remove excess body water, but
also may take out needed potassium in the process.

As an answer to this problem came the "potassium-sparing"
diuretics. These diuretics do their job without robbing the body of
potassium. Naturally, they seemed to be an important advance.
They were—except for those who combined their use with potassium supplements or salt substitutes. A number of those who did
developed high blood potassium, as the potassium-conserving
ability of these drugs is potent enough to disrupt the potassium
thermostat in some people.

Extra potassium—from supplements or salt substitutes—is generally not advisable for those who take potassium-sparing diuretics. The label of NuSalt salt substitute, for instance, advises that the product's "potassium content is significant for patients with advanced renal disease or those receiving potassium-sparing medication. For such patients, consultation with a physician before using is essential."

I am happy to see this labeling, but shudder to think that some people taking one of these drugs may know it only as a diuretic, not as a potassium-sparing agent. I hope you are not one of them, but just in case, here is a list of potassium-sparers. The brand names are listed first, with the generic name of the potassium-sparing ingredient in parentheses.

- Aldactazide or Aldactone (spironolactone)
- Dyrenium or Dyazide (triamterene)
- Midamor or Moduretic (amiloride)

Some of these drugs carry less risk of potassium overload than others. Aldactazide, Dyazide, and Moduretic, for example, contain two diuretics; one that conserves potassium and one that promotes potassium excretion. The actions of the two ingredients complement each other, making high blood potassium less likely than when the potassium-conserving ingredient is taken alone.

Please do not assume that everyone who takes these medications will develop high blood potassium. The manufacturer of both Midamor and Moduretic estimates that about 10 percent of Midamor users will develop high blood potassium. The estimate drops to only 1 to 2 percent for Moduretic because it contains both potassium-conserving and potassium-leaching ingredients. Regardless, the risk is highest in those with kidney impairment, diabetes, and in the elderly.

As mentioned earlier, those taking digitalis-type heart drugs should also use potassium only as directed by a doctor. Drugs in this category include Lanoxin and Lanoxicaps (digoxin) and Crystodigin (digitoxin).

THE BEST SUPPLEMENT OF ALL

"Get your nutrients from foods, not supplements" is the standard motto of my profession. I don't accept this attitude; my profession's own research makes clear that the vitamin A in supplements works just as well as the vitamin A in food. I could give a dozen similar examples.

In the case of potassium, however, I agree with those who say that food is usually the best potassium supplement. A convincing advocate of this position is the physician's newsletter *The Medical Letter*. Its editors point out that about 1,600 mg. of additional potassium is usually enough to prevent or treat the potassium deficiency associated with use of potassium-draining drugs. Two medium bananas and a cup of orange juice or 20 dried apricots will provide this amount—in a safer and better-tasting manner than prescription potassium supplements that are dissolved in liquid.

As for food versus over-the-counter potassium supplements, consider that these supplements have no more than 99 mg. of potassium per tablet. Every food listed in the potassium quiz starting on page 336 has at least 300 mg. per serving; some have twice that or more. Obviously, trying to match their potassium content with over-the-counter supplements requires swallowing pills in quantity. Doing so may not be as safe as relying on foods that are potassium rich. More often than not, the potassium in foods occurs in a different form than that used in supplements. Food-based potassium never has been reported to cause the digestive upsets sometimes associated with supplements.

Obviously, swallowing enough over-the-counter pills to match the amount of potassium in a potato or banana is not very cost-effective, either. Nor is it pleasant, unless you like to swallow a lot of pills every day.

THE STAR SYSTEM SHINES ON POTASSIUM

Side effects—Prescription potassium supplements have been associated with gastrointestinal upset, such as nausea, vomiting, and diarrhea. These effects have not been reported with over-the-counter supplements, but conceivably could occur—most likely if numerous tablets are taken at once. To minimize these side effects, take potassium supplements with a full glass of water, right after meals.

Acute ailments—Immediate reactions to potassium supplements have occurred almost exclusively from injected, not oral, doses. However, a few adults have developed ulceration of the digestive tract within one hour to three days of starting on prescription-strength potassium supplements. Infants and young children have suffered acute ailments, including one reported death, after being fed large amounts of salt substitutes. A second, accidental death occurred in a young child who swallowed numerous prescription slow-release potassium tablets that belonged to his grandmother. Acute high blood potassium from oral ingestion of potassium has not been reported in adults with normal potassium metabolism.

Long-term problems—The same types of reactions possible with acute ailments—gastrointestinal ulcers and high blood potassium—can occur with long-term use of supplemental potassium. In fact, such reactions are much more likely during long-term therapy. However, the cases reported so far have resulted from prescription strength supplements or use of salt substitutes by individuals with a predisposition to high blood potassium. (See page 350 for a list of these predisposing conditions.)

Patients taking prescription-strength potassium supplements are advised to report any of the following symptoms to their doctors:

- Black stools (a sign of gastrointestinal bleeding)
- Fatigue or weakness
- Heavy feeling in the legs
- Severe nausea, vomiting, or abdominal pain
- Tingling of hands and/or feet

These are possible warning signals of high blood potassium or injury to the gastrointestinal tract.

Two diagnostic tests that can reveal potassium overload are the ECG test of heart function and a measurement of the blood potassium level.

Finally, there have been reports of vitamin B_{12} malabsorption among some patients taking prescription potassium supplements in the form of either slow-release tablets or potassium citrate solutions. Again, no cases of this problem have been reported from use of over-the-counter supplements or salt substitutes.

Conflicting combinations—As I've already discussed at great length, caution with potassium supplements—or outright avoidance—is important for individuals who have certain conditions and/or use certain drugs. This applies particularly to those with heart, kidney, or liver ailments. Users of diuretics ("water pills") should also learn whether their particular drug conserves or depletes body potassium.

As with most nutrients, potassium nutrition is more likely to be reduced than enhanced by drugs. However potassium supplements can result in overload of the nutrient if combined with any of the potassium-conserving diuretics listed on page 351. A doctor's assessment of potassium status is also necessary before supplements are used by patients taking digitalis heart medications.

The list of drugs that may increase the body's need for potassium is far longer. At the top of the list, of course, are the diuretics that don't conserve potassium. The most common of these are the thiazides. An extensive list of both generic and brand name thiazides appears on page 321. Diuretics other than thiazides—excluding the potassium-conserving variety—are also risk factors for potassium depletion. Lasix (furosemide), Diamox (acetazolamide), and Edecrin (ethacrynic acid) are some of the most common ones in this category.

The remaining drugs that can cause loss of potassium are primarily antibiotics, particularly penicillin and its derivatives. Remember the general rule that long-term use, not a brief treatment, is the cause for concern. Some miscellaneous additions to the list of drugs that may adversely affect potassium nutrition include:

- Two antituberculosis drugs, capreomycin and p-aminosalicylic acid
- The antifungal drug amphotericin B
- Cortisone drugs
- The antigout drugs probenecid (Benemid); and colchicine, sold separately or in combination with probenecid under the brand name ColBenemid
- The antiparkinsonism drug, levodopa (Laradopa, Sinemet)
- The laxative phenolphthalein, found in many over-the-counter products

An interaction between potassium and high doses of aspirin has also been reported, but its significance remains uncertain.

Hidden consequences—A high potassium intake has not been accused of masking other illnesses. As for laboratory tests, potassium reportedly does have the potential to interfere with correct readings, depending on the procedure used and the quality of the equipment. If poor instruments are used, for instance, potassium in the blood may cause a falsely increased reading of the blood calcium level. I would lay blame here more on the laboratory using a poorly maintained or inaccurate instrument than on the potassium.

Potassium supplements may cause a false negative reaction in the acetaminophen screen test—a urine test that measures levels of the common over-the-counter pain reliever best known by the brand name Tylenol. False increases in blood uric acid levels may also occur if a certain method of testing is used.

Finally, measurement of Diagnex blue in the urine may be falsely elevated by potassium compounds. Diagnex blue is a dye sometimes used in tests of stomach secretion (gastric analysis). However, some experts consider the Diagnex blue method outmoded. If its use is decreasing as a result, so is the significance of this finding.

HOW MUCH IS TOO MUCH

Potassium may be the most restricted nutrient in the marketplace, but the fact remains that for a healthy person, an upper safe limit is absolutely undefinable. As the widely respected drug manual *Facts and Comparisons* states, "With normal kidney function, it is difficult to produce potassium intoxication by oral administration."

For healthy adults, then, the safety issue is not really the amount of potassium taken in, but the source of it. The evidence shows that potassium supplements prepared in certain ways may harm some people. So far, however, these cases have been limited to supplements available by prescription only.

Though I feel that no basis exists for setting a ceiling on the potassium intake of healthy adults, I would like to offer these guidelines for using potassium supplements safely:

• Use potassium supplements or salt substitutes only with a doctor's consent if you have any medical condition, such as heart, kidney, or liver diseases, that might put you at risk.

• Except as prescribed by your doctor, do not use potassium supplements or salt substitutes if you take a potassium-sparing diuretic ("water pill") or other drug known to make a potentially troublesome combination with potassium supplements.

• Do not use both a potassium supplement and a potassium chloride salt substitute without a doctor's approval. Small amounts of over-the-counter supplements combined with a blended salt substitute containing both potassium chloride and table salt (e.g., Lite Salt) have not been reported hazardous to healthy people, however.

• Do not administer potassium chloride salt substitutes to infants and children. No objections have been raised, however, to using a blend such as Lite Salt to replace table salt in day-to-day cooking for a healthy family. In fact, this may be preferable, but those with very young children may want to seek a physician's consent.

• Always use salt substitutes as a seasoning taken with food. Supplemental potassium in this or any other form should not be taken on an empty stomach; taking a large amount at once or in isolated form is the most likely way to experience any adverse reaction.

My last piece of advice is a familiar plea: as safe and beneficial as potassium can be for most of us, please, please, keep supplements containing it out of children's reach.

C   O   O   K   I   N   G
for Potassium

WHITE BEAN SALAD WITH TINY PASTA

(Makes 4 servings)

Potassium: 483 mg. per serving
Calories: 188 per serving

2 cups cooked Great Northern beans	⅓ cup minced sweet red peppers
1 cup cooked tiny pasta, such as ditilini, acini di pepe, or orzo	⅓ cup minced scallions
	juice of ½ lemon
⅓ cup minced celery	1 teaspoon olive oil
	½ teaspoon dried thyme

Combine the beans, pasta, celery, peppers, and scallions in a large serving bowl.

In a small bowl, whisk together the lemon juice, oil, and thyme. Pour the dressing over the bean mixture and toss well to combine. Serve at room temperature or chilled.

MASHED PLANTAINS IN THEIR JACKETS

(Makes 4 servings)

Potassium: 687 mg. per serving
Calories: 192 per serving

2 large green plantains, about 1¾ pounds total	¼ cup unsweetened pineapple juice
seeds from 3 cardamom pods, freshly ground	2 tablespoons maple syrup

Lay a plantain on its side and keep it steady by laying one hand on top. Use a sharp knife to cut it in half horizontally, using sawing motions. Repeat with the other plantain.

(continued)

C O O K I N G

for Potassium—continued

Scoop out the plantain meat using a melon baller or grapefruit spoon, leaving the plantain jackets intact. Place the scooped-out meat into a small saucepan and pour enough water over it just to cover. Boil for 25 minutes, then drain.

Preheat the broiler.

Mash the plantain meat until smooth using a potato ricer or electric hand mixer. You can also use a food processor but take care to process for only 15 to 20 seconds or the plantain could become gummy. Stir in the cardamom, pineapple juice, and maple syrup and scoop the mixture into the jackets. Broil for about 2 minutes, or until mottled brown on top. Serve immediately as a side dish.

ROAST POTATOES AND GREEN CHILIES

(Makes 4 servings)

Potassium: 994 mg. per serving
Calories: 160 per serving

1½	pounds red potatoes	½ teaspoon hot chili powder
2	teaspoons olive oil	
3	mild green chilies (about 4 ounces, fresh or canned)	½ teaspoon dried oregano
		2 scallions, minced

Preheat oven to 400°F.

Chop potatoes into 1-inch cubes. Set the potatoes in a single layer in a medium-size baking pan. Pour the oil over the potatoes and toss until well coated. Roast the potatoes for about 20 minutes, or until tender.

Meanwhile, mince the green chilies. When the potatoes are ready, scoop them into a medium-size serving bowl and add the minced chilies, chili powder, oregano, and scallions. Serve hot or cold.

Potassium and the Multiples Market

Relatively few multiple vitamin-mineral products contain potassium. And as the chart that follows shows, those that do contain very little. Federal restrictions on the potassium content of supplements and consumer demand for multiples containing other minerals are among the reasons.

Also, fitting a substantial amount of potassium in a pill also containing a dozen or more other nutrients would be difficult. We need far more potassium daily, in milligrams, than we do trace minerals, or B vitamins, for instance. In the latter cases, recommended intakes are often on the order of a few milligrams per day—and in some instances only a fraction of a milligram. Compare that to the recommended potassium intake in the four-figure range, and you can see the problem of adding a significant amount of potassium to a pill also containing the big-name vitamins and minerals. It would be too big to swallow.

Certainly these multiples may provide ample amounts of many vitamins and certain minerals. In the case of potassium, however, washing them down with a glass of orange juice will provide hundreds of milligrams more potassium than the pills themselves provide.

Dosage is one tablet or capsule unless otherwise indicated.

Supplement	Manufacturer	Mg.
Abdol with Minerals	Parke-Davis	5.0
Centrum	Lederle	7.5
Geritinic	Geriatric Pharm.	30.0
Gerizyme (per tbsp.)	Upjohn	10.0
Gevral Protein	Lederle	13.0
Gevral T Capsules	Lederle	5.0
Obron-6	Pfipharmecs	2.0
Paladec with Minerals	Parke-Davis	3.0
Unicap T	Upjohn	5.0
Vitagett	North American	5.0
Vitamin-Mineral Capsules	North American	5.0

Source: Adapted from the American Pharmaceutical Association, *Handbook of Nonprescription Drugs*, 7th ed. (1982), 240–57.

Note: This chart is intended only as a guide. Vitamin formulations change periodically; always read product labels for accurate and up-to-date information on their nutrient levels.

17

Iron

For decades, iron was the "king of minerals." In fact, it was the only mineral nutritionists considered worthy of special attention. Sold on its importance, they convinced the government to require food companies to add iron (and three B vitamins) to white flour destined for certain uses. Even those nutritionists who adamantly opposed use of nutritional supplements thought differently when it came to iron and advocated supplements for infants, pregnant women, and nursing mothers. And at one time, iron was the only mineral added to many multiple vitamin products.

But opinion has been changing in the mineral world. Calcium has replaced iron in the limelight. And calcium and zinc are sharing equal space with iron on multiple supplement labels.

But don't let this fool you into thinking that iron is any less important to your health. Recent years have brought even more knowledge about your iron needs—and your potential for getting too much.

FACTS AND FUNCTIONS

Iron first earned its claim to fame when nutritionists established it as a vital component of hemoglobin, a key substance in red blood cells. Hemoglobin has the life-sustaining responsibility of picking up oxygen in the lungs and transporting it throughout the entire body. Though extremely important, however, this is not iron's only function. Iron is also part of a number of enzymes. In addition, some iron is converted to myoglobin, a hemoglobin-like substance found in muscle fibers. Myoglobin is our iron bank, storing iron for future use. And, as you'll find out as you keep reading, "iron stores" are essential to iron nutrition. But first, a little iron background.

THE TWO FACES OF IRON

As is often the case in nutrition, the body may absorb more of a mineral from some foods than from others. In extreme cases, interfering factors may prevent the body from absorbing almost all of a nutrient in food. In other words, the nutrient can be there, but it is of no use to the body.

Such is the case with iron. First, certain substances in food—dietary fiber, phytates, the food additive EDTA—as well as coffee and tea, can reduce iron absorption. However, the greatest influence on absorption appears to be the type of iron itself.

Food contains two basic types of iron. The best-absorbed type, called heme iron, is found exclusively in flesh foods. Lamb, beef, and chicken contain the highest percentages of heme iron—about 50 to 60 percent of their iron is the heme form. Pork, fish, and liver contain a smaller percentage—about 30 to 40 percent.

Not surprisingly, the remaining iron in flesh foods is known as nonheme iron. Vegetables, grains, beans, nuts, fruits, eggs, and most important to our discussion—iron supplements—contain only the nonheme form. While the body absorbs a smaller percentage of this nonheme iron, less does not have to mean none. With a little help from some friends, nonheme iron can become more available to the body, contributing enormously to our iron needs.

VITAMIN C TO THE RESCUE

Like calcium, nonheme iron cannot be absorbed unless in a soluble form, meaning it needs a substance (such as water) in which to dissolve. Stomach acid lends a hand here, as do nutritional factors. Among these, vitamin C plays the leading role.

Vitamin C is nonheme iron's best friend. It combines with this iron to make a soluble partnership; absorbable iron results. In fact, as the box below shows, a meal that includes enough vitamin C can make nonheme iron highly available to the body.

Iron Forms and Formulas

Knowledge about iron absorption has changed dramatically in the past decade. I can remember well my professors' credo that the body absorbs only 10 percent of the iron in food. Back then, iron absorption was easy arithmetic. We believed that simply dividing the iron content of a diet by 10 would provide a good estimate of how much was absorbed.

Today, the simple notions of my graduate school days are but a distant memory. Estimating iron absorption now entails an elaborate set of calculations based on four factors: Intakes of heme iron (found in meat, fish, and poultry); nonheme iron (found in such things as vegetables, fruits, and grains, as well as flesh foods); vitamin C; and the amount of iron stored in the body. This last factor has proven important; barring certain abnormalities, the body absorbs less iron when its stores are good. Conversely, absorption rises when body stores are low. Depending on these four factors, iron absorption can vary from virtually 0 to 35 percent of the amount consumed.

This change in estimating iron absorption allows nutritionists to predict iron absorption more precisely. But precision has its price: Complicated calculations are bound to frustrate those concerned about their iron intake, especially when it requires spending hours on the necessary measurements and mathematics.

Nevertheless, I think this problem can be solved easily. The meals patterns that follow simplify the issue by classifying the absorbability of nonheme iron in meals as low, moderate, or high, depending on the amount of flesh food and vitamin C eaten in the meal. I think that understanding the factors that increase absorption of nonheme iron matters

Other factors also assist in the absorption of nonheme iron. Even tiny amounts of an unidentified substance in flesh foods, as well as the heme iron found in these foods, enhance absorption of the nonheme form. In addition, acidic foods cooked in iron pots

most when evaluating diets, for two reasons. First, this form of iron predominates in food. Second, absorption varies so much more with nonheme than with heme iron. Knowing how to vary nonheme absorption in your favor is the key.

The sample meals don't include heme iron, for you can expect its absorption to be good. Men absorb an average of about 15 percent of the heme iron in food. In women, the average rate varies between 23 to 35 percent, depending on their iron stores.

Elaine R. Monsen, Ph.D., of the University of Washington, along with coworkers from throughout the world, formulated the examples that follow. Published in the January 1978 edition of the *American Journal of Clinical Nutrition*, this method has become the standard for estimating absorption of nonheme iron.

All measurements for meat, poultry, and fish refer to the raw weight, before cooking.

A Low-Availability Meal
• Less than 1 ounce of lean meat, poultry, or fish or
• Less than 25 mg. of vitamin C

A Moderate-Availability Meal
• 1 to 3 ounces of lean meat, poultry, or fish or
• 25 to 75 mg. vitamin C

A High-Availability Meal
• More than 3 ounces of lean meat, poultry, or fish or
• More than 75 mg. of vitamin C or
• 1 to 3 ounces lean meat, poultry, or fish *plus* 25 to 75 mg. of vitamin C

pick up some of the cookware's iron. The acid factor converts the iron into a soluble form, adding another source of absorbable nonheme iron to the diet.

HEME ISN'T EVERYTHING

Studies show that distinct differences exist between the absorption of heme and nonheme iron. The differences look real, and I see no reason to deny that heme iron is more readily absorbed. Nonetheless, heme isn't everything. First, while heme wins for quality, nonheme wins for quantity. Most of the iron found in food is nonheme, making it an important contributor to our iron supply.

To me the proof is on the bottom line—the rate of iron deficiency between those who consume large amounts of heme iron (meat-eaters) and those who consume nonheme iron (vegetarians).

I have looked, but cannot find, any convincing evidence that vegetarians in industrialized countries suffer higher rates of iron deficiency than meat-eaters. In undeveloped areas where vegetarian diets are limited, iron deficiency remains a major problem. But, as a group, vegetarians who have access to a balanced diet seem to be doing well.

If some of us can do fine without heme iron, I have to ask whether this issue isn't of more academic than practical significance. Where the diet is varied enough to include substantial amounts of vitamin C and other factors enhancing iron absorption, I see no reason to be alarmed at the absence of heme-rich foods in the diet. Besides, since many heme-rich foods are high in fat, I can't help but believe we're better off limiting our intake of them.

ENTER IRON SUPPLEMENTS

Like the nonheme iron in food, supplemental iron can contribute mightily to iron needs. In fact, when iron deficiency sets in, it is supplemental iron that provides the cure. An iron-rich diet generally is not enough to do the job.

Like other supplements you've read about in this book, iron supplements come in more than one form. And, some forms of supplemental iron are better absorbed than others.

The list of iron-containing compounds is very long, but can be divided into three forms: the ferrous family, the ferric family, and reduced iron. This last form is powdered iron, unbound to other substances.

Differences in availability do exist within these families. As a general rule, however, ferrous forms are better absorbed than ferric. As for reduced forms of iron, absorption may vary greatly, depending on manufacturing methods. This matters little for our discussion since virtually all of the iron supplements contain one of three ferrous forms: ferrous fumarate, ferrous sulfate, or ferrous gluconate.

The ferrous forms of iron are either fairly soluble in their natural state or easily made soluble by stomach acid. Therefore, enhancing factors such as vitamin C probably are not needed for absorption. Differences in absorption among the three common forms appear insignificant. The biggest difference is probably price, with ferrous sulfate often being the least expensive.

FACTS AND FALLACIES

Now that you have read the basics about iron supplements, here are some additional facts. Also included are some myths that need refuting.

• Side effects of iron supplements include diarrhea, stomach pain, constipation, headache, heartburn, loss of appetite, gas, and vomiting. Of these, constipation is probably the most common, followed by stomach upset.
• Iron in supplements is best absorbed when taken on an empty stomach. Doing so is not recommended, however, because unpleasant side effects also are more likely under this condition.
• Side effects occur less frequently when iron supplementation begins at a low level and is increased gradually.
• Contrary to widely held beliefs, a 1979 study found no evidence that short-term iron supplementation discolors teeth. The study lasted eight weeks, and the supplement dosage was 60 milligrams (mg.) of iron daily.
• Side effects from supplemental iron are likely to be related to dosage, with the chances of ill effects growing as the dosage is increased.

(continued on page 368)

The Diet Detective Searches for Iron

The most accurate methods of estimating iron involve complicated calculations. You have to know how much iron your body already has stored, for instance, making a simple estimate impossible. However, the quiz I've devised will give you a good estimate of your total iron *intake*. As I have said, these results are meaningful, even though less precise than those based on the newer, more complex calculations that measure how much iron you actually absorb.

However, for those who would like some way to apply newer knowledge, foods that make nonheme iron moderately or highly absorbable in the body are highlighted with an asterisk. (The rating is based on the serving size, not simply the food.) Remember, however, that vitamin C can substitute for the enhancing power of these foods. Therefore, if your diet is low on the foods marked with asterisks, your iron absorption can be good nonetheless.

The procedure here is the same as for previous diet quizzes. Simply tally up the number of points assigned to each of the following foods you ate on the day you want to test. After the food list, you will find how to calculate and evaluate your score.

1 point
2 slices bread
1 English muffin
⅓ cup 100% bran cereal
⅔ cup Cracklin' Oat Bran cereal
1 cup speckled butter beans
1 large waffle
3 pancakes
4 ounces lamb roast or chop*
4 ounces tuna*
⅕ recipe Tuna Helper*
¼ cup Scramblers egg substitute
4 ounces broiled chicken*
4 ounces turkey*
4 ounces tofu
4 ounces veal scallopini*
3 ounces canned shrimp*
2 ounces corned beef*
½ cup peanuts
½ cup filberts, chopped

½ cup raisins
½ cup chestnuts, shelled
½ cup pecans

2 points
1 8-ounce can pork and
    beans
⅕ recipe Hamburger
    Helper*
2 ounces dried chipped
    beef*
4 ounces beef rib roast*
4 ounces ham roast*
1 Italian sandwich roll
4 ounces roasted duck*
1 veal chop*
1 cup black-eyed peas
2 tablespoons sturgeon
    caviar
4 ounces roasted goose*
4 ounces oil-packed
    sardines*
4 ounces ground beef*
4 ounces steamed scallops*
4 ounces sirloin steak*
1 cup Cheerios cereal
4 ounces pork roast*
4 ounces veal cutlet*
1 cup coconut milk
4 ounces beef round*
1 cup lentils
4 ounces veal roast*
1 serving frozen dinner
    with meat, chicken, or
    fish*

1 frozen pizza, meatless
2 slices fast-food pizza,
    meatless
1 fast-food sandwich*
1 fast-food egg breakfast
½ cup cashews
⅔ cup any of the following
    cereals: Crispy Wheats
    'n Raisins, Golden
    Grahams, Grape-nuts
    flakes, Honey Bran,
    Raisins, Rice & Rye,
    Special K, Wheaties
½ cup chopped almonds
½ cup chopped black
    walnuts
½ cup dried apricots

3 points
1 cup most children's
    cereals
⅔ cup any of the following
    cereals: 40% Bran cereal,
    Fruit 'n Fibre, Life,
    Wheat Chex
⅓ cup Bran Buds or
    granola
1 packet Quaker instant
    oats
1 cup kidney beans
1 cup canned clams*
1 cup Great Northern
    beans

(continued)

The Diet Detective—
Iron (continued)

1 cup soybeans
1 cup farina
2 slices braunschweiger*
4 ounces Cornish hen*
1 cup lima beans
⅔ cup regular or quick
   cream of wheat
½ cup dried peaches
½ cup sunflower seeds

4 points
1 cup King Vitaman cereal
⅔ cup Buc Wheats cereal
½ cup pumpkin seeds

5 points
1 cup Kix cereal
1 cup Body Buddies cereal
⅔ cup instant cream of
   wheat

1 packet Mix 'n Eat cream
   of wheat
1 cup chicken liver*
2 slices liver cheese*

6 points
4 ounces beef liver*

7 points
⅔ cup Total or Corn Total
   cereal

9 points
⅔ cup Product 19 cereal
4 ounces calf liver*

13 points
⅔ cup Most cereal

Scoring
   Add up your total points. Multiply the total by 10 to estimate the percent of the U.S. RDA for iron that you consumed from food on the test day. If you scored 9 points, for instance, multiply 9 by 10 for a score of 90 percent of the U.S. RDA.

• One of the largest studies of iron safety compared ferrous fumarate, ferrous sulfate, ferrous gluconate, and ferrous glycine sulfate. Rates and types of side effects proved almost identical for all four.
• As previously noted, coffee and tea can inhibit iron absorption. Therefore, iron supplements are best taken with a different beverage, and at least an hour before or after drinking either coffee or tea. Of the two, tea appears to be the worse offender.

Now for an important point. As I have discussed much earlier in this book, the FDA had to pick a single value as the U.S. RDA for each nutrient so that food manufacturers can provide nutrition information on food labels. Food labels simply cannot include the percentage of the RDA of each nutrient for every sex and age group. The FDA chose the highest RDA for any sex and age group (excluding pregnant and nursing women) as its U.S. RDA in order to keep nutrition labeling relatively simple.

For most nutrients the U.S. RDA is usually close enough to the RDA specific to your age and sex because the recommended allowances differ little from one sex and age group to another. For iron, however, recommended allowances for adult men and women over age 50 differ greatly from those of younger women. The 18 mg. RDA for women aged 11 to 50 is almost double the 10 mg. for men and older women. Under the FDA's rules, the higher value—18 mg.—is the U.S. RDA, roughly twice the amount recommended for certain adults.

What all this means is that if you are male or a woman older than 50 (postmenopausal actually would be a more specific marker than age 50), you need not score 100 on this quiz in order to satisfy the RDA for your sex and age group. To the contrary, a score of 55 suffices to cover the iron allowance designed specifically for you.

• From the standpoint of absorption, timed-release iron preparations offer no special benefits, nor do enteric-coated products. The latter are designed to prevent release of medication in the stomach, where irritation may occur. Standard supplements actually may be better absorbed than either of these special forms.
• Calcium and magnesium compounds in prenatal and other vitamin/mineral supplements may make iron in these tablets less

available. A pure iron supplement, taken at a different time, may prove preferable.

• Among those with iron deficiency, iron supplements have improved physical performance. In addition, iron-deficient children performed better on tests of psychological health after supplementation, leading one researcher to write an editorial in the *British Medical Journal* entitled "Happiness is: Iron."

• Iron supplements should not be used unless prescribed by a doctor if you have peptic ulcer, ulcerative colitis, diseases of the liver or pancreas, alcoholism, or any condition where iron overload may occur. (You'll hear more about iron overload later.)

THE ROAD TO ANEMIA

Although the terms iron deficiency and iron-deficiency anemia are commonly used interchangeably, there is actually quite a difference between the two.

Iron deficiency exists when the body's iron stores are inadequate. This is the first step in the process leading to iron-deficiency anemia. Anemia does not develop until the iron stores are depleted. As a result, blood tests for anemia can be negative even though iron deficiency exists.

However, a laboratory test of the blood ferritin level can diagnose iron deficiency in this preanemic state. Blood ferritin reflects the amount of stored iron, so a low level signals poor iron stores. Impaired physical performance can accompany this early stage. Psychological effects also have been noted in children having low iron stores, but no laboratory evidence of anemia.

Of course, iron deficiency left unchecked can progress to anemia. Once iron stores are gone, the conditions are ripe for its development. The following symptoms are associated with iron-deficiency anemia:

• Coldness or tingling in the hands or feet
• Craving for ice or for nonfoods such as dirt, clay, or laundry starch
• Irritability
• Overwhelming fatigue and weakness
• Sensation of a rapid or fluttering heartbeat
• Shortness of breath upon exertion

An observant doctor will probably notice paleness of mucous membranes, such as the eyelids.

Two familiar laboratory tests used in diagnosing anemia are the blood hemoglobin and the hematocrit. When anemia arrives, the values on these tests fall to abnormally low levels. Two lesser-known factors—the amount of iron in the blood (serum iron) and the percentage of iron bound to a substance called transferrin—also drop too low. (Blood transferrin is an iron-carrying protein to which iron is bound and transported in the blood.) In addition to the abnormal values found in these tests, microscopic examination of the blood reveals abnormally small and pale red blood cells.

MISTAKEN ANEMIA

Oddly enough, some people who test positive for anemia on hemoglobin or hematocrit tests may actually have *too much* iron in their bodies. The problem is that not enough iron is going into the blood's hemoglobin (hence the abnormally low test results). Instead, the excessive iron is being stored elsewhere. Such a pattern is called iron overload.

Based on current estimates, iron overload is not a common problem and is not mistaken for anemia very often. Nonetheless, the Iron Overload Diseases Association believes that tests to rule out iron overload are warranted before finalizing a diagnosis of anemia.

A simple way to distinguish between iron-deficiency anemia and iron overload is a blood iron level. The reading is abnormally low in anemia, but not in overload. As excessive iron accumulates, the iron-carrying protein, transferrin, is able to bind up unusually large amounts of iron. This latter factor is called the total iron-binding capacity, or TIBC, and it can be tested in a medical laboratory. When results on both tests are considered, it should be possible to distinguish between iron overload and anemia.

Finally, the blood ferritin test that provides an early means of detecting iron deficiency also helps in diagnosing iron overload. As you will recall, the blood ferritin level reflects the body's iron stores. In anemia, the ferritin level is abnormally low, due to dwindling iron stores. By contrast, the ferritin level is elevated when iron stores are too high.

We'll get into more facts about iron overload soon, under the section "When Supplements Are Risky."

RISK AND REALITY

In their campaigns against iron deficiency, both commercial interests and some nutritionists give the impression that iron deficiency is running rampant in the United States. I don't believe it is. However, over a lifetime there are certain times when we are most likely to be at risk.

INFANCY. At birth, an infant's iron stores are usually not large enough to last more than six months, if that. During these months, milk—a poor source of iron—is often the baby's staple food. As a result, infancy can be a high-risk period for iron deficiency. Vitamin and iron supplements or foods containing supplemental iron are commonly advocated.

GROWTH SPURTS. During times of rapid growth during childhood and adolescence, the body needs more iron to fill its expanding stores. Naturally, when iron needs are greater, so is the risk of deficiency.

MENSTRUATION. I hesitate to classify all menstruating women as high-risk, though many nutritionists do. Women lose iron during menstruation, to be sure. But I am not convinced that menstruation creates widespread deficiencies. Many menstruating women maintain adequate iron nutrition without supplementation or special attention to their iron intake.

I prefer the term "moderate-risk" for menstruating women. Mild iron deficiency due to menstrual losses sometimes responds to supplementation during the menstrual period alone. However, those who bleed heavily, diet regularly, or suffer frequent infections may risk serious deficiency requiring more aggressive treatment.

PREGNANCY AND NURSING. Nature protects the growing fetus by putting its iron needs before that of the mother. Though the baby is protected, the mother is not. Research has found that the mother's iron nutrition is likely to suffer in the later stages of her pregnancy if she does not take supplemental iron. Rare is the nutritionist who opposes use of supplemental iron during pregnancy.

After the baby is born, the mother's iron needs fall to levels resembling those of nonpregnant women. But the mother may have lost some of her stored iron during pregnancy, so continued supplementation for another two to three months is commonly recommended.

IRON AND THE ATHLETE

Iron deficiency can be a problem for a surprising number of athletes. This possibility received much attention back in 1983 when Alberto Salazar, holder of the world record in the marathon and who was virtually unbeatable at the time, inexplicably started showing poor results in races. Eventually, doctors made a discovery—Salazar was suffering from iron deficiency.

Why athletes—and I don't mean just Olympic-class runners—are more vulnerable to iron deficiency is a hot topic in research circles. Possible explanations involve all three of the factors considered most important to iron nutrition.

• Iron losses: Iron is lost in body excretions, including sweat. Athletes may lose large amounts of sweat, and therefore significant amounts of iron, during strenuous and frequent exercise.
• Iron absorption: Studies have shown that food passes through the digestive tract more quickly in runners. That's good in some ways, but perhaps not for iron nutrition. With food spending less time in the digestive tract, the body may have less opportunity to absorb iron.
• Iron intake: Because some exercise devotees work out to lose pounds or prevent weight gain, they limit their diets to low-calorie foods providing little iron.

More investigation is needed to establish the amount of iron advisable for athletes. One estimate, however, suggests that athletes should try to increase their Recommended Dietary Allowance (RDA) by 30 percent. For example, the RDA for adult males is 10 mg.; a 30 percent increase would mean an RDA of 13 mg. for men who exercise heavily.

Two final points: First, this type of iron deficiency differs from so-called sports anemia. Sports anemia appears to be a temporary condition that occurs during the first stage of physical training. No ill effects or need for treatment have been established for this transient condition.

Second, athletes need not be in the dark about their iron status. A quick check at the doctor's office can determine if iron nutrition is up to par.

WHEN SUPPLEMENTATION IS RISKY

In 1970, organizations representing American bakers and millers asked the Food and Drug Administration (FDA) to allow a substantial increase in the amount of iron added to bread. Originally, the FDA intended to approve the proposal. No doubt, the agency had been influenced by nutritionists who considered iron-deficient diets to be extremely common in the United States.

Seven years and a few new voices later, the FDA changed its mind and ruled against the proposal. In denying the bakers' request, the FDA stated that "there is a need for increased iron for 1 to 2 percent of the population ... but this need has not been proven by any surveys or studies to be greater than that."

The FDA was not claiming that the risk of iron deficiency in the U.S. population was only 1 to 2 percent. Rather, its figures estimated how many people needed, but were not receiving sufficient iron. When anemic individuals receiving treatment are also counted, the rate of iron-deficiency anemia rises. According to one study, this rate is about 8 percent in American women. The same study, however, found barely more than 1 percent of American men to be anemic.

Regardless, the FDA had made an unusual about-face. The change was not merely motivated by the conviction that few Americans truly needed more iron. Rather, credit was due to a small but persuasive group of physicians who convinced the FDA that increasing the iron content of bread might harm an undetermined number of individuals who have iron overload, the condition mentioned earlier.

Excessive storage of iron is not a single disease, but rather a characteristic of several disorders in which too much iron is absorbed and/or retained in the body. Regardless of the cause, however, the condition is serious. The stockpiling of iron slowly wreaks havoc with the liver, heart, or both. Naturally, impairment of either of these vital organs will cause serious trouble if left untreated too long.

The chances for recovery from iron overload vary, depending

partly on the underlying cause. Most important in many cases is early detection. The sooner treatment begins, the better the chances for a successful outcome. Sad to say, the condition can be fatal if treatment does not begin soon enough.

THE SIGNS OF IRON OVERLOAD

Unfortunately, some patients with iron overload have no obvious symptoms until the disease has progressed considerably. As it advances, the following symptoms may appear:

- Abdominal or joint pain
- Bronze coloring of the skin
- Fatigue or loss of libido
- Symptoms of diabetes, such as excessive urination and thirst; hunger; weight loss; and, in women, frequent yeast infections
- Weight loss

On examining the patient with iron overload, the doctor will often encounter an enlarged spleen; signs of damage to the heart or joints; pigmentation of the skin; loss of body hair; and in men, testicles reduced in size.

Consultation with a medical laboratory comes next. Blood tests almost certainly will be ordered to confirm a diagnosis of iron overload. If the condition is confirmed, or strongly suspected, a liver biopsy can help to determine the extent of excessive iron storage.

As noted earlier, iron overload is not a single disease. Some cases have an underlying cause, with iron overload being merely one result. Diseases that impair formation of red blood cells, such as sideroblastic anemia, thalassemia, and sickle cell or other hemolytic anemias predispose their victims to iron overload.

Under these circumstances, iron overload is less likely to escape early detection. These disorders themselves produce symptoms that cause those afflicted to seek medical attention. If one of these underlying conditions is diagnosed, the doctor will be on the lookout for signs of iron overload. Needless to say, affected individuals should never take supplemental iron (or vitamin C) except as their doctors direct.

Iron overload eventually damages the liver, but in some

cases, the liver disease comes first. Individuals who have liver cirrhosis from alcoholism or who have had surgery involving certain blood vessels of the liver are potential candidates for iron overload. Impairment of the pancreas is another possible risk factor. Again, patients with these conditions should avoid supplemental iron and vitamin C unless prescribed by their doctors.

Finally, iron overload sometimes occurs on its own, not because of an existing illness. Such cases are termed "idiopathic," meaning that no underlying cause can be found. In addition, physicians refer to iron overload involving damage to body tissues as hemochromatosis. Putting both terms together, you have idiopathic hemochromatosis: a long-winded term for iron overload in the absence of an underlying cause. For simplicity, I prefer the abbreviation, IHC.

IHC has long been considered a genetic disorder. Experts believe those affected to have a genetic abnormality that interferes with the body's iron thermostat. Without sensors to monitor iron absorption, IHC victims absorb and store excessive amounts of iron. The Iron Overload Diseases Association estimates that as many as 1 in 10 people carry one of the genes responsible for IHC, and that up to 3 per 1,000 have both genes. Only those with both genes seem at serious risk of IHC. The ill effects, if any, from having only one IHC gene remain undetermined.

For many years, prevailing opinion held IHC to be both exclusively genetic and extremely rare. A few dissenters, however, expressed concern that the disease might develop simply from prolonged intakes of iron at high doses. That possibility is attracting more attention in light of a few recent findings.

HEREDITY VERSUS ENVIRONMENT

To me, the most pressing issue in iron safety is determining whether IHC can develop in individuals who don't have the genetic traits but have taken high doses of iron for many years. Arguing against such a risk are several published reports attesting to the safety of long-term iron intake. By way of example, one woman reportedly took 120 mg. supplemental iron daily for about 18 years and 240 mg. daily for another year, with no sign of ill effects. A classic pharmacy text similarly advises that many adults have taken as much as 180 mg. daily of supplemental iron (from ferrous sulfate) for many years, without any signs of toxicity.

On the other hand, there are a few reports of iron overload in individuals who took large amounts of supplemental iron for long periods of time. Some consider these cases evidence that high iron intake alone can cause overload. However, unbeknownst to themselves and their doctors, these patients may have had the genetic traits that cause IHC. In retrospect, one simply cannot know.

Recent findings from Sweden, where iron has been added to food for almost 40 years, have raised some troubling questions. Owing to fortification, average iron intakes in Sweden are considerably greater than in the United States. In one area of this Scandinavian country, investigators tested almost all individuals between the ages of 30 and 39.

Since IHC rarely occurs this early in life, you may wonder about the purpose of this study. Because IHC often advances before symptoms appear, researchers were hoping to detect signs of the condition during its early, often silent, stage. To their dismay, they did. Early signs of the condition—as measured by blood tests—proved far more common than expected among the men, but not among the women.

These findings may mean only that IHC genetic factors were widespread among those tested. One cannot help but wonder, however, whether increases in the iron content of Swedish food may have contributed to more and earlier cases of overload.

ALCOHOL AND EXCESS IRON

Studies of alcohol provide another hint that diet itself may play a role in iron overload. The condition is common among South African Bantus, who commonly drink beer brewed in iron pots. Prepared this way, the iron content of the beer is extremely high.

At first, experts suspected the beer's iron to be the culprit. Evidence is accumulating, however, that alcohol itself greatly enhances the absorption of iron. High iron content also has been documented in some wines, particularly in samples from Italy and Portugal.

Whether overload in heavy users of these iron-containing

alcoholic beverages results from iron itself, alcohol-enhanced absorption, or genetic factors, one can only guess. Some patients with iron overload reportedly admit to heavy use of alcohol; others, however, clearly do not drink excessively.

THE LOWDOWN ON OVERLOAD

I have to stress that the causes of IHC need further study. However, the findings regarding alcohol and Swedes consuming an iron-rich diet have raised my concerns. I feel the belief that IHC results solely from a rare genetic disorder remains to be firmly established.

Clearly, IHC runs in families, confirming a major role of genetic factors. When one family member receives a diagnosis of IHC, all relatives should be tested. Even if heredity alone accounts for IHC, the genes responsible may be more common than presently realized.

Feeling that so many unanswered questions remain, I have become much more cautious about long-term use of iron supplements. Naturally, I am most concerned about long-term use of high doses simply as a preventive measure. However rare iron overload may be, why risk furthering its development with high-potency supplements unless medically necessary?

I also believe that the FDA's decision to revoke permission to fortify bread with increased levels of iron was a good one. Concerns that higher iron intakes would accelerate overload in those at risk are reasonable. I feel that the intake of additional iron should remain at our discretion, in the form of supplements, rather than forced on us by loading iron into a staple food such as bread.

My concerns are shared by Alexander Schmidt, M.D., the FDA commissioner who initially approved the proposal to fortify bread with more iron. After his successor revoked the increase, Dr. Schmidt wrote, "I heartily applaud this action by the [new] Commissioner, even though I signed the order he reversed . . . [After I approved the increase], it became apparent that the regulation, while supported by some who knew a lot about nutrition, was opposed by individuals knowing the most about iron metabolism . . . Those I judged most expert in the science of the matter ranged from unenthusiastic to violently opposed to the regulation!"

I heartily applaud Dr. Schmidt's open-mindedness in reconsidering his original position and his candor in labeling it a mistake. I also applaud the physicians concerned about iron overload who devoted time to convincing the FDA to think twice about this potentially harmful proposal.

(The Iron Overload Diseases Association publishes a bimonthly newsletter and other information about iron overload diseases. The address is Harvey Building, Suite 912, 224 Datura Street, West Palm Beach, FL 33041.)

SAD NEWS FROM
THE EMERGENCY ROOM

Obviously, adults who suffer at the hands of iron do so slowly, over the course of many years. In children, however, the story differs. Acute ailments account for most iron-related problems in childhood.

In fact, no supplement brings children to the emergency room more often than iron. Every year, hundreds, if not thousands, of children get their hands on iron supplements and swallow numerous tablets at once.

No doubt, the widespread availability of iron plays a role in the saga; mothers of young children are more likely to have supplements of iron on hand than any other mineral. But iron's effects on the body of a young child are also important. In children, iron possesses more toxic potential at high doses than do many other nutrients.

The outcome of iron overdose in children is no longer grim, as it once was. The numbers, however, are disconcerting. Estimates of iron poisonings among American children range from a low of 566 cases per year (a recent tally from the Centers for Disease Control) to a high of 2,000 from other sources. Most victims are four years old and under. Obviously, the acute toxicity of iron varies dramatically with age.

Having seen so many cases, experts have established that these iron poisonings generally involve four stages, each with its own symptoms and effects. The typical pattern after a young child consumes numerous iron tablets is as follows:

• First stage—within 1 to 6 hours: vomiting, diarrhea, passing of black stools, and possibly shock and coma. The color of the urine may resemble that of rose wine. Some doctors actually use the French term for such wine—vin rose—to describe the color of the poisoned child's urine.

• Second stage—6 to 12 hours after intake: a period of seeming, but short-lived, improvement.

• Third stage—12 to 48 hours after iron ingestion: abnormalities of the central nervous system, impaired liver function, signs of bleeding, and altered metabolism, creating a blood condition called acidosis.

• Fourth stage—days or weeks later: late complications, such as intestinal obstruction resulting from damage to organ tissue caused by the iron overdose.

Needless to say, these poisonings in children invariably result from failure to keep iron supplements out of their reach. Occasionally, children take large numbers of their own supplements—that is, a children's multiple vitamin with iron. In the vast majority of cases, however, children have swallowed large numbers of potent iron tablets intended for adults.

ADULTS AND ACUTE AILMENTS

Poisonings such as these are extremely rare in adults. The few incidents on record have been limited to patients with psychiatric problems who took numerous tablets. The handful of published cases suggest, however, that adult poisonings tend to follow stages similar to those observed in children. In addition to the symptoms commonly observed in children, fever and abnormalities in an electrocardiogram (a heart test) have been reported in affected adults.

Also on the record of adult poisonings is a very sad case involving the death of a fetus. The woman, six months pregnant, had taken enormous quantities of an iron supplement and an undetermined amount of an over-the-counter medication. She survived, though comatose on arriving at the hospital. Four days after admission, however, she gave birth to a stillborn baby. One cannot be certain that the iron alone was responsible, but the possibility is undeniable.

PREVENTION AND CURE

As recently as a few decades ago, up to 50 percent of childhood iron poisonings were fatal ones. Today, however, doctors have a better understanding of the poisoning process, much experience, and a useful new drug, deferoxamine. This drug—also known by the brand name Desferal—binds to the excess iron in the body, reducing its toxic power. Some doctors use Desferal primarily in severe cases, believing it unnecessary in mild poisonings.

Thanks to these improvements, childhood deaths from iron poisoning in the United States have fallen dramatically—almost to zero. Some victims are hospitalized only a few days. Testifying to these advances is the following report by John T. McEnery, M.D., professor of pediatrics at Loyola University. It is excerpted from *Clinical Toxicology*, a medical journal.

> *A 13-month-old male weighing [19 pounds] was admitted in shock with absent peripheral pulses, cold clammy skin, and dehydration three hours after being found with iron pills in his mouth . . . Blood pressure was not detectable on admission, but responded to intravenous fluids, which included whole blood. He was given deferoxamine [the iron-binding drug, after the staff washed out his stomach]. One hour after admission his vital signs were stable and he made an unevental recovery . . . He was discharged 4 days after admission.*

Cook County Hospital in Chicago, where this baby was treated in the late sixties, had not lost a single child to iron poisoning since 1962. Not that there weren't any possible candidates. Between 1967 and 1969, the hospital admitted 107 children suffering from iron poisoning. The 100 percent survival rate among these children and all those admitted for iron poisoning between 1962 and 1967 strongly testifies to advances in treatment.

Needless to say, full recovery most often occurs when treatment begins promptly. Time is precious here, and breakthroughs

Recommended Dietary Allowances for Iron

Group/Age	Mg.
Infants 0–6 mon.	10
Infants 6–12 mon.	15
Children 1–3 yr.	15
Children 4–10 yr.	10
Males 11–18 yr.	18
Males 19+ yr.	10
Females 11–50 yr.	18
Females 51+ yr.	10
Pregnant and nursing women	30–60*

Note: The U.S. RDA for iron is 18 mg. The U.S. RDA is designed solely for nutrition labeling purposes. If you are an adult male or a woman older than 50, your allowance is just a little over half of the U.S. RDA. Therefore, a serving of food, a meal, or a daily diet that contains 50 percent of the U.S. RDA almost meets the recommended allowance for your sex and age group.

*According to the Committee on Dietary Allowances, "The increased requirement [for iron] during pregnancy cannot be met by the iron content of habitual American diets nor by the existing iron stores of many women; therefore, the use of 30–60 mg. of supplemental iron is recommended." The Committee found that iron needs during nursing do not differ much from the needs of nonpregnant women, but recommends continued supplementation of mothers for two to three months after giving birth. This measure is favored to replace any losses in iron stores that may have occurred during the pregnancy.

in treatment will accomplish much less if medical attention is delayed too long.

Even when treatment fully succeeds, however, the experience is a traumatic one. Clearly, the ultimate success is prevention. This goal can be realized simply by keeping iron supplements out of children's reach. If you no longer take the iron tablets prescribed during your pregnancy, consider discarding them.

THE STAR SYSTEM SHINES
ON IRON

Now for a summary of iron safety.

Side effects—Constipation is the most common side effect associated with supplemental iron. A variety of other digestive complaints, and occasionally headache, may also occur. Black, tarry stools are a common consequence of supplemental iron. I hesitate to classify this as a side effect.

Acute ailments—Used as intended, no acute ailments from supplemental iron have been reported. However, young children who gain access to iron-containing supplements and take many tablets often wind up in the emergency room, as large doses are poisonous to them. Fatalities from iron poisoning, once commonplace, are now rare in the United States due to advances in treatment. Nonetheless, the importance of keeping iron supplements out of children's reach cannot be overemphasized.

Acute iron poisoning in adults is extremely rare and generally limited to patients suffering from psychiatric problems. A few deaths have occurred among them. Also recorded is the case of a stillborn baby, described earlier, born four days after his mother had ingested an enormous amount of supplemental iron and an unknown quantity of an over-the-counter drug.

Long-term problems—Iron overload, discussed earlier in much detail, accounts for most long-term problems related to iron. To what extent supplemental iron can contribute to the condition remains unknown. Given the seriousness of this condition and the possibility that high iron intakes might cause or accelerate the disease, unnecessarily high supplementation is unwise.

Those afflicted with peptic ulcer, ulcerative colitis, liver or pancreatic disease, alcoholism, and any condition associated with iron overload should use supplemental iron only if a physician prescribes it.

There is one report of iron supplementation provoking extreme sensitivity to sunlight in a woman who had a condition known as EPP (erythropoietic protoporphyria). Sensitivity to sunlight is a hallmark of this condition, but this patient had tolerated sunlight well for eight years. She suffered a relapse only after taking iron therapy for two months. Her renewed sensitivity to sunlight gradually subsided after discontinuing the iron therapy.

Conflicting combinations—Iron is known to interfere with the action of tetracycline, the common antibiotic. During short-term therapy with tetracycline, consider avoiding iron supplements unless your medical condition requires otherwise. In the latter case, take the drug at least an hour or two apart from iron supplements. Use this same method of staggering doses during long-term therapy with both tetracycline and iron.

Where antibiotics are unavailable, researchers have found an interesting effect of iron on infection. In African nomads, supplemental iron given to combat widespread iron deficiency adversely affected ability to fight infection. Without antibiotics to thwart the infection, the iron may have nourished both the patient and the infecting agent. Such a finding has not been reported among those with access to infection-killing antibiotics.

The following drugs may decrease iron absorption. (Brand names are shown in parentheses.)

• Antacids containing carbonates (e.g., sodium bicarbonate, calcium carbonate, magnesium carbonate) and/or magnesium trisilicate
• Cholestyramine (Questran), a cholesterol-lowering drug
• Dactinomycin (Cosmegen), an anticancer drug
• Neomycin, an antibiotic

Indomethacin (Indocin), a drug with anti-inflammatory and pain-relieving properties, may cause anemia.

Chloramphenicol (Chloromycetin), a little-used antibiotic, may increase blood iron content and total iron-binding capacity. This is not good news for those with iron overload.

Hidden consequences—Iron-deficiency anemia may be a symptom of an underlying disease, especially in those who rarely develop anemia (men and postmenopausal women). Diseases that cause internal bleeding may lead to anemia, because as blood is lost, so is iron.

Some opponents of increasing iron in bread contended that

higher iron intakes might prevent diagnosis of illnesses marked by bleeding, such as colon cancer. The FDA sided with the opponents, but not for this reason. Its experts concluded that the additional iron proposed for bread would be unlikely to boost intakes high enough to compensate for iron lost due to abnormal bleeding.

Supplements, however, can supply much more iron than the highly fortified bread would have provided. Therefore, the possibility remains that at some level of supplementation, masking of disease-induced anemia might occur. Unfortunately, no one knows how high an intake might cause this to happen.

From the standpoint of the example raised—colon cancer—the problem may be a small one. Improved methods of detection have made doctors less dependent on anemia as a warning signal. As for other diseases marked by bleeding, I also have found no reports of supplemental iron preventing an accurate diagnosis. Nonetheless, I would not consider this concern irrelevant in making decisions about long-term supplementation, particularly for middle-aged and older individuals.

As for effects of iron supplements on laboratory tests, I have two reports to share with you:

• Ferrous gluconate may interfere with the acetaminophen screen test. This urine test measures the presence of acetaminophen, the popular over-the-counter pain reliever best known as Tylenol.
• Ferrous sulfate may interfere with the ability of two products—Clinistix and Diastix—to give correct readings for sugar in the urine. An effect on Testape, a similar product, has not been found.

HOW MUCH IS TOO MUCH

The Committee on Dietary Allowances states that "the toxicity of food iron is low, and deleterious effects of daily intakes of 25–75 mg. are unlikely in healthy persons." The Committee restricts its comments to "food iron" and gives no estimate regarding supplemental iron.

By use of this wording, the committee stops short of endorsing intakes up to 75 mg. as safe if supplements supply a good part of this amount. However, the term "food iron" includes iron added to food such as bread. Many people obtain a fair amount of their dietary iron from these supplemented foods rather than from naturally occurring sources. Moreover, the forms of iron used to enrich foods may differ little in their safety from those used in supplements; sometimes, the same form is used in both. Therefore, I don't think the committee can insist that its estimate has no relevance to supplement safety.

I also am curious about the evidence to support such a broad range of "food iron" intakes. Diets containing 75 mg. of iron are rare to nonexistent in the United States. In fact, few Americans consume even half this much food iron.

One key survey found that 95 percent of men took in less than 32 mg. of iron daily; as for women, 95 percent consumed less than 20 mg. If diets that habitually contain 75 mg. of food iron don't even exist in the United States (or similarly industrialized countries), I don't see how their safety has been proven.

Accordingly, it seems that supplemental iron must have been considered in order to put the seal of safety on intakes as high as 75 mg. daily. If so, and if the committee's estimates are correct, a total intake of 75 mg. or less—from food and supplements combined—may very well be safe for most healthy people.

Regardless, I can accept this estimate for short-term use, but not for a lifetime. When it comes to long-term practices, I have little enthusiasm for even moderate doses of extra iron when not medically necessary. My reasons follow.

First, the committee based its estimates on information dating back to 1972. Since then, we have developed a better appreciation for the problem of iron overload. Chances are that most people will be spared iron overload even with long-term supplementation at high doses. But we can't predict who is safe with certainty.

Therefore, taking high doses of iron for many years is like a low-risk game of Russian roulette. You are likely, but not guaranteed, to emerge unscathed. Under these circumstances, I would rather not play—unless a medical condition so requires. If you have no iron deficiency, why risk a potentially life-threatening illness?

Of course, high iron intake may be but a minor factor, or one of several risk factors in the development of overload disease. It may even be irrelevant. Based on current knowledge, though, I remain concerned that high iron intakes may invite or worsen the problem.

Finally, while the rate of iron overload in the United States is miniscule when compared to disorders such as heart disease or cancer, it is nonetheless much higher than the risk of overdosing on other nutrients. The annual number of overdoses from all other nutrients may not even come close to the yearly rate of iron overload. Moreover, iron overload is likely to be more serious, as well as more difficult and time-consuming to treat, than excesses of most other nutrients.

SENSIBLE SUPPLEMENTATION

The issue of choosing a supplemental iron dosage is made simpler (but less flexible) by the realities of the marketplace. Most multiple vitamins with iron contain 18 mg. per tablet. This supplies the entire RDA for those with the highest need, except for pregnant and nursing women.

Though just satisfying the RDA for menstruating girls and women, these multiples with iron provide almost twice the recommended allowance of 10 mg. for men and postmenopausal women. Add to this the average iron intake from food among these two groups. The total far exceeds the amount that men and postmenopausal women need unless they are iron deficient. Most, of course, are not.

If you are among these groups whose RDA is but half the iron content of the typical multiple vitamin with iron, I see three options for setting a long-term intake. The first is simple enough: Forgo iron supplementation if you know your iron stores are adequate or if you know your intake from food is high.

A second option is limiting supplemental iron to the 18 mg. found in the typical iron-containing multiple. The third is a middle ground: seeking out one of the few multiple supplements containing less iron than the U.S. RDA (see page 391). Children's multiples with iron sometimes provide 100 percent or more of the adult RDA for vitamins, but less than 18 mg. of iron.

As for premenopausal women, I again would be most comfortable limiting long-term supplementation to the 18 mg. found in most multiples with iron—unless tests show a need for more. For those who insist on a higher dose, I would expect that 25 to 30 mg. daily should pose little risk unless combined with generous intakes of alcohol or an iron-rich diet. Needless to say, any predisposition to iron overload makes supplementation out of the question, except as prescribed by a doctor.

I realize that these recommendations are conservative ones. I know that, in time, I may become more confident about iron safety. I expect the next decade to bring an outpouring of knowledge about iron overload. From there, we will be better able to say whether the condition can develop in the absence of genetic factors. But until then, I prefer to play it safe.

If tests show that you are too low on iron, or if you are pregnant or nursing, playing it safe does not mean limiting iron as described above. To the contrary, it means taking supplemental iron as necessary for good health. As long as you have no adverse reactions, take with confidence the amount of supplemental iron your doctor prescribes.

C   O   O   K   I   N   G
for Iron

CORNISH HENS WITH A CREAMY MARINADE

(Makes 2 to 4 servings)

Iron: 3.2 mg. per hen
Calories: 630 per hen

1 cup buttermilk	2 Cornish hens, halved
½ teaspoon dried	down the backbone
rosemary	½ teaspoon dijon-style
1 clove garlic, minced	mustard

To prepare the marinade, pour the buttermilk into a 9-inch glass baking dish. Crush the rosemary in a spice grinder or mortar and pestle and add it and the garlic to the buttermilk. Set the hen halves in the marinade and bathe them in the marinade. Cover and let them marinate, refrigerated, for at least 1 hour, or longer.

Preheat the oven to 400°F. Set the hen halves, skin-side-up, on a lightly oiled broiler rack and bake for about 20 minutes, or until their tops are mottled brown and bubbly.

C O O K I N G
for Iron—*continued*

Meanwhile, prepare a sauce by pouring the marinade into a small saucepan. Add the mustard and bring the sauce to a boil slowly, whisking constantly. When the sauce becomes thick and reduced by one-quarter, remove from heat and serve it with the hens.

TOTAL MUFFINS

(Makes 1 dozen)

Iron: 2.7 mg. per muffin
Calories: 124 per muffin

1¼ cups whole wheat
     flour
2   teaspoons baking
     powder
½   teaspoon ground
     cinnamon
     pinch of freshly grated
     nutmeg
½   cup chopped dried
     apricots

½   cup raisins
1   cup Total cereal
1   cup buttermilk
2   eggs
2   tablespoons safflower
     oil
⅓   cup molasses

Preheat oven to 375°F.

In a large mixing bowl, sift together the flour, baking powder, cinnamon, and nutmeg. Add the apricots, raisins, and cereal and toss to coat the fruit and cereal with flour.

Combine the buttermilk, eggs, oil, and molasses in a large bowl. Add the buttermilk mixture to the flour mixture and fold until just combined.

Spray muffin tins with no-stick spray and fill each cup ⅔ full. Bake for about 20 minutes, or until the muffins test done when a knife is inserted.

(continued)

C O O K I N G

for Iron—*continued*

SILKY HERBED PÂTÉ

(Makes 6 servings)

Iron: 6.8 mg. per serving
Calories: 122 per serving

1 teaspoon olive oil	1 bay leaf
1 medium onion, chopped	1 pound chicken or calf's liver
2 cloves garlic, chopped	¼ cup part-skim ricotta cheese
½ teaspoon dried marjoram	sprigs of parsley, for garnish
¼ teaspoon dried thyme pinch of freshly ground nutmeg	

In a large no-stick sauté pan, heat the oil. Add the onions, garlic, marjoram, thyme, nutmeg, and bay leaf and sauté for about 5 minutes or until the onion has wilted. Add the liver (if using calf's liver, chop it into pieces first) and continue to sauté for an additional 10 minutes, or until the liver has cooked through.

Remove the bay leaf and scoop the liver mixture into a food processor or blender. Process the mixture until it forms a silky pâté. Then, while the motor is still running, add the ricotta and process until combined.

Refrigerate the pâté, covered, until it's chilled.

Garnish with sprigs of parsley, if desired. Serve with crusty bread, crackers, tiny sliced sweet pickles and coarse mustard.

Iron Content
of Selected Supplements

Dosage is one tablet or capsule unless otherwise indicated.

Supplement	Manufacturer	Mg.
Abdol with Minerals	Parke-Davis	15
Abron	O'Neal, Jones & Feldman	60
AVP Natal	A.V.P.	66
Becomco	O'Neal, Jones & Feldman	27
Belfer	O'Neal, Jones & Feldman	94
Beta-Vite with Iron Liquid (per tsp.)	North American	75
Bugs Bunny Plus Iron	Miles	15
Cal-Prenal	North American	50
Cebetinic	Upjohn	38
Centrum	Lederle	27
Cluvisol 130	Ayerst	15
Dayalets plus Iron	Abbott	18
Engram-HP	Squibb	18
Feminins	Mead Johnson	18
Femiron with Vitamins	J.B. Williams	20
Feostim	O'Neal, Jones & Feldman	20
Ferritrinsic	Upjohn	60
Filibon Tablets	Lederle	18
Flintstones Plus Iron	Miles	15
Geriamic	North American	50
Gerilets	Abbott	27
Geriplex	Parke-Davis	30
Geriplex-FS Kapseals	Parke-Davis	30
Geriplex-FS Liquid (per 2 tbsp.)	Parke-Davis	15
Geritinic	Geriatric Pharm.	195
Geritol Junior Liquid (per tsp.)	J.B. Williams	100
Geritol Junior Tablets	J.B. Williams	25
Geritol Liquid (per tsp.)	J.B. Williams	100
Geritol Tablets	J.B. Williams	50
Gerix Elixir (per 2 tbsp.)	Abbott	15
Gerizyme (per tbsp.)	Upjohn	5
Gest	O'Neal, Jones & Feldman	18
Gevrabon (per 2 tbsp.)	Lederle	15
Gevral	Lederle	18

(continued)

Supplements—*continued*

Supplement	Manufacturer	Mg.
Gevral Protein	Lederle	4
Gevral T Capsules	Lederle	27
Gevrite	Lederle	18
Iberet	Abbott	105
Iberet-500	Abbott	105
Iberet-500 Oral Solution (per tsp.)	Abbott	26
Iberet Oral Solution (per 0.6 ml.)	Abbott	26
Iberol	Abbott	105
Incremin with Iron Syrup (per tsp.)	Lederle	30
Livitamin Capsules	Beecham Labs	33
Livitamin Chewable	Beecham Labs	2
Livitamin Liquid (per tbsp.)	Beecham Labs	36
Multiple Vitamins with Iron	North American	15
Myadec	Parke-Davis	20
Natabec	Parke-Davis	150
Natalins Tablets	Mead Johnson	45
Norlac	Rowell	60
Obron-6	Pfipharmecs	33
One-A-Day Plus Iron	Miles	18
One-A-Day Vitamins Plus Minerals	Miles	18
Optilets-M-500	Abbott	20
Os-Cal Forte	Marion	17
Os-Cal Plus	Marion	17
Paladec with Minerals	Parke-Davis	5
Panuitex	O'Neal, Jones & Feldman	48
Peritinic	Lederle	100
Poly-Vi-Sol with Iron Chewable	Mead Johnson	12
Poly-Vi-Sol with Iron Drops (per 0.6 ml.)	Mead Johnson	10
Rogenic	O'Neal, Jones & Feldman	60
Simiron Plus	Merrell Dow	10
S.S.S. Tablets	S.S.S.	50
S.S.S. Tonic (per tbsp.)	S.S.S.	33
Stresstabs 600 with Iron	Lederle	27
Stresstabs 600 with Zinc	Lederle	115

Supplements—*continued*

Supplement	Manufacturer	Mg.
Stuart Formula	Stuart	18
Stuart Hematinic Liquid (per tsp.)	Stuart	22
Stuartinic	Stuart	100
Stuart Prenatal	Stuart	60
Surbex 750 with Iron	Abbott	27
Theragran-M	Squibb	12
Theragran-Z	Squibb	12
Tri-Vi-Sol with Iron Drops (per 1 ml.)	Mead Johnson	10
Unicap T	Upjohn	18
Vicon Iron	Glaxo	30
Vio-Geric	Rowell	18
Vitagett	North American	13
Vita-Kaps-M Tablets	Abbott	10
Vitamin-Mineral Capsules	North American	13
Viterra	Pfipharmecs	10
Viterra High Potency	Pfipharmecs	10
VM Preparation (per 2 tbsp.)	Roberts	50
Zymalixir Syrup (per tsp.)	Upjohn	15

Source: Adapted from the American Pharmaceutical Association, *Handbook of Nonprescription Drugs*, 7th ed. (1982), 240–57.

Note: This chart is intended only as a guide. Vitamin formulations change periodically; always read product labels for accurate and up-to-date information on their nutrient levels.

18

Zinc

Zinc's star is on the rise.

For more than a decade now, its talents have continued to unfold. Today, science has its eyes on zinc as never before, and hopes are high that it might bring relief from colds, certain skin troubles, and loss of one of life's great pleasures—the sense of taste.

Stunned by signs of marginal deficiencies among both poor and affluent Americans, nutritionists, too, have turned their attention to zinc. So have consumers. Today, this once-obscure mineral has become the main attraction for dozens of vitamin and mineral supplements. At last, zinc has come into its own.

But not without a price. For as zinc's benefits emerged, so did its ill effects. Attempts to tap its benefits occasionally went astray, bringing problems instead of solutions. Today, we know that overdoing zinc can harm even the most health conscious, especially if taken without attention to intakes of other minerals.

RECOGNIZED ROLES

The full story of zinc remains to be told. But parts of it are well known and beyond debate. Today, nutritionists agree that zinc:

- Is a component of dozens of enzymes, including some that metabolize protein, carbohydrate, and alcohol
- Plays a role in the body's synthesis of protein
- Helps to build bones
- Has a major effect on our senses of taste and smell
- Works to rid the blood of carbon dioxide
- Is involved in the making of DNA and RNA, keepers of the body's genetic information
- Provides invaluable help in the healing of wounds

Small supplemental doses of zinc also have been shown to benefit victims of acrodermatitis enteropathica, a rare inherited disorder associated with a defect of zinc uptake. The discovery was hailed as a turning point in the understanding and treatment of this unusual but serious disease. It had baffled medical experts for many years.

Nutritionists also consider zinc to be involved in the blood-making process. Much of the blood's zinc is found in its red blood cells. Though its exact role there remains unknown, chances are good that it is an important one.

THE COLD WAR

Obviously, zinc's list of credits is impressive. Yet by all indications, there will be more. Researchers are testing zinc's potential as therapy for a variety of health problems. Though these treatments remain experimental, I think you might like to know what's on the drawing board.

The most recent and memorable event in zinc research didn't come from a scientist working in the laboratory. Its origins were far humbler, in the Texas home of an urban planner, George Eby. On the day that made zinc history, Mr. Eby's 3-year-old daughter, a leukemia patient, refused to swallow her daily zinc supplement, due to a cold that made swallowing too painful. Instead, she kept the zinc gluconate tablet in her mouth, where it dissolved slowly, like a lozenge.

A few hours later, Mr. Eby was stunned to find that her symptoms seemed to have vanished. He attempted to duplicate the findings with his own colds, and asked family, friends, and medical experts to do the same. Intrigued and astonished by successful results, Mr. Eby mounted a full-fledged scientific trial.

Mr. Eby enlisted the help of William Halcomb, M.D., and nutrition scientist Donald R. Davis, Ph.D. Together, they recruited dozens of cold sufferers to test zinc gluconate. They gave some of the volunteers zinc gluconate tablets; others, zinc-free look-alikes. No one knew who had the real thing or the impostor.

The procedure was simple; at the start of a cold, the volunteers were to dissolve two tablets in their mouths, for 10 to 20 minutes. Thereafter, they sucked on one tablet every 2 hours—except during sleep. Each tablet contained 23 milligrams (mg.) of zinc (about 150 percent of the U.S. Recommended Daily Allowance). With the frequent doses, the supplemental zinc amounted to 100 to 200 mg. daily.

The results took the medical world by surprise. The unknowing users of zinc gluconate recovered from their colds an average of seven days sooner than recipients of the zinc-free tablets.

The gratified research team wants to conduct more studies and hopes others will also. If all goes well, a firm judgment may be possible within a few years.

Incidentally, the researchers say that their findings apply only to treatment, not prevention, of the common cold.

THE WORD ON WOUND HEALING

The skin holds 20 percent of the body's zinc. More likely than not, such a generous portion resides there for good reason. Hoping to uncover it, dermatologists have tried zinc therapy for a variety of skin disorders, especially in those patients responding poorly to conventional treatment.

So far, efforts to improve healing of burns with supplemental zinc have not succeeded. Researchers are still studying and debating, however, about the effect of zinc on other skin problems.

Everyone agrees, for instance, that the body needs a certain amount of zinc to assist in the process of wound healing. Whether zinc intakes that push the body's supply still higher can provide additional benefits remains unsettled. The six or so studies on record have yielded conflicting results. Some, but not others, have found zinc therapy to speed healing of surgical excisions and leg ulcers.

No one knows, of course, how to account for the conflicting

results. However, those who healed more quickly when supplemented with zinc may have had undiagnosed deficiencies. Their response to zinc may have occurred simply from restoring zinc nutrition to par.

One study, for example, found patients with leg ulcers to have lower blood zinc levels than a comparison group of ulcer-free subjects. With supplementation, blood zinc rose by at least 25 percent in 10 of the 15 ulcer patients, suggesting that positive responses to zinc resulted from correcting an underlying deficiency. Those who didn't respond to supplemental zinc probably had their fair share from the start.

Skeptics of zinc's role argue that leg ulcers come and go so unpredictably that the positive results were simply coincidence. I am not skeptical enough to agree.

MORE ZINC MAYBES

Later in this chapter, we will look closely at the all-important interaction between zinc and copper. As I will explain then, an appreciation of how these two minerals work together is essential before taking supplemental zinc. Otherwise, healthy individuals who take zinc to maintain their good health may actually jeopardize it.

However, this interaction between minerals may greatly benefit those with Wilson's disease. Victims of this rare, genetic disorder store too much copper. The excess copper accumulates in the liver and the brain, creating a life-threatening situation if left untreated.

Experimental treatment with zinc is now in progress; hopefully, this therapy will help to prevent the excessive storage of copper. I am happy that, so far, good results have been reported in a few patients treated with supplemental zinc.

If success continues, zinc therapy may prove to be a valuable alternative to conventional treatment. An effective drug, penicillamine, is available to treat Wilson's disease; however, its side effects may become severe enough to force some patients to abandon treatment. An effective but less toxic alternative would be a major advance. Let's hope that zinc therapy will win the distinction.

Researchers are also experimenting with zinc in the treatment of sickle-cell anemia. Again, the results look promising. However, the zinc must be coupled with copper and administered under special conditions in order to be effective.

Another exciting development involves zinc therapy in treatment of taste disorders. Some victims may be suffering from little more than zinc deficiency. Many of those affected are elderly, but in one case, the beneficiary was an anorexic teenager. It's not clear which came first—the anorexia or the zinc deficiency—but her sense of taste seemed impaired. With zinc therapy, her appetite and sense of taste improved.

According to *Facts and Comparisons*, a classic drug manual for physicians, experimental zinc therapy also has been attempted to treat acne and rheumatoid arthritis, and to strengthen the immune system in the elderly. The editors comment that "data are insufficient to recommend these uses." In other words, effectiveness against these conditions remains to be established. Even when zinc therapy has failed, however, invaluable information about its safety has come to light. In fact, without these pioneering efforts, the safety of zinc supplementation would be unknown.

WHAT DEFICIENCY DOES

The original zinc pioneers were those who documented the effects of deficiency. They searched the globe looking for naturally occurring zinc deficiency. Their search took them to Egypt and Iran, where they documented classic cases in young boys. The key symptoms included decreased growth, enlarged spleen, and delayed sexual maturation. Supplemental zinc reversed the symptoms, confirming zinc deficiency as their cause.

American diets almost always provide enough zinc to prevent symptoms such as these. Of course, individuals who have disorders interfering with zinc nutrition may succumb to serious deficiency. In these cases, however, the diet is rarely to blame.

Nonetheless, a milder form of dietary zinc deficiency does occur in the United States. It has been reported most commonly among children—both poor and affluent. Children affected have poor appetite, suboptimal growth, and reduced sense of taste and smell. Mood changes may also occur.

Adults also may suffer from marginal deficiencies affecting their appetite, mood, and senses of taste and smell. Other symptoms of zinc deficiency may include scaliness of the skin, delayed wound healing, depression, fatigue, hair loss, diarrhea, and reduced resistance to infection.

AN INTERNATIONAL IRONY

Zinc deficiency has the ironic distinction of afflicting both wealthy and poor nations. The reason, strangely enough, is that both too much and too little food processing can lead the way.

In the United States, where zinc deficiencies are generally mild, affluence has brought increased reliance on processed foods. Unfortunately, some manufacturing techniques involved can remove much of the naturally occurring zinc in foods.

As the zinc comes out at the factory, additives that interfere with its absorption may go in. Among these are EDTA, an additive commonly found in canned foods, beer, soft drinks, and products rich in vegetable oils. EDTA traps metal impurities that can migrate into food from processing equipment, protecting consumers from exposure to unwanted metals and preserving the taste, color, and shelf life of foods. But zinc happens to be a metal also, and EDTA should be able to trap it, too. In addition, a variety of phosphorus-containing additives that are widely used in food processing may reduce absorption as well.

The picture is not entirely bleak, however. Processing can also work in zinc's favor by removing naturally occurring substances that adversely affect absorption. Furthermore, diets rich in processed foods usually come with a second safety factor— ample intakes of animal products. Flesh foods such as meats and seafood provide generous amounts of zinc. Nutritionists are virtually certain that the zinc in flesh foods is better absorbed than the zinc in nonflesh foods.

THE FIBER AND PHYTATE DEBATE

Highly processed diets are one extreme; diets consisting almost exclusively of unprocessed whole grain foods are the other. Such diets often contain more zinc than American fare, yet are associated with more severe zinc deficiencies than found in the United States.

This puzzling situation results partly from substances in

whole grain foods that interfere with zinc absorption. The two best known are fiber and phytate. Fruits and vegetables contain fiber, of course, but as a group are not major sources of phytates.

I'll bet you think fiber and whole grain foods are good for you. Don't worry—you are right. The effects of fiber and phytates on zinc absorption are not grounds to abandon fiber-rich foods and their many health benefits. Let me explain.

First, fiber and phytate probably are not powerful enough to prevent absorption of all zinc in whole grain foods. Moreover, these two zinc-blockers are likely to do significant damage only when whole grain foods constitute an enormous part of the diet. In addition, the phytate problem may be limited to unleavened whole grain foods such as cereals and flatbreads. Research has found that yeast and fermentation can break down phytates. The vast majority of whole grain breads in the United States are yeast-leavened.

I also doubt that fiber and phytate alone account for severe zinc deficiencies in populations that rely heavily on whole grain foods. These diets also contain little, if any, of the meat and seafood that provide zinc in its best-absorbed form. I think that severe diet-induced deficiencies probably result from both the absence of animal products and an excessive intake of whole grains. Diets such as these are very uncommon in the United States and industrialized countries.

ABOUT BRAN THERAPY

That loaf of whole wheat bread on your table may threaten your zinc nutrition less than previously believed, thanks to its yeast-leavening. But unprocessed bran and bran cereals contain no yeast. These foods may pose a problem if used frequently.

Bran therapy has earned its place in the treatment of a variety of digestive disorders. If you have a condition that responds well to bran therapy, I feel that such treatment must take precedence over the hypothetical fear of zinc deficiency.

In my experience, high bran consumption is usually practiced for medical reasons. But whatever the reason, if your intake is high (more than one serving a day), a multimineral supplement providing the recommended allowance for zinc and copper may be all you need to have your bran and good zinc nutrition, too. To minimize any effect of bran on the supplement, try not to take them at the same time.

TESTING FOR ZINC

Defining zinc deficiency isn't always as easy as physicians and nutritionists would like. No one method is considered foolproof. Most professionals, however, measure the zinc content of the blood or hair to test for deficiency.

In research reports, I found blood zinc analysis to be used more commonly than analysis of hair. No one considers it a perfect measure, however—time of day, birth control pills, and various diseases can affect the reading. Nonetheless, a blood zinc level below 90 (micrograms per milliliter) is usually accepted as evidence of zinc deficiency.

Analyzing the zinc content of hair also has its limitations. Factors such as hair color, the environment, and how the sample is prepared can affect the results. Nevertheless, researchers still use hair analysis to study zinc. The reading is considered useful in assessing zinc nutrition, provided that the individual's hair is growing. When malnutrition already has affected hair growth, analysis of hair zinc may provide misleading information.

Is there a better way? Sometimes. The best proof of zinc deficiency is the presence of some of its typical symptoms, followed by their improvement or disappearance after supplementation with zinc.

THE LIFESTYLE FACTORS

Geography is but one factor in zinc nutrition. How we live also affects our chances of succumbing to deficiencies. Various lifestyle factors that may compromise zinc nutrition have been identified. The most important follow.

STRENUOUS EXERCISE AND HOT CLIMATES. Zinc is lost in sweat at a rate significant for even the average person. Those who exercise strenuously, losing large amounts of sweat in the process, may have increased zinc needs. Similarly, individuals who live in a very hot climate and spend much time outdoors also may have higher needs as a result of perspiring heavily.

INSTITUTIONAL DIETS. According to one report, the zinc content of meals served in institutions—such as boarding schools

(continued on page 404)

The Diet Detective
Zeroes In on Zinc

Zinc deficiency knows no boundaries; young and old, rich and poor may be affected. In the United States, of course, severe deficiency has proved unlikely. Nonetheless, laboratory evidence of marginal deficiencies—particularly among children and the elderly—have prompted many to wonder about the zinc content of their own diets.

Although information about the zinc content of basic foods has become available in recent years, only a handful of food companies include zinc with the nutrition information on their product labels, for doing so is optional under FDA regulations. As a result, few manufacturers have measured zinc when analyzing the nutritional value of their products.

Nonetheless, you can estimate your daily intake from the zinc information available for basic foods. Of course, your result will be less precise than one considering the zinc in brand name foods, especially if you frequently eat the packaged combination meals that are so popular today. If your diet consists mostly of basic foods, however, your estimate won't be affected much by the missing information.

The method here is the same as for previous diet quizzes. On a day that you are eating as you normally do, jot down the number of points for any of the following foods that were included in your daily menu. Please keep in mind that, unless otherwise noted, the point values for fresh meats refer to cooked, not raw, portions.

1 point

⅓ can clam chowder
⅓ can cream of mushroom soup
⅓ can cream of tomato soup
½ medium avocado, peeled
1 cup green beans
1 cup cabbage
1 cup carrots
1 cup chick-peas
½ cup creamed corn
1 medium baked potato
1 cup raw spinach
1 cup canned tomatoes
½ cup tomato sauce with meat

½ cup tomato sauce with mushrooms

1 cup frozen mixed vegetables

1 ounce granola

1 ounce puffed rice cereal

1 ounce Total cereal

1 ounce Wheat Flakes cereal

1 ounce imported Camembert cheese

1 slice cheddar cheese

1 ounce low-fat processed cheese

2 medium oatmeal cookies

½ cup bread pudding

½ cup rice pudding

1 large whole egg

4 ounces gefilte fish

4 ounces trout, breaded and fried

4 ounces smoked fish

½ medium mango

1 cup noninstant white rice

1 medium bagel

2 slices corn-molasses bread

2 slices Italian bread

2 slices pumpernickel bread

2 slices white bread

1 ounce corn chips

1 cup macaroni

1 dinner or hard roll

1 cup cranberry-apple juice

1 cup pineapple juice

½ chicken breast

1 frankfurter (pork and beef blend)

1 ounce roasted almonds

6–8 cashews

10–12 filberts

2 points

⅓ can beef noodle soup

1 medium baked potato with skin

1 cup instant mashed potatoes

1 cup spinach

1 ounce puffed oat cereal

1 ounce 40% Bran cereal

1 tablespoon toasted wheat germ

1 ounce shredded wheat

1 cup creamed cottage cheese

1 ounce Gouda cheese

1 ounce mozzarella cheese

1 ounce Muenster cheese

1 ounce cheese spread

1 cup frozen macaroni and cheese

1 slice frozen pizza

7 ounces canned beef ravioli

4–5 hard-shell clams

4 ounces canned salmon

(continued)

The Diet Detective—
Zinc (continued)

4 ounces whitefish fillet
1 cup oatmeal
1 cup brown rice
2 slices rye bread
2 slices whole wheat bread
3 medium pancakes
4 ounces white meat chicken
½ chicken breast, with skin
1 chicken leg, with skin
2 slices bologna
1 beef frankfurter
1 cup milk
1 cup plain yogurt
4 medium Brazil nuts
¼ cup roasted peanuts

3 points
1 cup dry beans, red or white
1 cup lima beans
1 cup lentils
1 cup peas
1 ounce Parmesan cheese
½ cup corned beef hash
2 ounces braunschweiger

7 ounces frozen cheese ravioli
7 ounces canned spaghetti and meatballs
6 medium shrimp
4 ounces corned beef

4 points
4 ounces white meat turkey
½ cup chopped chicken liver
1 cup canned shrimp
1 8-ounce can surf clams

5 points
1 cup lobster meat
4 ounces dark meat chicken

6 points
4 ounces lean pork
4 ounces ham

7 points
4 ounces lean veal
4 ounces ground beef
4 ounces lean roast lamb
4 ounces dark meat turkey

and orphanages—sometimes falls short of the usual American intake of 10 to 15 mg. daily. One survey found the average institutional diet to provide about 9 mg. of zinc daily.

VEGETARIANISM. As a group, vegetarians have slightly lower, but still normal, blood zinc levels as compared to meat-eaters. However, subnormal blood zinc levels have been found

8 points
4 ounces beef liver

9 points
1 cup black-eyed peas
1 cup crabmeat
4 ounces lean roast beef
1 cup chicken gizzards

10 points
1 cup chicken hearts
1 cup calf liver

11 points
4 ounces London broil
   (beef)

20 points
½ 12-ounce can raw
   Pacific oysters

170 points
½ 12-ounce can raw
   Atlantic oysters

Scoring
Calculate your total number of points; multiply it by 5. The result is an estimate of the percentage of the U.S. RDA for zinc in your diet on the test day. If you scored 12 points, for instance, multiply 12 by 5 for a score of 60 percent of the U.S. RDA.

Because the zinc content of many foods remains unavailable, keep in mind that your score is a very approximate one. There is no simple way to account for unlisted sources of zinc in your diet, though you can assume that your zinc intake probably exceeds your score. However, if your estimate comes to only 40 percent or 50 percent of the allowance, even the uncounted zinc is unlikely to bring your true intake up to 100 percent.

among some vegetarians in the United States. Those who restrict their diets primarily to fruits and vegetables are most likely to be affected.

Female vegetarians chose this type of diet more often than vegetarian men. Male vegetarians are more likely to include generous amounts of grains, legumes, nuts, and dairy products in their diet—a pattern that provides a better zinc intake. I believe that vegetarians who do include a wide range of nonflesh foods in their diet do not have a significantly higher risk of deficiency than meat-eaters.

HIGH-FIBER DIETS. Vegetarians aren't alone in consuming fiber-rich diets. Meat-eaters who insist on whole grain cereals and breads and/or fiber-rich fruits and vegetables can consume as much fiber as some vegetarians.

As I explained in the earlier sections about fiber, phytate, and bran, I don't think that many Americans risk zinc deficiency by eating this way; actually, I think the benefits outweigh the risks. The fiber content of such a diet is more likely to be moderate than high, and I have yet to see moderate fiber intakes linked to zinc deficiency.

Whole grain foods provide much more zinc than refined grains. Despite interference from fiber and phytate, this higher zinc content may still cause us to come out ahead. To date, I have found no reports of declining zinc nutrition in the United States due to increased consumption of fiber-rich foods such as bran cereals and whole wheat bread.

When unleavened breads and cereals are eaten in large quantities, or if bran is used throughout the day, a significant risk of zinc deficiency probably exists. I would suggest a multimineral supplement, preferably taken apart from the fiber-rich foods, to be safe.

ALCOHOL-RICH DIETS. You hear much about alcohol these days, but little about its effect on zinc. Whether talked about or not, an alcohol-laden diet nonetheless is a major threat to zinc nutrition. In fact, I consider alcoholics to be at much higher risk of zinc deficiency than vegetarians who eat a wide variety of foods. Read the next section and you will know why.

ZINC AND SPECIAL CONDITIONS

Both acute and chronic illnesses may cause the body to lose excessive amounts of zinc. Surgery, burns, and multiple injuries are examples of acute problems that may cause unusually high losses.

The number of chronic conditions associated with too little zinc in the body is larger. Here is a list of disorders that may lead to low blood zinc, even when dietary intake is good.

- Alcoholism
- Chronic infections or inflammatory diseases
- Diabetes
- Kidney disease
- Pancreatic disease
- Psoriasis
- Sickle-cell anemia
- Thalassemia

Excessive losses of zinc in urine may accompany low blood zinc. In some alcoholics, zinc metabolism seems to be impaired severely, and large amounts of the mineral are excreted. Similarly, excessive losses sometimes occur with cirrhosis of the liver. Preliminary findings link diabetes with high losses as well.

Needless to say, if you have any of these conditions, periodic monitoring of your zinc levels is often recommended. With this information, your physician can best determine whether you need supplemental zinc, and if so, how much.

ZINC BY ANY OTHER NAME

That's everything that I have to say about food zinc. From here on, supplements are the issue.

Like other supplemental minerals, zinc is available in several forms. To start our discussion of supplements, let's look at those most commonly used.

ZINC SULFATE. To say that zinc research has really been zinc sulfate research is to exaggerate, but not much. Zinc sulfate accounts for almost all the supplemental zinc used in experimental therapies. As a result, we know much about this form, but little about the others.

About 22 percent zinc by weight, zinc sulfate is available in both prescription and over-the-counter supplements. Drug companies catering to the medical profession tend to favor zinc sulfate. By contrast, companies that sell supplements directly to consumers seem to offer zinc gluconate more often.

ZINC GLUCONATE. Scientific research has shunned zinc gluconate, probably because it is less concentrated than zinc sulfate. Zinc gluconate is about 14 percent zinc by weight. Supplements containing zinc gluconate are available widely through mail-order supplement companies, health food stores, and other sources serving consumers directly.

So far, this source of zinc has earned one distinction. Zinc gluconate tablets used as lozenges have been found to help speed recovery from the common cold. Zinc sulfate has not been tested to determine whether it has similar potential.

ZINC ACETATE. I have yet to see zinc acetate in the drugstore. If some leading researchers are right, however, it may appear there soon. Ananda S. Prasad, M.D., one of the world's leading zinc researchers, and his coworkers have reported that this form of zinc causes less gastrointestinal upset than zinc sulfate—at least at the high doses studied so far. Dr. Prasad, a professor of medicine at Wayne State University in Indiana, and his colleagues have switched some of their zinc-supplemented patients to this form.

CHELATED ZINC. Medical journals contain virtually no information about the safety of chelated zinc. Though the gluconate or acetate form of zinc has replaced zinc sulfate in a few studies, chelated zinc has not. As a result, we have no specifics about its side effects or the often-heard claims that this type of zinc is better absorbed.

Nonetheless, if you prefer this form of zinc, I see no reason to insist that other forms are better, or vice versa. If price matters to you, however, note that chelated minerals often cost considerably more than supplements made from other sources.

ZINC PYRITHIONE. This form of zinc, also known as zinc pyridine or ZPT, *is not for oral use*. Accordingly, supplements do not contain it. ZPT is an antidandruff agent found in dandruff shampoos and medicated hair conditioners. A few users have developed irritated, dry skin after using these products. Tests have confirmed ZPT to be the cause.

Cases such as these are extremely rare. One manufacturer has estimated that 100 million people in the United States and the United Kingdom have used products containing ZPT. Yet, you can count on one hand the number of adverse reactions that have been published in medical journals.

ZINC SAFETY: AN OVERVIEW

Just how safe are the forms of zinc available in supplements? And at what doses?

"The range between usual dietary levels and toxic levels of zinc is wide," says mineral expert Harold H. Sanstead, M.D., of the U.S. Department of Agriculture. "For practical purposes, zinc is nontoxic when compared to copper, selenium, lead, cadmium, and mercury."

Dr. Sanstead notes that most cases of toxicity have been job-related, the result of workers inhaling zinc in an industrial environment. Just as supplements given by injection usually pose much greater risks than those taken orally, so may occupational exposure. Evaluating the safety of zinc supplements based on the effects of constant on-the-job exposure to zinc-containing fumes is difficult, to say the least.

Regardless, whether you agree with Dr. Sanstead's assessment of zinc safety depends on your definition of "toxicity." If you consider only serious reactions observed within a few days to several years of supplementation, you will have no argument. But if you include annoying side effects or the threat of mineral imbalances during long-term use, you will find yourself ready to debate.

A SAGA OF SIDE EFFECTS

Without a doubt, zinc researchers have gone about their work with remarkable consistency. Whether trying to help patients with acne, surgical wounds, or leg ulcers, most of these zinc pioneers adhered to a standard dose of three 50 mg. doses per day, each taken with food or milk. On such a regimen, supplements provided a total of 150 mg. of zinc daily, in addition to the 10 to 15 mg. usually supplied by food.

Despite the consistent approach, the side effects recorded in the process could hardly be less consistent. In the best case, only 1 of 37 members of the U.S. Air Force suffered any side effects from the zinc therapy just described. Better still, the zinc had a positive effect on their recovery from surgical excisions. The one airman who complained of stomach discomfort failed to follow directions not to take the supplement before eating. His distress disappeared when, like the others, he took the zinc after meals or with milk.

A few facts about this study stand out. First, the subjects were young adults, an average of 25 years old. Second, the physicians in charge monitored their zinc therapy for only 2 to 3 months, a rather short period for making firm conclusions. The doctors do mention, however, that some of their patients have received this treatment for as long as 22 months, with no complaints of side effects or signs of toxicity.

Several other studies also have reported impressive tolerance to 150 mg. daily of zinc, with ill effects generally limited to a minority of patients who experienced mild nausea. But probing further, some far poorer results come into view.

THE YOUNGEST AND THE OLDEST

Some time ago, zinc sulfate became a household word among teenagers plagued with acne. Hopes were high that it would prove useful in treating this adolescent scourge.

But when its ability to fight acne was tested, the side effects stood out far more than the success rate. Though one key study found that zinc sulfate helped alleviate one of the half dozen or so lesions characteristic of acne, the side effects greatly outweighed the one benefit. Fully half of the participants experienced nausea, vomiting, or diarrhea. About 20 percent of the subjects, whose ages ranged from 14 to 25, found the side effects too severe to continue the zinc treatment.

In a second similar study, the drop-out rate was still higher; 30 percent of patients stopped taking zinc therapy due to severe side effects. One small consolation emerged; the severity of acne lessened in about 10 percent of those who took zinc treatment for four months.

Turning from these youngest users to the oldest, the picture does not change much. In an important test of its safety, almost 40 percent of elderly subjects who took zinc therapy had digestive complaints, predominately diarrhea. More often than not, the severity of side effects subsided as treatment continued, but 2 of 16 patients had to stop taking the zinc.

No other significant side effects occurred in these elderly patients, but their blood cholesterol levels increased an average of 7 mg. after 23 weeks of zinc. Later on, we will look in more detail at zinc's effects on blood fats and heart health.

Though various digestive upsets account for almost all side effects during zinc therapy, restlessness also has been reported. A far worse outcome, however, occurred in a 21-year-old acne patient. Though known to have an ulcer, it was causing no symptoms, so he and his doctors decided to try zinc therapy. Before long, the ulcer was perforated, and he ended up in the operating room. Surgeons there repaired the damage, which no doubt resulted from the irritating properties of zinc taken at high doses.

SULFATE VERSUS GLUCONATE

Obviously, zinc sulfate has had a virtual monopoly in medical research. Every study mentioned in the two preceding sections involved zinc sulfate. Other forms of zinc may or may not be equally troublesome at similarly high doses. As mentioned earlier, one research team has found zinc acetate to be better tolerated than zinc sulfate.

But zinc acetate isn't an option that I currently see on the supplement shelf. Zinc gluconate is, and whether it might cause fewer or less severe side effects than zinc sulfate needs to be determined—as soon as possible. I have searched for even one study comparing the two, but unfortunately, to no avail. However, a few reports of zinc gluconate used to treat special conditions shed some light on its safety. However, the earliest reports involved much lower doses than the 150 mg. daily provided in most studies of zinc sulfate.

A leukemia patient, for instance, reportedly took zinc gluconate in doses providing about 43 mg. of zinc daily, without signs of trouble. Two infants also seemed to tolerate this form well when given in three divided doses that provided a total daily dosage of 30 to 45 mg. of zinc.

Experience with zinc gluconate at higher levels is limited to findings from the common cold study described earlier in this chapter. About 25 percent of participants complained of one or more digestive complaints (nausea, stomach discomfort, vomiting, and diarrhea). This rate is much better than found in some studies of zinc sulfate, but much worse than recorded in others.

Unlike many who tried zinc sulfate, though, few zinc gluconate users actually stopped taking the supplements. This hints that the severity of digestive upsets was milder than experienced by those who started on zinc sulfate but stopped due to severe side effects.

On the other hand, the zinc gluconate tablets had only half the potency of the zinc sulfate, and doses were spread throughout the day (every 2 hours as compared to three times daily for zinc sulfate). The smaller but more frequent doses alone may account for any milder side effects. Regardless, the zinc gluconate users found, to no one's surprise, that taking their zinc "lozenge" with food prevented nausea and vomiting.

To make a definitive judgment as to whether zinc gluconate has fewer side effects than zinc sulfate, both would have to be administered the same way. Until put to such a test, no one can be certain that one is preferable to the other.

Moreover, the issue may become moot if other sources of zinc prove to have fewer side effects than either of these two. And when dosages are much smaller—in the range of the Recommended Dietary Allowances (RDA)—many, if not most, users may experience little or no differences in side effects regardless of the source of zinc.

LIFE WITH THE LOZENGES

Digestive complaints aside, zinc gluconate tablets used as lozenges produced a unique set of side effects. About 15 percent of subjects complained of mouth irritation, distorted sense of taste, or the unpleasant taste of the lozenge. When zinc is swallowed, rather than dissolved in the mouth, such complaints are rarely, if ever, heard.

However, these complaints about mouth irritation and the taste of zinc gluconate tablets must be viewed in perspective. The tablets taken were plain ones designed for swallowing. Instead, users sucked on them for 10 to 20 minutes.

Manufacturing the zinc specifically as a lozenge—either with a coating or in the familiar form resembling hard candy—might help alleviate such complaints. Regardless, most of those affected willingly tolerated these side effects as a small price to pay for the reported benefits to their colds.

THE DOSAGE DECISIONS

Regardless of the form used, I think a few facts about zinc supplements are obvious. First, tolerance to high doses varies dramatically from one person to another. Second, the available information hints that side effects are more likely to occur in adolescents and the elderly than in young adults. Finally, taking supplemental zinc with food minimizes side effects.

Reducing the risk of side effects by taking zinc with food probably comes at the expense of lesser absorption. But once again, less does not mean none. Increases in blood zinc levels have occurred in individuals who took zinc therapy with food, making clear that some was absorbed. Therefore, the recommendation to take these high-potency supplements with food stands—unless your physician feels that you need to sacrifice the protective effect of food for better absorption.

Of course, this advice to take zinc with meals grew out of patient experience with 50 mg. doses taken three times a day. At a lower dose, some individuals may have no problems taking supplemental zinc without food. Unfortunately, no one knows how low a dose is required to avoid the need for food. The answer, if known, would certainly vary from one person to another.

Nonetheless, I have found no reports of side effects caused by standard multiple vitamin tablets also containing zinc. Surely some users take these tablets at bedtime, without food. As these products generally contain 15 mg. of zinc (the U.S. RDA), I have a hunch that doses on this order, taken once a day, may be unlikely to bother an empty stomach.

GOING OVERBOARD

If you think that 150 mg. of zinc daily sounds high, I have a story you must hear. It's about a 16-year-old boy, Randy, who took 25 to 50 times the already sizable therapeutic dose of 150 mg. Fortunately, he took only two doses, on two successive days.

The following excerpt tells the tale. It is taken from a report that Jerome V. Murphy, M.D., published in the *Journal of the American Medical Association*.

> A 16-year-old boy was admitted to the U.S. Air Force Hospital ... complaining of lethargy which had lasted for five days. Nine and eight days before admission, the patient had ingested 4 and 8 grams [4,000–8,000 mg.] respectively of elemental zinc mixed with peanut butter. He had intended to promote the healing of a minor laceration as suggested in a then recent magazine report.
> Five days prior to admission, the patient had diffi-

culty in awakening after a full night's sleep, and later that day, he slept during school. The lethargy increased over the ensuing days. On the morning of admission he was difficult to arouse. Once awakened, he consumed a normal breakfast, and then returned to sleep, while sitting on a kitchen stool. Other symptoms included light-headedness, slight staggering of gait, and difficulty in writing legibly.

Dr. Murphy immediately suspected zinc poisoning. The diagnosis was confirmed with a test of Randy's blood zinc level; it was abnormally high. Randy was started on treatment with a zinc-binding drug 6 hours after being admitted to the hospital. Within 12 hours, his alertness improved. The next day he awoke at 6 A.M., his normal waking time.

A month later, Randy was reexamined; no consequences from his zinc overdose were found. Of course, he had been lucky. His excessive sleeping, staggering, and trouble writing after taking the zinc suggested ill effects on the areas of the brain controlling coordination and sleep. Were it not for prompt treatment, the excessive zinc might have accumulated and remained in his brain. The consequences of this are unknown; however, I feel that any potential effect on the brain is a serious matter.

THE COPPER ROBBER

At the time of Randy's experience, the record had shown that some adults suffered no adverse effects from a daily dose of 150 mg. taken for a few months to two years. That dosage was fully ten times the recommended allowance, yet it seemed to agree with many who took it.

For years, all looked well with those who could tolerate 100 to 150 mg. daily. But a silent storm was brewing. No one had anticipated that improvement of zinc nutrition with high-potency supplements could deplete the body's supply of a different but equally essential mineral.

The lesson was learned the hard way. Physicians had prescribed high doses of zinc in hopes of helping their patients, but several who followed the regimen for more than a year grew increasingly ill. The cause was copper deficiency induced by zinc therapy.

Those affected developed severe anemias, marked by inadequate blood copper levels and abnormal results on tests for iron deficiency. Fortunately, recovery followed after copper supplementation, and/or withdrawal of the offending zinc. In the three cases detailed below, copper nutrition returned to normal in a month or two.

TRUE TALES OF TOO LITTLE COPPER

The stories are true ones, taken from medical journals. The first two cases, both reported in the late 1970s, resulted from zinc therapy prescribed by doctors. The lesson learned—the importance of balancing zinc and copper—traveled quickly in medical circles.

Unfortunately, the new findings did not reach all consumers. In 1985, the *Annals of Internal Medicine* published the third case described here. This time, the damage had been done by a well-intentioned but uninformed consumer who had decided himself to take high-potency zinc supplements. Needless to say, he had not taken any additional copper.

The histories that follow are excerpted from reports submitted to medical journals by the patients' doctors. The first case, reported in 1977, concerns a woman referred to as Mrs. L. G.:

> *This 59-year-old woman had had several admissions to hospital for investigation of malabsorption and symptoms of nerve disease. Zinc (150 mg. daily) had been prescribed in November, 1975, for non-responsive celiac disease, and the patient had continued to take this oral supplement.*
>
> *In January, 1977 [14 months later], she presented with symptoms of severe anemia [extremely low hemoglobin and hematocrit, too few white blood cells, and abnormally low levels of copper in both blood and hair].*
>
> *She was treated [with blood] transfusion, the zinc supplements were withdrawn, and oral copper given daily. After 12 days, the blood copper had risen [to a normal level]. After 4 weeks she was discharged with a normal blood picture.*
>
> K. G. Porter, M.D., and coworkers
Queens University of Belfast

A 26-year-old black man with sickle cell anemia was admitted in February 1973 for [routine testing]. Results of his laboratory studies were compatible with anemia due to sickle cell disease.

The patient received 150 mg. zinc daily. Initially it was given because of possible zinc deficiency and for possible benefit to [a] leg ulcer. The ulcer healed by November 1973. [He continued to take 150 mg. of zinc daily, though the dose schedule was changed from 50 mg. three times a day to 25 mg. six times a day.]

In January 1975, the patient complained of considerable [stomach] distress attributed in part to the zinc sulfate. He was readmitted, and his treatment was changed to zinc acetate tablets, 25 mg. six times a day. He also complained of right leg and midback pain, which was attributed to his sickle cell disease. His temperature spiked to about 100.4 degrees almost every day. In an effort to control his symptoms, he was given 25 mg. of zinc every three hours [200 mg. daily] for 40 days of hospitalization, but his clinical status did not improve.

Between February 22, 1975 and March 8, 1975, [the white blood cell count] gradually decreased. All therapies except [a pain-killer] were stopped. Bone marrow examination results showed...changes suggestive of iron deficiency.

Copper deficiency due to zinc therapy was suspected.

On April 12, 1975, one milligram of copper was administered daily. By May 6, 1975, [signs of copper nutrition] became normal.

Ananda S. Prasad, M.D., and coworkers
Wayne State University
and University of Michigan

We report the case of a patient taking more than 30 times the usual daily mixed diet content of 10 to 15 mg. of zinc for over 2 years as a treatment for "prostate trouble" ... Our patient developed sideroblastic anemia [an unusual form of anemia marked by high rather than low iron levels. Iron-laden red blood cells surrounded by *rings of iron granules also may accompany the condition. These blood cells are called ringed sideroblasts. The details follow.]*

A 57-year-old white man presented with a 6-month history of malaise and easy fatigability. Five weeks before admission, after a viral upper respiratory infection, he noted the onset of [chest and leg pain and shortness of breath after physical exertion]. Examination by his personal physician showed profound anemia, and the patient was referred to another hospital.

The patient's previous medications included zinc supplements, 450 mg./day for 2 years, and vitamin B_{12}, 2,000 mcg. during the previous 5 weeks.

The history of massive zinc ingestion suggested a connection with his sideroblastic anemia, as zinc interferes with copper absorption and copper deficiency is a known cause of sideroblastic anemia. We requested that the patient discontinue zinc supplements, and he was discharged . . . [He improved gradually, and 3 months later, appeared to have recovered fully.]

William Patterson, M.D. and coworkers
University of Missouri

Mineral experts recognized that these cases might have been isolated and atypical ones. More evidence—based on groups of people rather than single individuals—was sought.

One of the first reported victims of zinc-induced copper deficiency, for instance, had been taking high doses of zinc to combat his sickle-cell anemia. He was but 1 of 14 sickle-cell patients receiving supplements under the supervision of Dr. Prasad. Almost certain that this zinc therapy had caused the first patient's copper deficiency, Dr. Prasad tested his other 13 patients taking high doses of zinc. Seven of them tested positive for copper deficiency.

Of course, those patients already had a significant illness. No one could be sure that healthy individuals would react the same way. A few years later, Peter W. F. Fischer, Ph.D., and coworkers at the Canadian Department of Health and Welfare recruited healthy men and tested their response to daily supplementation with 50 mg. of zinc. After six weeks, the men showed signs of

Recommended Dietary Allowances for Zinc

Group/Age	Mg.
Infants 0–6 mon.	3
Infants 6–12 mon.	5
Children 1–10 yr.	10
Males 11+ yr.	15
Females 11+ yr.	15
Pregnant women	20
Nursing women	25

Note: The U.S. RDA for zinc, designed solely for nutrition labeling purposes, is 15 mg.

declining copper nutrition. It was obvious that high intakes of zinc could inhibit copper absorption in healthy people, too.

Meanwhile, another storm was approaching. It was one that would require decades—not just a year or two—to do its damage. But it was not one to be taken lightly, for at stake was America's number one killer: heart disease.

MORE SUBTLE TROUBLE

I am sure you remember the headlines of a decade ago heralding the discovery of "good cholesterol" in the blood. Who coined the term "good cholesterol," I don't know, but given its real name—high-density lipoprotein-cholesterol—I can see why. In research circles, the term HDL-cholesterol was adopted for simplicity, and study after study found those who had higher levels of it were less likely to succumb to heart disease.

Overjoyed to find a protective factor rather than a harmful one, researchers sought for ways to increase its presence. In the process, they also discovered factors that worked against HDL-cholesterol, causing blood levels to fall. Among the villains was a high intake of supplemental zinc.

Philip Hopper, M.D., and coworkers at the Albuquerque Veterans Hospital were among the first to document zinc's effect. The men who participated in their classic study took 80 mg. of supplemental zinc daily. Over the course of five weeks, their HDL-cholesterol fell by an average of 25 percent. Unfortunately, only men were tested, and logical as it may seem to expect women to react similarly, a reasonable assumption differs from hard facts.

No one has determined whether the zinc alone or an imbalance of zinc to copper causes the HDL-cholesterol to fall. Only a handful of studies are available, and, frankly, we have more questions than answers. In particular, the effect of zinc intakes in the 30 to 80 mg. range on HDL-cholesterol are not known. But one study of low-dose supplementation found that adding about 30 mg. of zinc daily did not harm HDL-cholesterol levels in either active or sedentary men.

HDL-cholesterol is only one aspect of heart health that may be affected by zinc. The zinc-copper balance so important to prevention of copper deficiency has been at issue in relation to other risk factors for heart disease. Some interesting, but preliminary facts stand out:

• A higher zinc-to-copper ratio has been found in the heart muscle of patients with confirmed heart disease. Increasing zinc intake, of course, widens the unwelcome gap between these two minerals.
• Physical activity is linked to reduced risk of heart disease, partly because exercise increases HDL-cholesterol. Exercise also may benefit the heart by narrowing the gap between zinc and copper. Zinc is lost is sweat, thereby allowing a better balance between it and copper.
• High blood pressure, also known as hypertension, promotes heart disease. Some hypertensive patients apparently excrete large amounts of copper. This, too, furthers the imbalance between zinc and copper that may affect heart health.

I have to stress that these are only leads, not conclusions. The adverse effects of high zinc intakes on HDL-cholesterol and copper deficiency are more certain. But if you combine all the possibilities, and consider, too, the high rate of heart disease in the United States, the case for maintaining a better balance between zinc and copper becomes a strong one.

A THREAT TO IMMUNITY?

Several years ago, R. K. Chandra, M.D., of Canada's Memorial University, reported that high doses of zinc can impair the body's ability to fight infection. His research, published in the *Journal of the American Medical Association*, received widespread attention.

Dr. Chandra asked 11 men to take the typical doses used in experimental zinc therapy: 50 mg. three times a day, for six weeks. Their blood was analyzed in the laboratory, where several tests designed to measure its infection-fighting ability were performed. On some of these tests, scores declined over the six weeks of zinc supplementation.

Obviously, these tests took place outside of the body, under "test-tube" conditions. Such approaches can be meaningful, and the results admittedly are intriguing. However, Dr. Chandra did not report that the men actually suffered more infections while taking supplemental zinc.

For a broader perspective, I compared these results to previous work with zinc therapy. Though these earlier studies tested zinc's therapeutic ability against problems such as acne and wound healing, their authors watched carefully for any signs of toxicity. Many side effects (and some serious reactions) were reported, but increased susceptibility to infection was not among them. Yet, similar doses of zinc were taken longer than in the test-tube study.

With such conflicting results, I feel that commenting now on this aspect of zinc safety would be jumping to unjustified conclusions. Regardless, decisions about sensible supplementation can be made without more information about zinc's effect on immunity. Its impact on copper nutrition and heart health factors already has convinced me that long-term supplementation with high doses should be practiced only when medically necessary. Otherwise, you will serve your health better by taking more moderate doses of supplemental zinc.

THE STAR SYSTEM SHINES ON ZINC

Side effects—Like some of its fellow minerals, zinc is most likely to cause trouble in the digestive tract. The list of complaints runs the gamut, including nausea, vomiting, stomach pain, and diarrhea. Complaints such as these were voiced by up to 50 percent of those who took 150 mg. of zinc daily (from zinc sulfate).

Taking each dose with meals or milk often lessens or eliminates the side effects. Also, side effects subside gradually in some patients as treatment continues.

Zinc gluconate, another commonly available source, may produce less severe digestive upsets, but knowledge of its side effects is extremely limited. Zinc acetate—a newcomer to zinc therapy—reportedly shows less potential to upset the gastrointestinal tract than zinc sulfate, but is not yet widely available to consumers.

Under some circumstances, taking zinc on an empty stomach has been prescribed to improve absorption. However, you should do so only at your doctor's recommendation.

Acute ailments—Many prescription insulin products contain zinc, and after using them, some diabetics have had allergic reactions. Their symptoms have included pain and swelling around the injection area and hives over a large area of the body. Testing confirmed the insulin's zinc to be the offending substance in some patients. The body's greater sensitivity to injected substances may account, at least in part, for these allergic reactions. As I have said time and again, injecting a nutrient poses far more risk than taking it orally.

When taken orally, zinc has caused a small number of acute ailments. In one test group, for example, almost 30 percent of patients had to stop therapy after a week or less of the standard regimen. Though few of them reacted within hours, I feel these cases are better classified as acute ailments than as long-term problems.

Unknown, of course, is whether at least some of these individuals might have adjusted to therapy with time. And no doubt, a lower dose would have spared some victims. Needless to say, neither of these approaches would have been advisable for the young man who suffered a perforated ulcer from zinc therapy.

The one other acute ailment to note was that of the 16-year-old boy who took two astronomical doses of zinc—4,000 mg. on the first day and 8,000 mg. the second. Though he recovered, he had exposed himself to a serious hazard offering no benefits at all.

Long-term problems—To me, the most important problems related to supplemental zinc are those that develop slowly. In terms of symptoms, some of these reactions will resemble acute ailments, differing only in the time required for development of symptoms. A more insidious problem, however, is zinc's ability to interfere with copper absorption. The threat of copper deficiency should be taken seriously whenever high-potency supplementation is practiced for more than a few months.

Most worrisome of all is zinc's potential to reduce levels of HDL-cholesterol—the "good cholesterol" that helps to prevent heart disease. The impact on heart health would be slow and gradual, but ultimately could be very serious. And as also discussed earlier, altered zinc-copper balance due to excessive zinc intake may harm the heart in other ways as well. Limiting long-term supplementation to modest levels is best; if that's not possible, the blood pressure and cholesterol profile should be monitored.

Conflicting combinations—Clearly, zinc can interfere with absorption of copper; the interaction is beyond dispute. But calcium, in turn, may have a similar effect on zinc. Much less is known about this possible interaction, particularly whether it is potent enough to affect zinc absorption significantly.

Actually, authorities differ as to whether calcium alone can interfere with zinc. Some believe that calcium must be accompanied by phytates (as in whole grain foods) to do so; others believe that calcium alone can reduce zinc absorption. I have found no reports of zinc deficiencies in healthy people resulting from high intakes of calcium alone or calcium with phytates. After all, healthy meals are more likely than poorly balanced ones to contain significant amounts of calcium, zinc, and phytates.

For most of us, worrying about taking zinc at the same time as calcium or calcium and whole grains appears unnecessary. I also would not want to make a blanket statement against use of multiminerals containing both calcium and zinc. However, if you need to maximize absorption of either mineral, I would try to separate some of your zinc from calcium.

If you want to enhance calcium absorption, for example, you might be taking supplemental calcium several times daily. If you also are taking a zinc supplement, you might do best by taking the zinc at breakfast, with calcium supplements at other meals or at bedtime. (Depending on the form of calcium, its potency, and your tolerance to it, you may need to take food or milk with a bedtime dose to prevent stomach upset.)

As for drugs that interact with zinc, tetracycline heads the list. Like calcium and iron, zinc can reduce absorption of this common antibiotic. The labels that the pharmacy puts on tetracycline bottles, unfortunately, don't include zinc among the foods, supplements, and medicines that should not be taken within an hour of the antibiotic. When tetracycline treatment is short-term, and if your doctor agrees, you can make things simpler by suspending these supplemental minerals until you finish the drug.

The zinc-tetracycline connection works both ways; tetracycline inhibits the absorption of zinc, too. Here is a more complete list of drugs that may interfere with zinc nutrition in some way. Words in parentheses are brand names.

• Antibiotics—Tetracycline (Achromycin V, Mysteclin F, and Sumycin) and its relatives, chlortetracycline (Aureomycin) and oxytetracyline (Terramycin), can decrease zinc absorption.
• Anticancer drugs—There is one published report of zinc deficiency in a patient treated with mercaptopurine (Purinethol) and methotrexate.
• Cortisone medication—This class of drugs may increase excretion of zinc. One source reports persistent wounds—a sign of zinc deficiency—in six cortisone-treated patients. Zinc supplementation restored the normal healing process.

Cortisone-containing skin creams and ointments, as well as eye or ear drops, are best known by their brand names. Tablets taken orally, however, are more often identified by their generic name. There are many types of oral tablets; among the most common are dexamethasone (Decadron), prednisone, and prednisolone (Deltasone). Additional forms include betamethasone (Celestone), desoxycortisone (Percorten), and methyl-prednisolone (Depo-Medrol, Depo-Predate).

Note that the last syllable or two of these generic names are "sone," or "solone." Such endings on a drug's generic name are a clue that it might belong to the cortisone family.
• Diuretics ("water pills")—Chlorthalidone (Combipres, Hygroton, Regreton) increases zinc excretion, as do thiazide diuretics.

See page 321 for a comprehensive list of commonly prescribed thiazides.
• Metal-binding drugs—Penicillamine (Cuprimine), used to treat the copper accumulation of Wilson's disease, binds to zinc as well as copper. Long-term use may cause zinc deficiency, with loss of taste a likely symptom.
• Oral contraceptives—Birth control pills may increase the amount of zinc in red blood cells. The significance, if any, of this change is unknown.

Finally, I would like to mention a very unusual case of zinc aggravating a syndrome referred to as drug-induced lupus. This condition should not be confused with systemic lupus erythematosus (SLE), a disease of the immune system. In drug-induced lupus, rashes and skin ulcers commonly occur. However, the syndrome frequently disappears after the offending drug is discontinued.

In the one case on record, the patient had been taking two drugs to control her blood pressure: a diuretic, hydralazine (Apresolin), and propranolol (Inderal), a drug commonly used to treat certain heart (and occasionally other) conditions. She had taken the two drugs for several years, with no clear signs of drug-related lupus. However, she had a problem with chronic leg ulcers, and her doctor eventually prescribed a large dose (135 mg. daily) of supplemental zinc as treatment for the ulcers.

Within a week, she developed a fever, severe rash, blotches of red skin, and mouth ulcers. Her doctor withdrew the zinc therapy, and her mouth ulcers and fever disappeared a few days later. Her skin eruptions and leg ulcers, however, healed only after the drugs, too, were stopped. A year later, she tried the original zinc regimen for a week and did not have a similar reaction.

Obviously, her symptoms occurred only when she took the drugs and supplemental zinc together; neither factor alone could be held responsible. Therefore, her doctors concluded that the supplemental zinc aggravated—but did not directly cause—her reaction. Rather, it made her more sensitive to the drugs, enough so to cause the lupus-like symptoms.

Hidden consequences—I have not found any reports of a high zinc intake masking the signs or diagnosis of any health problem. The mineral may affect a few laboratory tests under certain conditions. Levels of blood calcium and urine magnesium, for example, may be falsely increased if the laboratory uses a technique susceptible to interference from zinc.

In addition, zinc may falsely reduce the reading for alkaline phosphatase, an enzyme in the blood. Though commonly performed as part of a multitest health profile (such as the so-called SMAC test), the alkaline phosphatase level itself has no specific meaning. An abnormal level indicates the need to test further for any of a number of conditions that affect levels of this enzyme.

HOW MUCH IS TOO MUCH

The record is clear; some people have tolerated 150 mg. of zinc daily without the slightest side effect. Others reacted so severely to the same dose that treatment could not continue. Regardless of the outcome, however, the reporting physicians always stressed one point: *that the long-term effects of high doses are unknown.*

Of the many commentaries that have been published about zinc supplementation, I found most thoughtful some remarks by Dr. Sanstead. Looking back at many years of research at doses of 150 mg. daily, he wrote these words:

> In retrospect it does not seem reasonable to give ten times the recommended allowance for zinc (15 mg.) to patients who have a normally functioning gastrointestinal tract . . . It seems more reasonable to be therapeutically conservative and not give more than two to three times the recommended allowance for zinc [that is, 30 to 45 mg. daily] where the condition under therapy is probably nutritional in origin and not due to metabolic inhibition, intestinal malabsorption, or excessive losses caused by impaired [zinc]-conserving mechanisms . . . If amounts greatly in excess of the recommended allowance are necessary, the copper status of the individual should be carefully monitored.

I doubt that anyone would disagree. I certainly don't.

Dr. Sanstead's comments appeared several years before the discovery of zinc's potential to lower the HDL-cholesterol levels.

These and other findings relating to heart health further support the need for careful attention to dosage during long-term supplementation. Caution is especially important when one or more enemies of heart health (especially high blood cholesterol, high blood pressure, or smoking) already exist. Under these circumstances, I think you should consider skipping supplementation if your diet provides ample zinc. Otherwise, limit your dose to the recommended allowance of 15 mg. Should you need or insist on a higher dose, have your cholesterol profile monitored for your own safety.

If you have a clean bill of health and your diet contains 5 to 15 mg. of zinc, I feel that supplementation with an additional 15 to 25 mg. (for a total of 30 mg. intake per day) is unlikely to be hazardous. The risk of total intakes in the 40 mg. range has not been tested, but probably is not high.

A SECOND OPINION

At the National Research Council, the Committee on Dietary Allowances also has taken a position on long-term zinc supplementation. Citing the potential for copper deficiency, the committee advises that "chronic ingestion of zinc supplements of more than 15 mg./day, in addition to the dietary intake is not recommended without medical supervision."

I don't really object to this recommendation, though I do disagree with the reasoning. I have some doubts that supplementation with two or three times the recommended allowance for zinc would cause copper deficiency. The cases on record involved doses of 10 to 30 times the adult RDA.

I vote for caution during long-term supplementation because of our knowledge gap. In my opinion, the effect of long-term zinc intakes in the 40 to 75 mg. range are unknown. I would rather be a little cautious than too adventurous until this knowledge gap is narrowed. Until then, I admit that my conclusions are tentative. And I wouldn't be surprised if the effect of doses in this range were to vary from harmless to harmful—depending on the copper intake.

That brings me to my final point. The commercials extolling zinc as "more valuable to your health than gold" are true enough. Of the two, only zinc is essential to the body. But copper deserves lavish praise, too. Without copper, high doses of zinc can make for a bad investment.

For the best return, insist on a supplement that contains both copper and zinc in good balance. A multimineral product that provides 15 mg. of zinc and 2 to 3 mg. of copper is a good choice.

C O O K I N G
for Zinc

WARM GRILLED BEEF WITH CRACKED WHEAT SALAD

(Makes 5 servings)

Zinc: 8 mg. per serving
Calories: 411 per serving

1 pound top round of beef, about 1 inch thick	1 teaspoon black peppercorns
1 tablespoon coarse mustard	4 bay leaves
¼ cup red wine vinegar	1 cup cracked wheat
	⅓ cup minced scallions
	2 teaspoons olive oil

Set the beef in a large glass baking dish and poke some holes in it with a skewer or long-tined fork. In a small bowl, combine the mustard, vinegar, peppercorns, and 3 bay leaves. Pour the marinade over the beef, cover, and let it marinate in the refrigerator overnight.

When ready to cook, pour the cracked wheat into a large heatproof bowl and add the remaining bay leaf. Cover with boiling water and let it sit uncovered for about 25 minutes.

Meanwhile, preheat the broiler. Set the beef on a broiler pan (reserving the marinade) and broil for about 8 minutes, turning once, for medium rare. Remove it from the broiler and let it sit for a few minutes before slicing.

(continued)

C O O K I N G
for Zinc—*continued*

To assemble the salad, drain the cracked wheat and add the scallions. Strain the reserved marinade into a small saucepan and heat through. Add the olive oil, pour over the cracked wheat, and toss well. Then mound the cracked wheat in the center of a serving dish.

Slice the beef as thinly as possible and arrange it around the cracked wheat. Serve warm with ripe red tomatoes and coarse mustard.

THAI OYSTERS

(Makes 4 servings)

Zinc: 72 mg. per serving
Calories: 119 per serving

3   cups shucked oysters
½   cup oyster liquor (juice)
1   teaspoon lemon grass, minced
3   tablespoons minced fresh basil
¼   teaspoon grated lime rind
¼   teaspoon crushed red pepper

Preheat oven to 375°F.

Scoop the oysters into a 1-quart baking dish. Combine the liquor, lemon grass, basil, lime rind, and pepper in a small bowl. Pour over the oysters and toss until well coated. Cover tightly and bake for about 10 minutes or until the oysters are opaque. Serve with rice.

C O O K I N G

for Zinc—continued

STRAWBERRY CREAM WITH CRUNCH

(Makes approximately 1 cup)

Zinc: 1.6 mg. per ⅓ cup
Calories: 235 per ⅓ cup

1 cup low-fat cottage cheese
2 tablespoons strawberry jam
¼ cup chopped Brazil nuts

Scoop the cottage cheese into a blender or food processor and process until completely smooth and creamy. Add the jam and process just enough to combine, then fold in the nuts by hand. Serve immediately or refrigerate until ready to use.

Zinc Content
of Selected Supplements

Dosage is one tablet or capsule unless otherwise indicated.

Supplement	Manufacturer	Mg.
Abdol with Minerals	Parke-Davis	0.5
Centrum	Lederle	22.5
Cluvisol Syrup (per tsp.)	Ayerst	0.5
Feminins	Mead Johnson	10.0
Gevrabon (per 2 tbsp.)	Lederle	2.0
Gevral Protein	Lederle	0.2
Gevral T Capsules	Lederle	22.5
Myadec	Parke-Davis	20.0
Norlac	Rowell	15.0
Obron-6	Pfipharmecs	0.4
One-A-Day Vitamins Plus Minerals	Miles	15.0

(continued)

Supplements—*continued*

Supplement	Manufacturer	Mg.
Optilets-M-500	Abbott	2.0
Os-Cal Forte	Marion	0.5
Os-Cal Plus	Marion	0.8
Stresstabs 600 with Zinc	Lederle	23.9
Surbex 750 with Zinc	Abbott	22.5
Theragran-M	Squibb	1.5
Theragran-Z	Squibb	22.5
Unicap T	Upjohn	15.0
Vicon-C	Glaxo	80.0
Vicon Iron	Glaxo	10.0
Vicon Plus	Glaxo	80.0
Vio-Geric	Rowell	15.0
Vitagett	North American	1.4
Vita-Kaps-M Tablets	Abbott	7.5
Vitamin-Mineral Capsules	North American	1.4
Viterra	Pfipharmecs	1.2
Viterra High Potency	Pfipharmecs	1.2
Vi-Zac	Glaxo	80.0
Z-Bec	Robins	22.5
Zinkaps (25)	Ortega	25.0
Zinkaps (110)	Ortega	110.0
Zinkaps (220)	Ortega	220.0

Source: Adapted from the American Pharmaceutical Association, *Handbook of Nonprescription Drugs*, 7th ed. (1982), 240–57.

Note: This chart is intended only as a guide. Vitamin formulations change periodically; always read product labels for accurate and up-to-date information on their nutrient levels.

19
Selenium

Every new decade brings evidence that a food element long considered unimportant provides benefits never imagined. Consider the subject of cancer prevention. Until recently, no one would have guessed that fiber, carotene, or indoles (obscure factors found in foods of the cabbage family) could provide important protection from the disease.

Rarely, though, does a food substance once considered poisonous rise to a position of great esteem. But, in some professional circles, selenium has earned this distinction. With each year, its fan club grows, and while foes remain, their ranks are dwindling.

If you have been following the reports of selenium's cancer-fighting potential, you may wonder why anyone would harbor hostility toward such a valuable mineral. But for decades, selenium had bad press. It left the mineral with a notorious reputation that has been difficult to live down.

THE PLAGUE OF THE PLAINS

Had you been a farmer in earlier times and watched with bewilderment as your horses, for instance, first lost the hair on

431

their manes and tails, then became crippled by cracking and loss of their hooves, you might not want to forgive the culprit either. Not knowing the cause, the farmers called the affliction the "alkali disease." In its later stages, the disease attacked the animals' vital organs, causing rapid deterioration and death within a few months.

Even worse was another disease that attacked cattle, sheep, and horses. The afflicted would wander aimlessly, walk in circles, or stumble directly into objects blocking their way. Owing to its initial symptoms, the disease was dubbed "blind staggers." But as it progressed, the name no longer described the problem. The stricken animals lost their appetite, became paralyzed, and died.

Alkali disease and blind staggers plagued thousands of livestock in the Great Plains for decades. Their causes remained unknown, but were assumed to be unrelated. In the 1930s, however, animal experts established that their cause was one and the same: selenium poisoning. The afflicted animals had been grazing in pastures where the soil—and forage growing in it—contained enormous levels of the mineral. In no time at all, selenium's name became mud.

THE TABLES TURN

A few decades later, the winds of change set in. Scientists had been on the trail of a substance vital to animal health in minute amounts. But its identity had eluded them. In 1957, two researchers at the National Institutes of Health (NIH) isolated some material that seemed to be rich in the mystery substance.

As they were trying to identify it, the chief of the NIH walked into their laboratory. Detecting a garliclike odor in the air, he suggested that selenium had pervaded the room. Sure enough, he was right; the mystery nutrient was the long-despised mineral, selenium. Though clearly toxic in high doses, small amounts proved essential.

By the end of the 1960s, nutritionists had accepted selenium as an essential nutrient for both animals and humans. But while acknowledging its vital role, they did not embrace selenium with open arms. Damning it with faint praise, some dubbed it "the essential poison." For years, the Committee on Dietary Allowances declined to set recommended intakes. In 1980, the Committee finally offered some numbers for guidance—not a Recommended Dietary Allowance (RDA), but a so-called safe and adequate range.

After reading this chapter, I think you will agree that the upper limit of the "safe and adequate" range is unjustifiably overcautious. Yet, the Committee on Dietary Allowances is not alone in its conservatism. Many, if not most, nutritionists also exaggerate the amount of selenium likely to be toxic. To this day, only a few scientists—usually cancer researchers who have studied selenium in depth—have freed themselves completely from the old prejudices.

COMBATING CANCER WITH SELENIUM

Ironically enough, selenium once was suspected to be cancer-causing. In fact, the Food and Drug Administration took steps to prevent its addition to animal feed. That was years ago, when selenium had such a bad name that the slightest hint of another harmful characteristic was accepted readily. This school of thought is now history, overwhelmed by evidence that selenium helps to prevent cancer. The change of heart came slowly, but here are a few of the facts responsible for it:

BLOOD SELENIUM AND CANCER RATES. Two decades ago, a survey of 19 American cities found the fewest number of cancer deaths where blood selenium levels were highest. Rapid City, South Dakota, was the luckiest of the 19, with the highest blood selenium and the lowest cancer death rate. Twice as many cancer deaths occurred where the blood selenium level was lowest. Similar findings were found worldwide. The average level of selenium in human blood banks of 27 countries showed an "inverse relationship" with cancer deaths. In other words, cancer death rates decreased as the average blood selenium level increased.

The most common studies compared blood selenium levels between cancer patients and healthy people—often finding higher levels in nonvictims. Some believed that cancer had caused blood selenium levels to fall, but optimists believed that the low levels came first, lowering victim's resistance to the disease.

Support for the optimists' view came in 1983, when Harvard

scientists analyzed blood samples taken from hundreds of volunteers a decade before. Originally, none had cancer, but 110 developed it during the five years that followed. Analysis of their original blood samples showed that those stricken had lower blood selenium levels before their cancers were diagnosed than the 210 subjects who remained free of the disease. Those who started the project with the highest blood selenium levels proved only half as likely to develop cancers as those who began with the lowest levels.

SOIL SELENIUM AND CANCER RATES. Lower rates of cancer also have been found among people living where the soil is selenium rich. This comes as no surprise, as high-selenium soil and higher blood selenium levels go hand in hand. The evidence for a protective effect of selenium is strongest for cancers of the digestive tract. These organs, of course, are most likely to come into direct content with the selenium in food.

ANIMAL RESEARCH. As early as 1949, research in animals suggested that selenium helped protect against chemically induced cancers. Dozens of studies have followed, more often than not supporting the protective effect observed decades ago.

INTERPRETING THE FINDINGS. Selenium deficiency almost certainly does not cause cancer directly. Rather, low selenium intakes probably lower our defenses against the substances that do. On a low-selenium diet, sufficient amounts of the key selenium-containing enzyme, glutathione peroxidase, may be lacking, depriving us of this important substance that helps protect our cell walls from cancer-causing troublemakers.

Though individual scientists are convinced of selenium's value in cancer prevention, official recognition has yet to come. In 1982, the National Research Council's Committee on Diet, Nutrition, and Cancer released a two-year study of relationships between food and cancer. In summarizing findings on selenium, the committee wrote:

> Both the epidemiological and laboratory studies suggest that selenium may offer some protection against the risk of cancer. However, firm conclusions cannot be drawn on the basis of the present limited evidence. Increasing the selenium intake to more than 200 micrograms [mcg.] a day (the upper limit of the range of Safe and Adequate Daily Dietary Intakes published in the

Recommended Dietary Allowances) by use of supplements has not been shown to confer health benefits exceeding those derived from the consumption of a balanced diet.

But neither had a balanced diet been shown preferable to a supplemented diet. No research comparing the two had ever been conducted, nor had the "safe and adequate" level that the committee defended been proven optimal either. (I'll be saying more about this "safe and adequate" range later.)

The committee did advise daily consumption of foods rich in two of selenium's cousins: carotene and vitamin C. Both are antioxidants, substances widely regarded as important factors in cancer prevention. Yet, despite its impressive antioxidant properties, selenium received no similar endorsement.

Were it not for selenium's past as a bad guy and exaggerated fears of its toxicity, I believe that the committee would have acknowledged its role in cancer prevention more strongly. But old notions die hard, and it will probably be another decade before fear of selenium is put behind us. When that day comes, I believe selenium will get the credit it deserves.

A CINDERELLA STORY

Selenium's story basically began in a chimney. In 1817, Swedish scientist Jon Jacob Berzelius was working with flue dust left behind after the burning of sulfuric acid. Noticing a familiar odor on his breath, his housekeeper warned him that he must have been eating too much garlic.

Actually a then-unknown mineral left behind in the chimney deposits had made its way into the scientist's body, imparting the "garlic breath." Sidetracked from his original pursuits, Berzelius analyzed the garlic-scented substance. Selenium was discovered, and it earned his place in scientific history.

Knowledge of selenium's effect on health, however, did not emerge for another century. For all Berzelius knew, selenium affected only one part of his body: his breath. Here are a few other interesting tidbits from the annals of selenium history:

• The name selenium comes from a Greek word meaning "the moon."
• In 1295, Marco Polo became the first to report a mysterious

animal disease ("hoof rot") in western China. Today, however, the malady is known to be selenium poisoning.
• The plant popularly known as locoweed has long been recognized as poisonous to horses. Among its notable characteristics is a special talent for hoarding selenium. Rumor holds that horses poisoned by the plant prevented relief troops from arriving at General Custer's Battle of Little Big Horn.

SELENIUM SECRETS

Before turning to selenium safety, I would like to mention a few basic facts about this newly appreciated mineral.

• Selenium helps maintain the health of muscle, red blood cells, and keratins—the tough proteins of our hair and nails. It also lends a helping hand to the pancreas and immune system.
• Selenium helps reduce the toxicity of mercury, silver, and cadmium—all potentially harmful if the body accumulates too much.
• A selenium-containing enzyme, glutathione peroxidase, has detoxifying properties.
• Vitamin E and selenium work together as antioxidants. Possibly, each may boost the power of the other. If so, their combined effects on health would exceed the sum of their individual contributions. This concept, of course, is known as synergy.
• When selenium deficiency exists, too little vitamin E can aggravate its severity.
• For two decades, selenium has been used successfully in the Keshan province of China to prevent potentially fatal degeneration of the heart muscle (cardiomyopathy). "Keshan's syndrome," as the disease has been called, primarily struck children of the province, where both soil and diets are selenium deficient. Originally discovered in Keshan in 1935, this form of congestive heart failure also had affected women of childbearing age.
• Selenium has been linked to other aspects of heart health. In some surveys, fewer heart disease deaths were found where drinking water, diets, or human blood contained higher levels of selenium. Experts are still debating whether the selenium itself, or another factor present where the mineral abounds, confers protection to the heart.

• Selenium occurs in many forms: in compounds called selenites or selenates, in complexes with other minerals, or in combination with an amino acid. The selenium bound to amino acids appears to be best absorbed. Though soil does not contain this form, plants make it from other forms of selenium that they take up from soil. Animal foods also provide selenium in this best-absorbed form. The selenium supplements I have found contain a related yeast-bound form that should be absorbed well.

• Selenium plays important roles in both health and industry. Ceramic, rubber, and electronic industries are among its many users. Red in color, selenium is used to tint paints, inks, and even car taillights. Its leading industrial use, however, is in the manufacturing of photoelectric cells that sense light or turn it into electricity.

THE ERRATIC ELEMENT

Selenium is abundant in the earth's crust, enough so to rank as one of its ten most common minerals. But though the total amount is large, its distribution is uneven. As a result, the amount of selenium in soil varies dramatically throughout the world.

Within a small area—a state such as Arizona, for instance—some pockets of land have selenium-rich soil, while others have soil so selenium poor that livestock grazing on forage there have developed selenium deficiency. Of course, the selenium content of our food, too, depends greatly on the soil where it is grown.

Grains can be excellent sources if grown in high-selenium soil. Eggs and dairy products also vary in selenium content, depending on the animal's diet. Cows grazing on selenium-rich pastures produce milk with more selenium than those grazing on selenium-poor soils. The mineral can be added to animal feed, however, so that the selenium content of meat and poultry is no longer determined solely by the amount in the local soil.

Burning coal also produces selenium that may wind its way into the food chain. No effects of this selenium on community health have been documented in the United States. In combination with other factors, however, it may have contributed to an outbreak of toxicity that I will tell you about soon.

In short, selenium's erratic ways have led to both extremes. Life-threatening deficiencies have occurred in some parts of the world, while overdoses have haunted others. And those who have suffered toxicity rarely had taken a single supplement; selenium-rich food alone had done the deed.

Two tales of Mother Nature's own overdoses follow.

SOUTH DAKOTA SOIL

Imagine you're a farmer who has just learned that selenium-rich forage in your area has been killing your livestock for decades. In no time, you would probably wonder about your family and neighbors. After all, their food had been growing in the same high-selenium soil.

Soon after selenium poisoning was discovered as the cause of alkali disease and blind staggers in livestock, public health officials had the same thoughts. They dispatched experts to check on the welfare of the citizens eating food grown in "seleniferous" (selenium-rich) soil. Parts of South Dakota were best known for seleniferous soil, so a team of researchers headed there.

Their findings became classic, and a half century later, remain among the few reports of dietary selenium toxicity in Americans. Among the symptoms observed:

- Bad teeth
- Brittleness of fingernails
- Discoloration of skin
- Dizziness
- Fatigue and tiredness
- Garlic odor of breath
- Gastrointestinal complaints
- Hair brittleness or loss
- Irritability
- Jaundice
- Skin inflammation

Elevated levels of selenium in the urine often accompanied the symptoms. The syndrome became known as "selenosis."

Since the mid-1930s, when these studies were done, America's food supply has changed dramatically. In those days, most food was grown and sold locally; today food is shipped from coast to coast—even imported from other continents. As a result, selenium intakes in the United States appear to be evening out, no longer depending heavily on the selenium content of local soils. In the selenium-rich areas of South Dakota, intakes no doubt have fallen since the days of selenosis.

Nonetheless, if you thought that the symptoms found in South Dakota a half century ago were striking, brace yourself for the story that follows.

THE CHINA SYNDROME

Selenium has been both a miracle worker and major trouble-maker in China. In its Keshan Province, selenium supplementation has brought enormous relief from the plague that threatened the heart health of countless children. Selenium deficiency had been rampant there for decades.

But China's Hubei Province had a selenium plague of the opposite extreme. In fact, the disease that struck the province's Enshi County during the 1960s is the worst outbreak of selenium toxicity on record. Many scientists in the West first became aware of it in 1983, when experts at the Chinese Academy of Medical Sciences published a detailed report in the *American Journal of Clinical Nutrition*. It is excerpted below:

> In Enshi County of Hubei Province an endemic human disease of unknown origin, characterized by loss of hair and nails, appeared more than 20 years ago and reached a peak prevalence during the years 1961 to 1964. The average incidence in five [heavily affected villages with 248 inhabitants was almost 50 percent]. In the most severely affected village, incidence reached 82.5 percent and only one elderly man of 82 years and three breast-fed infants were unaffected. All residents were evacuated from their homes to nearby places of safety; they recovered as soon as their diets were changed, except those with symptoms of the nervous system who needed a longer time.
>
> Research showed that the corn from this area was toxic. Because of a pink coloration in the tip of the corn embryo and of fungus spores in the seed, fungal intoxication was suggested as the cause of the disease. Later work from our laboratory, however, demonstrated that the toxicant in the corn was selenium. The pink color indicated the presence of elemental selenium.

The most common symptoms among the afflicted villagers resembled those observed in South Dakota 30 years before. Disturbances of the nervous system also were found in the most heavily affected village, no doubt because the severity of selenium poisoning there was greater than in the United States. Victims had "pins and needles" sensations and diminished sense of touch in their limbs. Numbness, convulsions, paralysis, and impaired coordination sometimes followed. One woman eventually became paralyzed on one side of her body and died. As her previous medical history was unknown, no one could determine whether the selenium toxicity had caused her death or had simply made an existing condition worse.

The research team found extraordinary levels of selenium in the local vegetables and grains. Corn grown in the affected villages of Enshi, for instance, contained about 1,500 times as much selenium as the corn of Keshan, where the soil is selenium deficient. Selenium intakes of the Enshi villagers were estimated to range from 3,200 to 6,690 mcg. daily. The average intake was estimated at 4,990 mcg.—25 times the upper limit of the "safe and adequate" range set by the Committee on Dietary Allowances.

Eventually, the research team pinpointed selenium-rich coal burned nearby as the primary source of the selenium. Nonetheless, they considered it but one contributing factor. The villagers also had been using lime fertilizer, which encouraged crops to take up more selenium from the soil. And a drought had caused the local rice crop to fail, forcing the villagers to eat far more vegetables and corn than usual. The corn contained about twice as much selenium as the rice it replaced.

NO PROBLEMS HERE

After determining the mysterious disease in Enshi County to be selenium toxicity, the researchers expanded their investigation to other parts of China. They found both selenium-rich and selenium-poor areas. But contrary to conventional wisdom, they found no signs of selenium toxicity in an area where estimated intakes averaged 750 mcg. daily, and went as high as 1,500 mcg. Yet these levels were three to seven times the upper limit of 200 mcg. set by the RDA Committee.

Long-term experiences such as these are the most meaningful, but some findings from brief studies are noteworthy. The Chromalloy American Company, for instance, recruited seven volunteers who took a total of 87,000 mcg. of selenium over a 70-day period (daily doses varied from 50 to 20,000 mcg. per day). Seven other volunteers received dummy pills, though no one involved knew who had the selenium and who did not. Neither the doctors, nor assisting personnel, nor the subjects detected any differences between the two groups, with the exception of increased blood selenium levels in the mineral-treated volunteers.

Similarly, no medical or laboratory abnormalities were found in two individuals who took selenium supplements of 350 and 600 mcg. respectively for 1½ years—in addition to the 90 to 170 mcg. in their diets. The supplements were high-selenium yeast that probably is one of the best-tolerated forms.

SELENIUM ON THE JOB

Naturally, those who work with selenium are exposed to an additional source of the mineral. The amount of exposure varies and is difficult to measure. Most often, selenium in the work environment is inhaled, so that it enters the body differently than food does. The type of selenium in workplace settings also differs; it is not the selenium-amino acid complex commonly found in food, nor the related selenium-yeast compound used in most supplements.

If I had no other information about selenium, I might be tempted to make judgments about supplementation based on its safety in industrial settings. But reports on the safety of selenium-rich food and a few experiences with supplements are available. I have considered these a better barometer of supplement safety than reports based on selenium in the workplace.

Though I judge supplements mostly by the safety of the selenium in food, occupational exposure to the mineral should be considered before using supplements. Such exposure can occur during the refining of metals or sulfur compounds. Selenium is produced in the process of refining copper, for instance. Of course, workers in some plants refine selenium itself, and still others may be exposed to it while manufacturing products in which the mineral is used. On-the-job exposure may also occur in scientific laboratories where selenium may be used to grow bacteria for research.

Regardless of the setting, however, only the workers exposed to selenium on the job—not consumers who buy their final products—are considered at risk. Of course, precautions are taken to limit on-the-job exposure to selenium, but it cannot be prevented entirely. As a result, the breath or urine of exposed workers

(continued on page 446)

Guesstimating Your Selenium Intake

Whether grown in Florida or California, the vitamin C content of oranges differs but slightly. But location has enormous influence on the selenium content of foods. Vegetables grown in selenium-rich South Dakota soil, for instance, have been found to contain 50 to 1,500 times as much as those purchased (and presumably grown) in a low-selenium area outside of Washington, D.C.

With selenium content so variable, I can't offer you a simple test to measure your intake of the mineral. I've looked hard for alternatives, however, and have come up with those that follow:

REGIONAL AVERAGES. In the mid-1970s, the Food and Drug Administration analyzed the selenium content of a typical "market basket" of foods purchased in various parts of the country. Here are the results, expressed as an average daily selenium intake for each region:

- Northeastern states: 147 mcg.
- Southern states: 154 mcg.
- North central states: 198 mcg.
- Western states: 191 mcg.

This method has one advantage; it couldn't be simpler. I'm a big fan of simplicity as long as a reasonable degree of accuracy comes with it. These numbers can qualify as such, but barely.

More often than not, this approach overestimates intakes by not allowing for selenium lost when food is prepared or discarded. Chemical analysis of the food actually eaten by individuals in North Carolina and in Beltsville, Maryland (a suburb of Washington, D.C.), showed significantly lower selenium intakes, averaging 93 and 88 mcg. respectively.

Moreover, how well these estimates apply to you depends on how much your diet resembles the standard fare used in the study. If your diet is very different—in terms of food choices or total calories—these averages may be a poor estimate of your intake. Calories and selenium intakes often are closely related.

Dividing the country into a handful of regions has another pitfall. Within each of these regions are areas where soil selenium greatly exceeds or falls short of the regional average. If you live in one of them and depend heavily on locally grown foods, your selenium intake is unlikely to resemble these average intakes.

The accompanying map illustrates selenium variation throughout the country. Your local Cooperative Extension Service, Soil Conservation Office, agricultural university, or farm organizations may have more specific and up-to-date information about the selenium content of your area's soil.

The selenium content of soil varies dramatically in the United States. Selenium deficiency has afflicted animals grazing in areas colored black—a good sign of selenium-poor soil. By contrast, vegetation growing in areas shaded gray has proven selenium rich. Fruits and vegetables grown in these lands presumably will provide more selenium than those from other areas.

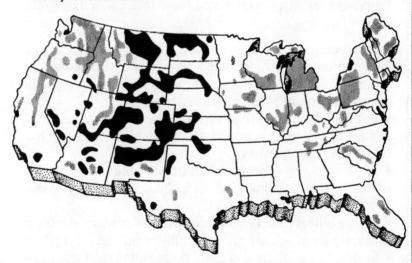

PREDICTIVE NUTRIENTS. In a recent study, researchers at the U.S. Department of Agriculture (USDA) found that higher selenium intakes tended to be accompanied by higher

(continued)

Guesstimating Your Selenium
Intake—*continued*

intakes of iron and magnesium. To a lesser extent, zinc intake also corresponded to selenium intake.

This method offers a more personal approach to evaluating your selenium intake than using the regional averages listed above. Review your results from the diet quizzes in the magnesium, iron, and zinc chapters. If your intakes of these other minerals tend to be generous, you are likely to be consuming a selenium-rich diet also.

FOODS THAT FAVOR SELENIUM. As a third alternative, consider your consumption of the foods that most readily take selenium from the environment. As long as the soil, sea, or feed provides sufficient amounts of selenium, these foods are likely to be the best sources.

USDA researchers have analyzed the selenium content of packaged foods and produce sold near their Beltsville, Maryland, facility. On an ounce-for-ounce basis, they found that:

• Mushrooms and radishes topped other vegetables for highest selenium content, followed by carrots and cabbage.
• Green beans, corn, and mushrooms had about the same selenium content whether fresh or canned.
• Canned carrots had half as much selenium as fresh, but canned tomatoes and canned potatoes had twice as much as their fresh counterparts.
• Most fruits were low in selenium, and the selenium content of canned versus fresh did not differ among apples, peaches, pears, or pineapples.
• Whole wheat bread and whole wheat flour contained significantly more selenium than white bread and white flour.
• Brown rice contained slightly more selenium than white rice.
• Brown sugar contained more selenium than white sugar, though neither was a notable source of the mineral.

- Corn flakes and puffed rice had very low levels of selenium, while hot barley cereal and ready-to-eat oat cereal (Cheerios) were the richest sources among cereals tested. Hot wheat cereal (Wheatena) and whole wheat flakes (Wheaties) had intermediate levels.
- The selenium content of milk products varied dramatically, with skim milk supplying the most and table cream providing very little. Skim milk contained about four times as much selenium as whole milk.
- Among cheeses, Swiss had the most selenium and cottage cheese the least. The selenium content of American cheese was in between the two, though fairly close to Swiss.
- Fresh meats and seafoods proved to be very good sources of selenium. Chicken had less selenium than red meats or fish, but still significant amounts. Excluding organ meats, round steak scored higher than other cuts and types of meat or chicken. When organ meats were included, however, kidneys and beef liver topped the list.
- As a group, seafoods contained more than twice as much selenium as meats. Though shellfish such as oysters, shrimp, and lobster outranked cod and flounder for selenium content, the latter two nonetheless contained more than red meat or chicken.

While the selenium in these foods will vary from place to place, the rankings relative to similar foods probably will remain the same. Therefore, if you favor the richer sources, you are more likely to consume ample amounts of selenium.

These findings make obvious that a diet of minimally processed foods is far more likely to provide generous amounts of selenium than a highly processed one. If you eat mostly fresh, natural foods and also live in a seleniferous area, you are probably among one of the highest consumers of dietary selenium in the United States.

usually is tested for signs of excessive selenium. Such measures are designed to prevent cases like the following one, excerpted from a report by Charles J. Diskin, M.D., and his colleagues at Roger Williams General Hospital in Providence, Rhode Island.

> A 71-year old man was admitted to the Roger Williams General Hospital with chest pain and ECG evidence of [a heart attack]. History disclosed no prior medical problems or evidence of heart disease in his family. He had been employed in selenium refining for 50 years, working until the day of admission. Although he had risen to company ownership, he continued to supervise the work daily and personally handled the selenium and inhaled its fumes. Because of this exposure he had reddish orange hair and red fingernails, but denied any respiratory or gastrointestinal symptoms . . .
>
> During his hospital course the patient was treated with [a variety of heart drugs, but heart] shock developed and he died eight days after admission.

Severe congestion in the lungs, spleen, and liver were found on autopsy. Tests also revealed extraordinary levels of selenium in his lungs, hair, and nails—as much as 250 to 500 times normal limits.

This is the most dramatic case I have found and is by no means typical of selenium-exposed workers. Those who do suffer from excessive exposure to selenium more commonly develop a condition called "rose cold," marked by sore throat, cough, inflamed nose, and bronchitis. But whether the usual or the highly unusual, these symptoms and test results make clear that workers exposed to selenium can accumulate too much selenium in their bodies.

In addition, one laboratory has reported an unusual rate of spontaneous abortions ("miscarriages") among women working with sodium selenite powder. This is a common form of selenium, though not the usual form in food or supplements.

According to the report, four definite and one possible pregnancy occurred among eight women working in the laboratory. All but one ended in spontaneous abortions; the woman who completed her pregnancy gave birth to a baby with clubfeet. Numerous other laboratories doing similar work were contacted, but only one worker who had experienced a spontaneous abortion was found. Whether these problem pregnancies were due to chance or selenium exposure cannot be determined based on these few experiences.

According to one authority, "occupational selenium poisoning is mostly accidental and rare." With the precautions in effect today, I have no reason to doubt it. But as infrequent as these problems might be, I generally would not recommend selenium supplements for those exposed to the mineral on the job. Workers who insist on supplementation should have tests to ensure that body selenium levels are well within normal limits.

SELENIUM AND CYSTIC FIBROSIS

About a decade ago, a veterinarian got some public attention when he advocated selenium as a promising treatment for cystic fibrosis. This proposal gathered enough notice to be a subject of debate at a workshop conference sponsored by the NIH. Most participants agreed that good evidence was lacking that selenium deficiency caused CF or that supplementation aided in its routine treatment.

Some CF patients nonetheless continued supplementation, usually given by their parents. A year after the NIH meeting, serious complications in two selenium-treated patients were reported. One 17-year-old victim experienced a dramatic worsening of his CF symptoms after taking 200 mcg. of supplemental selenium for two weeks. He spent the following two weeks in a hospital, and fortunately, he recovered. But the second victim, an 11-month-old girl, was not as lucky. Sad to say, she died after several months of selenium supplementation.

In both children, selenium supplementation was associated with abnormally low levels of chloride in the blood. Excessively hot or cold weather is known to deplete CF victims of this important substance, but neither child had been exposed to extremes in temperature.

Without any other explanation for the low chloride levels, it appeared that the selenium supplements may have been to blame. Both the baby and the teenager had taken only small to moderate amounts of selenium that healthy individuals no doubt would have tolerated well. But physicians involved with these two cases speculated that CF may predispose its victims to selenium toxicity, perhaps due to its impact on related nutritional factors that affect tolerance to the mineral.

In light of this possibility, I feel that selenium supplementation should *not* be administered to those who have cystic fibrosis, except as directed by the physician treating the disease.

A FALSE ALARM?

A few years before the selenium-CF connection surfaced, two investigators reported a "cluster" of four cases of Lou Gehrig's disease (officially known as amyotropic lateral sclerosis, ALS, or motor-neuron disease) within a small area of South Dakota. The four victims lived within a 10-mile radius of each other.

Considering the number of cases to be unusually high for such a sparsely populated area, the research team proposed the high-selenium environment as a likely cause. Originally published in the *Journal of the American Medical Association*, the findings were widely publicized in the press, spreading alarm among residents of seleniferous areas.

I hope that all who heard the first report also learned of the commentaries that followed. Klaus Schwarz, M.D., of the UCLA School of Medicine was among those who analyzed the findings and discussed them with others in the field. He summarized his results in a letter to the journal. Here is an excerpt of his response:

> I would like to point out that clusters of ALS occur elsewhere in areas with normal or low selenium levels [in the soil]... Since the article [reporting the four cases in South Dakota] appeared, I have communicated with departments of neurology in the Pacific Northwest, an area which is notoriously selenium deficient, and in Boston (also situated in an area where the selenium supply is low) and with experts at the National Institutes of Health and elsewhere. The consensus is that the frequency of ALS is at least as high, if not higher in areas that are selenium deficient compared to those with normal or elevated levels.
>
> From an economic as well as a health point of view, selenium deficiency appears to be a much more serious problem in the United States than selenium toxicity.

"Safe and Adequate" Intakes for Selenium

Until 1980, a nutrient either had an RDA or it didn't. Many minerals had attained status as essential nutrients, but the Committee on Dietary Allowances insisted that information was insufficient to set RDAs for them.

Eventually, a compromise emerged: the "safe and adequate" range. In theory, or according to the committee, these ranges fully meet our needs without exceeding safe limits. It sounds as though the recommendations have been based on research designed to determine optimal intakes.

In some cases, I believe this to be so. The sodium range, for instance, clearly rests on research into the health effects of sodium. I cannot convince myself that the selenium range—50–200 mcg. for adults—was developed in a similar way. It is obvious that many individuals can tolerate intakes greater than 200 mcg. (and also likely that higher intakes may be beneficial). I believe that the "safe and adequate" range represents little but the current range of American intakes expressed in round numbers.

That's my opinion, of course. Most nutritionists still toe the 200 mcg. maximum line. However, I doubt that this limit is based on hard facts. At any rate, here are the "safe and adequate" ranges set by the Committee on Dietary Allowances in 1980.

Group/Age	Mcg.
Infants 0–6 mon.	10–40
Infants 6–12 mon.	20–60
Children 1–3 yr.	20–80
Children 4–6 yr.	30–120
Children 7–10 yr.	50–200
Males 11+ yr.	50–200
Females 11+ yr.	50–200

Leonard T. Kurland, M.D., of the Mayo Clinic in Rochester, Minnesota, echoed these sentiments. His letter to the journal, published alongside Dr. Schwarz's, included these comments:

> *The ALS death rates for previous years have been described in detail and comparison reveals remarkably even distribution, state by state and region by region, throughout the United States. The distribution of selenium levels in soil varies greatly ... Thus there is not an obvious relationship between levels of selenium available to man in his food and water and the death rates from ALS in the United States.*

Dr. Kurland expressed deep concern about fear that the news reports had engendered among residents of Rochester, where selenium soil levels tend to be high. These fears were unfortunate, for I found the rebuttals more convincing than the original report. Also, no further reports linking ALS and seleniferous areas have followed. All things considered, I agree with Dr. Kurland that the four cases in South Dakota were most likely "a chance occurrence," better known as a false alarm.

AN ISOLATED ACCIDENT

In 1984, a manufacturing error resulted in the marketing of some ultrapotent selenium tablets. The label stated the potency as 150 mcg., but the tablets actually contained about 30,000 mcg. each—almost 200 times the amount intended.

Thirteen cases of toxicity were officially reported. At least one patient noticed ill effects within less than 11 days: loss of hair, white streaks on a fingernail, followed by swelling of her fingertips and a discharge around her nails. After three weeks, all of her fingernails were affected, and one fell off entirely. From time to time, she felt nauseous and tired, and her breath had a sour odor.

Some of the others took the product for several months; all had gastrointestinal symptoms. Eight of the 13 suffered adverse effects on their hair, from dry and brittle texture to loss of large amounts. A similar number became more irritable. Nails were damaged in all but two. Five had skin inflammation. As I have found no follow-up reports, I have no reason to suspect permanent damage to any of those affected.

The manufacturer voluntarily recalled the product, of course. As best as I can determine, this was an isolated instance. Just as an isolated recall of a drug, food, or other product due to a manufacturing error has no bearing on the safety of the product when made properly, this incident in no way reflects on the safety of accurately formulated selenium supplements.

THE STAR SYSTEM SHINES ON SELENIUM

Side effects—High levels of selenium in food or at the workplace account for virtually all cases of adverse reactions; selenium in supplemental form has not been tested the way that zinc, vitamin C, or other nutrients have been. As a result, few opportunities to assess side effects of supplemental selenium exist.

One of the few reported ill effects from supplements occurred in a Chinese man who took a 1,000 mcg. supplement daily for a year and a half. Whether his symptoms—garlic odor on his breath and damaged fingernails—should be classified under toxicity or as side effects is a matter of opinion. If a drug were to cause streaked fingernails and breath odor, these would invariably be called side effects. Nonetheless, nail changes resulting from high selenium intakes have long been labeled as a toxic reaction. Regardless, the man's nails and breath returned to normal soon after he stopped taking the supplement.

Though little else is known about supplement side effects, more information is expected. The National Cancer Institute, for instance, is sponsoring research on selenium's ability to prevent cancer. Participants are receiving either a 100 mcg. selenium supplement or a dummy pill. Regardless of the outcome on cancer rates, this research will give us facts about side effects that we currently lack. Of course, the results at the dose level studied—100 mcg. daily—may differ from side effects that would occur with higher-potency supplements.

Acute ailments—The early signs of selenium toxicity—such as lethargy, irritability, dry hair—are vague and easily attributed to other causes. Those affected often haven't suspected anything until their symptoms worsened or other family members and neighbors reported similar complaints. As a result, the problem of selenium toxicity usually fits the pattern of a long-term problem better than that of an acute ailment.

Except for two cases in cystic fibrosis victims discussed earlier in the chapter and the experience of the Chinese man mentioned above, I have found no reports of acute ailments after very brief exposure to selenium in the workplace or from properly manufactured supplements.

Long-term problems—We have looked at the symptoms experienced by those who live or work in high-selenium environments. From exploring their symptoms, we now know that selenium toxicity most commonly affects four body systems:

THE LUNGS AND RESPIRATORY SYSTEM. Workers who inhale selenium on the job are most likely to suffer adverse effects on these organs. They experience the so-called rose cold and garlic breath described earlier. Of course, selenium-exposed workers presumably are more likely to accumulate too much of the mineral from supplementation than unexposed workers.

THE SKIN, HAIR, AND NAILS. Burns, red skin lesions, itching, hives, brittle or streaked nails, and dry, brittle hair are classic signs of selenium toxicity. If the condition progresses, nails and hair may be lost.

THE DIGESTIVE TRACT. Nausea, vomiting, stomach or abdominal pain commonly occur in selenium toxicity. The symptoms may be mild at first, then worsen as the amount of selenium in the body increases.

THE CENTRAL NERVOUS SYSTEM. Ever since the days of blind staggers, selenium toxicity has been known to affect the nervous system in animals. In humans, such reactions appear to occur only in the most severe cases; odd or diminished sensations in the limbs as well as paralysis may occur. Weakness and depression noted in milder cases may be an early sign of effects on the central nervous system.

Finally, I have read of four studies that found higher rates of tooth decay among children raised in seleniferous areas (as well as of two that did not confirm these findings). Concern seems to have faded on this issue, but were selenium to affect dental health, it probably would do so only while teeth are developing. Adults are long past this stage and generally suffer little tooth decay. Moreover, who wouldn't be willing to tolerate some selenium-related tooth decay if the mineral is helping to prevent cancer?

Conflicting combinations—No interactions between selenium and drugs are known, mostly because researchers have had too few people to test. The last outbreak of selenium toxicity in the United States occurred almost a half century ago. Obviously, we can't go back with the thousands of new drugs that have been developed since to determine whether those with high selenium intakes suffer unusual reactions.

At the levels of selenium in the current American diet, I have found no reports of reactions with drugs (or other substances). At the same time, I have found no reports that actually tested for such interactions. Still, it is reassuring that none have popped up unexpectedly among those who eat selenium-rich diets or use supplements.

Vitamin C occasionally has been advocated as a treatment for selenium poisoning, based on a belief that it makes selenium less usable to the body. In researching vitamin C safety, I found no cases of compromised selenium nutrition resulting from its use. I also have found no hard numbers that show how much vitamin C is required to affect a given amount of selenium. Until I have more information, I am reserving judgment on this interaction.

There has been speculation that zinc and selenium interact. However, what, if anything, goes on between the two remains to be seen.

Hidden consequences—I have found no reports of selenium masking the signs of any illness or interfering with accurate readings in laboratory tests.

ENTER THE FOOD AND NUTRITION BOARD

Four years before its Committee on Dietary Allowances set "safe and adequate" intakes for selenium, the Food and Nutrition Board's Committee on Nutritional Misinformation issued a position paper on selenium in general—and supplements in particular. Applying knowledge of levels toxic to animals, this committee calculated that "overt chronic selenium intoxication would be expected in human beings after long-term consumption of 2,400 to 3,000 micrograms daily."

Two pages later, the committee concluded that "there is no justification at this time for the use of selenium supplements by the general population. Should selenium supplements eventually be considered desirable for those persons living in low-selenium areas, or for those consuming vegetarian diets, a daily supplement of 50 to 100 micrograms could probably be taken safely."

Assuming that the committee would consider a diet containing less than 100 mcg. to be low in selenium, adding this "probably safe" supplement of 50 to 100 mcg. would make for a total safe intake of 150 to 200 mcg. daily.

How the committee reduced its definition of danger from the 2,400 to 3,000 mcg. range down to less than a tenth as much within three pages remained a mystery that has never been explained. Nor was it questioned for many years.

In fact, others supported the committee's harsh view toward selenium. Thomas H. Jukes of the University of California, for example, noted that "The difference between nutritional and toxic levels of selenium is only about 20-fold. This is a very narrow margin of safety."

HOW SAFE IS SAFE?

Depending on how you define a "nutritional level" of selenium, you may or may not agree that levels 20 times greater are safe. If you think of 150 mcg., for instance, as a healthy intake, 20 times that—3,000 mcg.—hardly falls within my notion of a safe range.

Nor do I consider a 20-fold margin of safety for a nutrient to be "very narrow." I would be delighted if every nutrient had a 20-fold margin of safety, but I would not make such a claim for vitamin A, vitamin D, or zinc—among others. I suspect that selenium has been singled out as most toxic simply because, unlike other nutrients, its toxicity was recognized before its nutritional value.

Regardless, I think a distinction needs to be made between desirable margins of safety for nutrients as compared to toxic chemicals. As I first discussed in chapter 11 (vitamin C), experts in chemical toxicity often want a 100-fold margin of safety. I feel that this classic approach—setting safety levels at $1/100$ of the lowest-known hazardous level—makes sense for toxic chemicals, but not for nutrients.

During my years of researching nutrient safety, I noticed an important difference between high doses of essential nutrients and toxic chemicals having no nutritional value. Our bodies have thermostats for many nutrients that reduce the risk of overdoses by regulating how much we absorb. Such a thermostat does not evolve with each new chemical that comes along.

THE RECOVERY FACTOR

I have another reason for feeling that nutrients can be judged less stringently than toxic chemicals. Brief exposure to certain troublesome chemicals can cause irreversible damage. But much to my surprise, I have found that victims of nutrient overdoses are far more likely to recover fully than to be harmed permanently.

For all the fear that selenium's reputed toxicity has caused, the fact remains that most cases on record ended in recovery. As an extreme example, consider the case of a 15-year-old girl who had consumed, at once, a liquid supplement for sheep feed estimated to contain more than a million mcg. of selenium. Her parents rushed her to the hospital; there she received vigorous treatment similar to that used in severe cases of iron poisoning. Seventeen days later, she left the hospital, and the doctors did not observe any further consequences.

No doubt, selenium poisoning might have ended the girl's life, were it not for prompt medical attention and advances in treating mineral overdoses. Nonetheless, her story shows that full recovery is also possible, though certainly no one would recommend repeating her experience to confirm this.

As noted earlier, most of the villagers in Enshi County also recovered from their selenium poisoning soon after changing their diets. Similarly, in 1941, selenium toxicity was suspected as the cause of irritated skin, fatigue, dizziness, and depression among residents of North and South Dakota. A low-selenium diet reportedly relieved their symptoms, just as withdrawal of extra selenium restored normal nail growth in a man who had been taking a 1,000 mcg. supplement daily for a year and a half.

INFORMED DISSENT

I am not the only one who believes that the dangers of selenium have been exaggerated. The rumblings of dissent are growing louder. Some scientists had already calculated higher levels to be acceptable before the Committee on Dietary Allowances set its "safe and adequate" range at 200 mcg. Here are three examples:

After careful review of studies worldwide and some elaborate calculations, two researchers wrote:

> In the previous sections we concluded that the [average] normal daily intake of selenium may be around 50–150 mcg. in man, and that the range of the margin of safety may be 10–200 times the normal level. Taking the lower values of both these estimates, the lowest level of potentially dangerous daily intake of selenium is estimated to be about 500 mcg.

They found support from a team at the Toxicological Evaluation Division of Canada's Health and Welfare department, who says that "based . . . on observation and considering the normal levels in foods, 500 mcg./day may be regarded as a maximum tolerable level [of selenium for adults]."

Moreover, as Donald Buell of the National Cancer Institute points out, the 200 mcg. limit "contrasts with an earlier statement of the Food and Nutrition Board that said that, 'overt toxicity would be expected in human beings after long-term consumption of 2,400 to 3,000 mcg. daily.' The upper limit of 200 mcg. of selenium per day is a conservative one." I think he's right.

HOW MUCH IS TOO MUCH

My first recommendation is that pregnant and nursing women use selenium supplements cautiously, if at all. I'm among those who believe that drugs or unnecessarily high doses of nutrients should be avoided during pregnancy, if possible. I also feel that too little is known about the effect of selenium on the growing fetus.

As for healthy individuals, I feel that the proposed maximum safe intake of 500 mcg. rests on firmer scientific ground than the

200 mcg. limit recommended by the Committee on Dietary Allowances. Nonetheless, the 500 mcg. limit was based mostly on studies of men. Maximum recommended levels for women may need to be lower.

On the other hand, the 500 mcg. guideline may be conservative; Chinese villagers consumed as much as 1,500 mcg. daily from dietary sources without signs of trouble. But the diets and health problems of Americans differ enough from those of the Chinese farmer that I am hesitant to assume that we would react the same way to intakes in the 750–1,500 mcg. range.

ABSOLUTE SAFETY OR ALERT SUPPLEMENTATION?

Here are my final thoughts.

In setting a safe intake for selenium, I think one fact is often forgotten. Though no one likes the thought of toxicity, the need to define an absolute safe dose has not been proven for those who are alert for signs of too much. The record shows that full recovery is the rule if excessive intakes are stopped at the first signs of toxicity. Therefore, making a major issue over a maximum safe dose is not as crucial as it has seemed.

Of course, when the first signs of toxicity occur, supplementation should be stopped until all nails, hair, and affected organs return to normal. Supplements then should not be taken for several months. If supplements are later consumed, lower doses should be taken.

As for drawing the traditional lines between safe and unsafe, I agree with those who consider the 200 mcg. limit of the "safe and adequate" range to be rooted in "selenophobia." The proposed alternative—500 mcg.—seems sound, but I am concerned that women and those who weigh much less than the average adult male may need lower limits.

For these individuals, and for those who want to play it very safe, I would recommend a total intake of no more than 350 mcg. daily. If you eat primarily unprocessed foods, your diet probably ranks at the upper end of customary U.S. intakes—160 to 200 mcg. per day. A supplement of 150 mcg. daily would not bring your total intake above 350 mcg. I find that most supplements contain 50 or

100 mcg. of selenium. It is difficult to believe that American adults would be harmed by taking one of these tablets daily.

In fact, the federal government allows daily supplements of up to 200 mcg. daily to be used in human cancer research. The diets of participants probably contain 60 to 200 mcg.; supplementation with 200 mcg. would bring their total intakes to 260 to 400 mcg. daily—beyond the "safe and adequate" range set by the Committee on Dietary Allowances. Obviously, those who have studied the matter carefully don't share the committee's phobia over selenium.

A few years from now, the results of these cancer prevention studies with selenium will be in. I am optimistic that the results will confirm the safety of sensible supplementation, enabling selenophobia to be cured once and for all.

C   O   O   K   I   N   G
for Selenium

MAPLE BREAD PUDDING

(Makes 4 servings)

Selenium: 31 mcg. per serving
Calories: 262 per serving

6 slices whole wheat bread	½ cup apple juice
1½ cups skim milk	2 eggs
	¼ cup maple syrup

Preheat oven to 375°F.

Spray a 1½-quart baking dish with no-stick spray. Cut the bread into 1-inch pieces and place them in the dish.

In a medium bowl, whisk together the skim milk, apple juice, eggs, and maple syrup. Pour it over the bread and bake for about 55 minutes. Serve immediately.

C　O　O　K　I　N　G
for Selenium—*continued*

MARINATED PORK WITH ASPARAGUS

(Makes 4 servings)

Selenium: 28 mcg. per serving
Calories: 287 per serving

¾ pound boneless pork
　　loin, center cut
1　tablespoon white grape
　　juice
1　tablespoon soy sauce
¼ teaspoon minced fresh
　　ginger
　　pinch of freshly grated
　　orange rind

1　pound asparagus
1　cup snow peas, about 4
　　ounces
2　tablespoons orange
　　juice
2　teaspoons soy sauce
1　teaspoon cornstarch
2　teaspoons peanut oil

Use a sharp knife to trim the pork of fat, then slice it against the grain as thinly as possible. Slice these pieces into strips. Put the pork into a small bowl. In a cup, combine the grape juice, 1 tablespoon soy sauce, ginger, and orange rind and pour over the pork. Cover the bowl and let the pork marinate in the refrigerator for 3 hours.

Meanwhile, clean and trim the asparagus and cut it diagonally into 2-inch pieces. String the peas, if necessary, and put them and the asparagus into a strainer. Blanch them by pouring boiling water over them. Then pat them dry and refrigerate until ready to cook.

Mix the orange juice, 2 teaspoons soy sauce, and cornstarch in a small bowl, and set aside.

Heat the peanut oil in a wok or 10-inch sauté pan. Add the pork and stir-fry until the meat is cooked through, about 5 minutes.

continued

C O O K I N G

for Selenium—*continued*

Add the asparagus and peas to the pork and toss to heat through. Make a well in the middle of the pork and vegetables and pour in the orange juice mixture. Stir constantly until it is thick and shiny, then toss quickly to combine it with the pork and vegetables.

Serve immediately with rice or thin Chinese noodles.

SEA SALAD WITH GARLIC AND ROSEMARY

(Makes 3 servings)

Selenium: 108 mcg. per serving
Calories: 174 per serving

½ pound shrimp
½ pound sea scallops
2 scallions, cut into
   julienne strips
2 tablespoons minced
   sweet red pepper
¼ teaspoon dried
   rosemary

1 clove garlic
2 tablespoons cider
   vinegar
1 teaspoon olive oil
   pinch of dried mustard
2 tablespoons crumbled
   feta cheese

Set a steamer over boiling water and add the shrimp. Steam for 1 minute, then add the scallops and continue to steam another 3 minutes.

Peel the shrimp, slice them in half down the vein, and set them in a medium-size mixing bowl. Add the scallops, scallions, and pepper and toss to combine.

Using a mortar and pestle, grind the rosemary, then add the garlic and grind to a paste. Scrape the paste into a small

C   O   O   K   I   N   G
for Selenium—continued

bowl and whisk in the vinegar, oil, and mustard. Pour the dressing over the salad and toss to combine. Sprinkle with the feta cheese and serve on a mound of shredded lettuce. Serve warm or cold.

Selenium Content of Selected Supplements

You may have some trouble finding selenium in common multiple vitamin products. Supplements containing selenium alone, however, are readily available and most companies offer a choice of potencies. Some typical options are listed below.

Manufacturer	Available Potencies (mcg.)
Arco	50, 200
General Nutrition Center	25, 50, 100, 200
Lee Nutrition	50, 100
Nutrition Headquarters	50, 100, 200
Puritan's Pride	50
SDV Vitamins	50, 100
Stur-dee	25, 50, 100

20

More about Minerals

In addition to the six minerals spotlighted so far, others, too, are essential to our health. Like selenium, most of them are trace minerals, needed in extremely small amounts. Important as these nutrients may be, however, precious little is known about their safety in supplement form.

For some of these minerals, such as copper, lack of experience with supplements is the problem. With the exception of multimineral products that rarely provide more than the "safe and adequate" recommended intake, supplemental copper is a rare commodity. Many companies don't offer it at all—probably with good reason. As a result, there is little basis to judge the safety of dosages exceeding recommended intakes.

For other minerals, we know little about their safety simply because little is known about the nutrient at all. In this category are certain minerals so obscure that recommended intakes remain undetermined. In other cases, such as manganese, a "safe and adequate" intake has been established, though other details about safety remain sketchy.

At the opposite extreme is a mineral understood so well as to

462

make clear that supplementation generally is unadvisable. This mineral is phosphorus.

Though research doesn't exist to offer detailed chapters on all the other minerals, I would like to offer some basic information and general facts about four remaining nutrients that may be familiar to you: the trace minerals chromium, copper, and manganese; and the major mineral phosphorus.

THE CHROMIUM CHRONICLE

Chromium is a valued trace mineral most recognized for its essential role in glucose tolerance. Impaired glucose tolerance is found in diabetes and hypoglycemia. Chromium deficiency is not considered the leading cause of these conditions; however, glucose tolerance has improved in some chromium-deficient individuals after supplementation with brewer's yeast, one of the richest sources of biologically active chromium.

The term "biologically active" is important to the subject of chromium nutrition, for only this active form—known as glucose tolerance factor (GTF)—participates in maintaining health. GTF is actually a complex of substances that includes chromium, nicotinic acid (a form of niacin), and amino acids. Apparently, it assists the action of insulin, the familiar substance long recognized for its role in sugar metabolism.

Severe chromium deficiency is extremely rare in the United States, but nutritionists now believe that many Americans may have borderline deficiencies. The risk of these marginal deficiencies probably increases with age, as our bodies store less chromium as we grow older.

Food choices, too, affect our chances of deficiency. Diets containing large amounts of refined grain foods (white bread, refined cereals) and sugar are likely to be low in chromium. These foods contain carbohydrates that cannot be metabolized without the mineral, yet the chromium contained in their unrefined state has been removed. As a result, these foods cause the body to use chromium, but do not replace what is lost. Polished rice, butter, and margarine are also poor sources of chromium. As the amount of these foods in a diet increases, the more likely it is to be chromium poor.

Facts about the chromium content of other foods are few. The richest known sources are liver and brewer's yeast, but not other forms of yeast. Beef, poultry, whole grain cereals, bran, wheat germ, and cheese are generally good sources. In addition, chromium that migrates into food from stainless steel cookware, utensils, and metal cans may contribute greatly to our chromium intake.

USING CHROMIUM SUPPLEMENTS SAFELY

Fortunately, a few studies with chromium supplements are available. From these, we have learned the basics of supplement safety.

First, not all chromium supplements are created equal. The chromium in supplements other than brewer's yeast must be converted into the biologically active form. Most of us can convert chromium from chelated supplements or from chromium chloride into a usable form, but some people apparently cannot. Without testing, you cannot be sure that you can readily convert to the active form. Therefore, relying on a biologically active form is the best bet.

Though supplements of "glucose tolerance factor" sound like the active form, their resemblence to the real thing has been challenged. According to one researcher who tested a number of different brands, "none was biologically active." That leaves brewer's yeast as the only supplement with definitely active properties. As the chart that follows shows, the chromium content of these yeasts varies among brands.

Though potentially beneficial to many of us, chromium supplementation must be taken only under a doctor's supervision for those with impaired glucose tolerance. A diabetic may benefit from supplements, but because insulin requirements may change as a result, supplementation must be monitored by a physician.

In addition, there are a handful of reported allergies to chromium. Most cases involve forms of chromium used industrially, rather than the forms found in supplements. However, at sufficiently high doses, some of those allergic to industrial forms of chromium may also react to the "trivalent" form—usually chromium chloride—found in some supplements.

Chromium Content of Brewer's Yeast

Here are some estimates of chromium content of brewer's yeast supplements, the most reliable source of usable chromium.

Reliable and palatable, unfortunately, don't always go together. Many people find the taste of brewer's yeast powders, flakes, and buds to be far from acceptable. You may find one brand tastes better than another; also, try mixing the yeast with juice or soup to reduce its strong, bitter taste.

The 10-gram measure used in these estimates translates into just slightly more than a level tablespoon.

Brand	Mcg. (per 10 g.)
KAL	22
Lewis Labs	60
NatureAde	60
NatureMost	60
Plus	16
Solgar	60
VitaFood	6

Source: *Nutrition Action*, January/February (1985): 12.

Note: As product formulations may change, check labels or with manufacturers for the most current information on the nutrient levels.

Now for some facts about dosage.

• Toxicity from supplementation with brewer's yeast or chromium chloride has not been reported. There is one case on record of a hidden consequence, however, in a young man who had been taking at least 30 tablets (about one-third of an ounce) of brewer's yeast daily. Something in the yeast apparently caused him to have a false-positive reading on a test for porphyria, a rare genetic disease that his doctors thought could explain his nagging abdominal pain. Fortunately, further study revealed that he did not have the disease and his pains relented after he stopped taking the supplements.

● Poor absorption of chromium may account for the low potential for toxicity. Average absorption is estimated to be no more than 2 percent of intake.

● While no toxic effects are known from safe forms of chromium, lack of experience with high doses may account for the clean record. The safest approach is to limit chromium intake to 200 micrograms (mcg.) daily—a level that has been tested without signs of toxicity. The Committee on Dietary Allowances notes that "the safety of 200 mcg. has been established in long-term supplementation trials in human subjects receiving 150 mcg./day in addition to the dietary intake."

In making this conclusion, the committee obviously assumes that the diet provides no more than 50 mcg. This is a fair assumption for the average diet, though some will provide more. Nonetheless, the 150 mcg. supplement is likely to be safe for a healthy adult.

Chromium—"Safe and Adequate"

Although there are no RDA for chromium, the Committee on Dietary Allowances of the National Research Council set these "safe and adequate" allowances in 1980.

Group/Age	Mcg.
Infants 0–6 mon.	10–40
Infants 7–12 mon.	20–60
Children 1–3 yr.	20–80
Children 4–6 yr.	30–120
Children 7–10 yr.	50–200
Males 11+ yr.	50–200
Females 11+ yr.	50–200

Note: There is no U.S. RDA for chromium.

KUDOS FOR COPPER

Thanks to copper, our bodies are able to make many of the enzymes that keep us healthy. Copper is part of superoxide dismutase, an in-the-news enzyme whose detoxifying properties have won the attention of cancer researchers. Another important copper-containing enzyme assists in making hemoglobin. This explains why impaired copper nutrition leads to low hemoglobin levels and iron-deficiency anemia. When this form of anemia appears, care must be taken to determine whether its root cause is inadequate iron or inadequate copper.

Most of the copper in our blood is bound to a protein called ceruloplasmin. Levels of this copper-protein complex are commonly measured when testing for copper deficiency.

Oysters, liver, dried yeast, and lobster are among our best food sources of copper. Other good sources include crabmeat, nuts, seeds, legumes, and fresh vegetables and fruits. Refined sugars, cereals, and milk—except mother's milk—generally are poor sources of this important mineral.

Fortunately, reports of copper deficiency caused by inadequate diets have been few. The condition has afflicted premature babies fed low-copper formulas. Infants suffering from protein-calorie malnutrition who were treated with milk-rich diets also have been victims.

A rare genetic disease, Menkes' syndrome, is marked by copper deficiency. Failure to absorb copper rather than inadequate intake, however, is to blame. Similarly, kidney disease may also impair copper nutrition. And as discussed in earlier chapters, high intakes of zinc and vitamin C impair copper absorption. However, with intakes of zinc and vitamin C typically found in our diets—or with supplementation at levels recommended in this book—copper deficiency should not be very likely.

COPPER SUPPLEMENTATION

If you want to take copper supplements, your choices are fairly limited. Multimineral products containing copper are often the only supplements available, and their copper content per tablet rarely exceeds the maximum recommended intake of 3

"Safe and Adequate" Intakes for Copper

Although there are no RDA for copper, the Committee on Dietary Allowances of the National Research Council set these "safe and adequate" allowances in 1980.

Group/Age	Mg.
Infants 0–6 mon.	0.5–0.7
Infants 6–12 mon.	0.7–1.0
Children 1–3 yr.	1.0–1.5
Children 4–6 yr.	1.5–2.0
Children 7–10 yr.	2.0–2.5
Males 11+ yr.	2.0–3.0
Females 11+ yr.	2.0–3.0

Note: There is no U.S. RDA for copper.

milligrams (mg.) daily. Higher-potency supplements are probably not marketed because of serious reactions that occurred years ago when copper sulfate was used medically to induce vomiting.

As for safe amounts, the Committee on Dietary Allowances states that, "It can be assumed that an occasional intake of up to 10 mg. is safe for human adults. However, in order to include an extra margin of safety, it is recommended that the copper intake in adults over extended periods of time be in the range of 2–3 mg./day."

Since 1966, most American diets have provided less than 1.3 mg. of copper daily. Though combining the 3 mg. provided by some supplements with such a dietary intake would exceed the limit set by the RDA committee, such a total intake is unlikely to be unsafe. As acknowledged by the committee, a group of experts convened by the Food and Agriculture Organization/World Health Organization came up with a very different estimate. In 1971, this group calculated upper limits to be about 0.23 mg. per pound of body weight. In other words, this estimate puts the tolerable limit for a 100-pound individual at 23 mg. I am not comfortable with an intake this high, however.

Rather than concern yourself with which safety estimate is most accurate, keep in mind that copper needs can be low even in extreme situations. In severe copper deficiency caused by excessive zinc intake, 1 mg. of copper daily was enough to restore copper balance. (Chapter 18 discusses some of these cases in detail.)

Supplements of the copper-containing enzyme superoxide dismutase have become popular in recent years. These supplements have not proven to be useful. Apparently, only the superoxide dismutase made by the body is active. Your best bet, then, is to have adequate copper in your diet or supplement program.

Needless to say, individuals afflicted with Wilson's disease—a genetic condition marked by overaccumulation of copper in the body—should not take copper supplements.

MANGANESE AND SUPPLEMENT SAFETY

Manganese has proven to be an essential mineral for many different animals. Nutritionists assume that humans require it, too, for certain enzymes involved in protein and calorie metabolism contain manganese.

The usual adult diet provides an estimated 2 to 9 mg. of manganese daily. Whole grains, nuts, and especially tea are among our best food sources. Fruits and vegetables are moderate sources; meats, milk, and seafood are poor ones.

Fortunately, there are no cases on record of manganese deficiency in man.

Manganese supplements are another rare commodity. The most likely sources are multimineral combinations that provide much less than the upper limit of the "safe and adequate" range. Supplements containing manganese alone are uncommon.

Now for some facts about intakes and toxicity.

• The Committee on Dietary Allowances has concluded that in light of "the low toxicity of manganese, an occasional intake of 10 mg./day can be considered safe. However, in order to include an extra margin of safety, it is recommended that the manganese intakes of adults over a long period of time be in the range of 2.5 to 5 mg./day."

• The toxicity of manganese supplements is probably low because, like chromium, only a small percentage is absorbed. There are no cases of toxicity from diet on record.

• A clear danger exists for workers who mine manganese ore, inhaling the mineral in the process. Body movement disorders and psychiatric diseases have occurred in these workers and are potentially permanent. For this reason, supplementation is unadvisable for them.

Recommended "Safe and Adequate" Allowances for Manganese

Although there are no RDA for manganese, the Committee on Dietary Allowances of the National Research Council set these "safe and adequate" allowances in 1980.

Group/Age	Mg.
Infants 0–6 mon.	0.5–0.7
Infants 6–12 mon.	0.7–1.0
Children 1–3 yr.	1.0–1.5
Children 4–6 yr.	1.5–2.0
Children 7–10 yr.	2.0–3.0
Males 11+ yr.	2.5–5.0
Females 11+ yr.	2.5–5.0

Note: There is no U.S. RDA for manganese.

A FLOOD OF PHOSPHORUS

Phosphorus plays many roles in nutrition; it contributes, for instance, to healthy bones, normal muscle contraction, and activation of the B vitamins. Though we need phosphorus in so many places, our diet more than manages to take care of demand. The average American diet contains at least twice the recommended allowance.

But having enough of this mineral on hand is just a first step. Also important is balancing phosphorus with calcium. On this count, we are slipping.

The balance between these two minerals is called the calcium-phosphorus (Ca:P) ratio. In animals, for instance, equal intakes of calcium and phosphorus—a Ca:P ratio of 1—seems optimal for building and maintaining healthy bones. According to the Committee on Dietary Allowances, "Current evidence... supports the recommendation that in infancy the Ca:P ratio of the diet be 1.5:1, decreasing to 1:1 at 1 year of age."

Though an equal balance between phosphorus and calcium is accepted as ideal, nutritionists also believe that we can adjust to diets containing up to twice as much phosphorus as calcium. If so, a phosphorus intake of 1,500 mg. and a calcium intake of 750 mg. would be safe.

But many of us consume neither equal amounts of the two minerals nor diets containing at most twice as much phosphorus as calcium. This imbalance isn't evident at first glance; government surveys quoted by the Committee on Dietary Allowances put our phosphorus intake at 1,500 to 1,600 mg. daily, a level that does not exceed the corresponding calcium intake twofold.

But appearances are deceiving. This estimate includes the phosphorus that occurs naturally in foods, but ignores the phosphorus-containing additives in processed foods. These additives are used widely to flavor colas and root beers, leaven breads, and bind water and prevent discoloration in many packaged goods. Estimates of our intake of phosphorus from these sources range from 400 to 1,800 mg. daily. Adding the lowest estimate, 400 mg., to the amount occurring naturally in a typical diet would bring our average phosphorus intake to about 2,000 mg. daily. This forgotten phosphorus alone places our calcium-phosphorus balance in a new light.

There is another factor to consider—the major difference in calcium intakes between men and women. Women who don't take calcium supplements often consume much less calcium than men—on the order of 500 mg. daily. Compare this to a typical phosphorus intake of at least 2,000 mg., and you realize that many American women probably have been consuming not merely twice as much phosphorus as calcium, but four times as much.

Many nutritionists are "on the fence" about the effects of this imbalance heavily weighted in favor of phosphorus, but I am not. With osteoporosis so common in the United States, I cannot help but be concerned that our lopsided intake of phosphorus is part of the problem. And mainland Americans are not alone here. Poor bone health afflicts Eskimos more commonly and at earlier ages than many other populations. Their heavy consumption of seal and walrus meats makes for a diet containing far more phosphorus than calcium, quite possibly the explanation for their troubles.

Admittedly, no one has proven that our high phosphorus intake plays a major role in osteoporosis. But neither has any benefit from our current high intakes emerged. Therefore, supplementation is at best a waste of money.

FACTS ABOUT PHOSPHORUS SUPPLEMENTS

The issue of calcium and phosphorus balance has received too little attention, but fortunately, no one has taken to the airwaves urging us to consume more phosphorus. As a result, supplements of phosphorus itself rarely grace the advertising pages or drugstore shelves. Our diet alone—not supplementation—generally is responsible for excessive intakes of the mineral.

A few medical uses for phosphorus supplements do exist. Such supplements sometimes are prescribed to reduce urinary calcium in those prone to form kidney stones. Supplements also may be used to correct phosphorus deficiency due to long-term overuse of antacids; such depletion is marked by muscle weakness, bone pain, and loss of appetite. Otherwise, however, phosphorus deficiency is extremely rare, and nutritionists consider deficiencies caused by diet alone to be unknown.

Because of these therapeutic uses, a few drug companies do manufacture phosphorus supplements. Given their purpose, these products are generally marketed to doctors rather than the general public. Nonetheless, the informed supplement user will want to be aware of these facts:

• Many phosphorus supplements also contain sodium and potassium. Those who are restricting intake of either of these two

Recommended Dietary Allowances for Phosphorus

Group/Age	Mg.
Infants 0–6 mon.	240
Infants 6–12 mon.	360
Children 1–10 yr.	800
Males 11–18 yr.	1,200
Males 19+ yr.	800
Females 11–18 yr.	1,200
Females 19+ yr.	800
Pregnant and nursing women	
18 yr. or less	1,600
19+ yr.	1,200

Note: The U.S. RDA for phosphorus is 1,000 mg.

additional minerals should use such products only with a doctor's consent. (If sodium but not potassium poses a problem, sodium-free phosphorus supplements are available.)
• Phosphorus supplements should not be used when high blood potassium or Addison's disease is present.
• Supplementation with phosphorus sometimes causes a laxative effect. The problem may be mild or may subside within a short time. Sometimes, however, the supplement must be reduced or stopped entirely.
• Multiminerals or calcium supplements providing phosphorus usually pose no problem. Often, multiples that contain the mineral have but small amounts and/or a good balance between calcium and phosphorus. Virtually all calcium supplements that also supply phosphorus do so because the source of their calcium is calcium phosphate. As discussed in chapter 15, this source of supplemental calcium contains a favorable balance between the two minerals.

A JOURNEY'S END

The Right Dose has been the most enormous undertaking of my career. I have learned far more than I ever dreamed possible about supplements, so much so that this book is three times as long as I originally had expected it to be. Now that I have told you everything that I have found during my years of research, it is time for me to sign off.

But though I close here, I do so with eyes open to the future. In the months and years that follow, I plan to keep my files open, staying on top of new developments. I hope these new findings will grow into future editions containing the latest information about both the supplements included here and new ones that become available. So though my journey seems to be ending here, it isn't.

This is only a beginning. I sense that vast changes in attitudes toward supplements now are under way. In coming years, I believe that supplements no longer will be scorned or merely tolerated, but credited for what they can do. I am sure that research on their value and safety will multiply. Most importantly, I feel certain that nutritionists soon will agree that supplements taken safely are among the best tools we have for protecting the good health that we value so much.

C O O K I N G
for Chromium

SALAD NICOISE WITH BELL PEPPER

(Makes 4 servings)

Chromium: 23 mcg. per serving*
Calories: 197 per serving

8 crisp romaine lettuce leaves	2 tablespoons red wine vinegar
1 can (12½ ounces) water-packed tuna, drained	2 tablespoons lemon juice
	2 tablespoons fruity olive oil
2 medium waxy-type potatoes	½ teaspoon dried tarragon
1 large green bell pepper	pinch of dried mustard
1 large ripe tomato	pinch of chervil
4 black olives, thinly sliced	

Select a large round platter and begin to build the salad by arranging the romaine in a starburst pattern and mounding the tuna in the center. Dice the potatoes and steam them for about 7 minutes, or until tender. Meanwhile, slice the pepper into thin strips and arrange them on the platter. Cut the tomato into wedges and arrange them, too. When the potatoes are ready, arrange them, while warm, with the other ingredients and sprinkle the olives over all.

In a small bowl, whisk together the vinegar, lemon juice, olive oil, tarragon, mustard, and chervil. Pour it into a small pitcher to drizzle on individual servings of the salad.

*Based on incomplete data.

(continued)

```
C     O     O     K     I     N     G
```

for Chromium—continued

WATERMELON SORBET

(Makes 7 servings)

Chromium: 8.9 mcg. per serving
Calories: 60 per serving

2 pounds watermelon, coarsely chopped
½ cup apple juice
½ cup white grape juice
1 tablespoon freshly squeezed lemon juice
¼ teaspoon vanilla extract

In a food processor or blender, process the watermelon until smooth. You should have about 4 cups of puree. Add the juices and the vanilla and process to combine.

Process in an ice cream maker according to the manufacturer's directions. If you don't have an ice cream maker, chill in the refrigerator for about 30 minutes. Pour the mixture into a flat glass baking dish and freeze until it just begins to set. Process in a food processor or blender for approximately 3½ minutes before serving.

PEAR AND CURRANT SODA BREAD

(Makes 1 loaf, 10 slices)

Chromium: 47 mcg. per slice*
Calories: 246 per slice

4 cups whole wheat flour
¼ cup high-chromium brewer's yeast
¼ teaspoon baking soda
1 tablespoon baking powder
⅓ cup dried currants
1 pear, grated
pinch of freshly grated orange rind
1 tablespoon maple syrup
2 cups plain low-fat yogurt

C O O K I N G
for Chromium—*continued*

Preheat oven to 425°F.

In a large bowl, combine the flour, brewer's yeast, baking soda, baking powder, currants, pear, and orange rind. Add the maple syrup and yogurt and combine. Turn the dough out onto a floured surface. It will be a bit sticky, so flour your hands.

Shape the dough into a round loaf and set it on an oiled and floured cookie sheet. Use a sharp knife to cut a ½-inch X into the top of the loaf, which will keep it from breaking as it expands. Sprinkle a bit of flour over the top and bake for 45 to 50 minutes. Let it cool before slicing with a serrated knife.

*Based on incomplete data.

Copper Content of Selected Supplements

Dosage is one tablet or capsule unless otherwise indicated.

Supplement	Manufacturer	Mg.
Centrum	Lederle	3.0
Gevral Protein	Lederle	0.4
Gevral T Capsules	Lederle	1.5
Livitamin Capsules	Beecham Labs	0.7
Livitamin Chewable	Beecham Labs	0.3
Livitamin Liquid (per tbsp.)	Beecham Labs	0.7
Myadec	Parke-Davis	2.0
Norlac	Rowell	2.0
One-A-Day Vitamins Plus Minerals	Miles	2.0
Optilets-M-500	Abbott	2.0
Os-Cal Forte	Marion	0.3
S.S.S. Tablets	S.S.S.	1.0
Stresstabs 600 with Iron	Lederle	3.0
Theragran-M	Squibb	2.0
Theragran-Z	Squibb	2.0
Unicap T	Upjohn	2.0
Vio-Geric	Rowell	2.0
Vita-Kaps-M Tablets	Abbott	1.0
Viterra	Pfipharmecs	1.0
Viterra High Potency	Pfipharmecs	1.0

Source: Adapted from the American Pharmaceutical Association, *Handbook of Nonprescription Drugs*, 7th ed. (1982), 240–57.

Note: This chart is intended only as a guide. Vitamin formulations change periodically; always read product labels for accurate and up-to-date information on their nutrient levels.

Manganese Content
of Selected Supplements

Dosage is one tablet or capsule unless otherwise indicated.

Supplement	Manufacturer	Mg.
Abdol with Minerals	Parke-Davis	1.0
Centrum	Lederle	7.5
Cluvisol Syrup (per tsp.)	Ayerst	0.5
Gevrabon (per 2 tbsp.)	Lederle	2.0
Gevral Protein	Lederle	0.4
Myadec	Parke-Davis	1.3
Obron-6	Pfipharmecs	0.3
Optilets-M-500	Abbott	1.0
Os-Cal Forte	Marion	0.3
Os-Cal Plus	Marion	0.8
Theragran-M	Squibb	1.0
Theragran-Z	Squibb	1.0
Unicap T	Upjohn	1.0
Vitagett	North American	1.5
Vita-Kaps-M Tablets	Abbott	1.0
Vitamin-Mineral Capsules	North American	1.5
Viterra	Pfipharmecs	1.0
Viterra High Potency	Pfipharmecs	1.0
VM Preparation (per 2 tbsp.)	Roberts	2.0

Source: Adapted from the American Pharmaceutical Association, *Handbook of Nonprescription Drugs*, 7th ed. (1982), 240–57.

Note: This chart is intended only as a guide. Vitamin formulations change periodically; always read product labels for accurate and up-to-date information on their nutrient levels.

Phosphorus Content
of Selected Supplements

Dosage is one tablet or capsule unless otherwise indicated.

Supplement	Manufacturer	Mg.
Abdol with Minerals	Parke-Davis	34
Calcium, Phosphate, and Vitamin D	Squibb	156
Calciwafers	Nion	137
Centrum	Lederle	125
Di-Calcium Phosphate Tablets	North American	58
Di-Cal D Capsules	Abbott	90
Di-Cal D Wafers	Abbott	228
Di-Cal D with Vitamin C Capsules	Abbott	90
Geriplex	Parke-Davis	46
Geriplex-FS Kapseals	Parke-Davis	46
Gevral	Lederle	125
Gevral Protein	Lederle	53
Gevral T Capsules	Lederle	125
Nutra-Cal	Anabolic	125
One-A-Day Vitamins Plus Minerals	Miles	100
Paladec with Minerals	Parke-Davis	17
Stuart Formula	Stuart	125
Sugar Calcicaps	Nion	42
Vio-Geric	Rowell	125
Vitagett	North American	166
Vitamin-Mineral Capsules	North American	35
Viterra	Pfipharmecs	70
VM Preparation (per 2 tbsp.)	Roberts	94

Source: Adapted from the American Pharmaceutical Association, *Handbook of Nonprescription Drugs*, 7th ed. (1982), 240–57.

Note: This chart is intended only as a guide. Vitamin formulations change periodically; always read product labels for accurate and up-to-date information on their nutrient levels.

Bibliography

REFERENCES AND HOW TO USE THEM

The pages that follow list many, though not all, of the sources used in this book. In the interest of space, I have included primarily those sources concerned specifically with nutrient safety.

If you would like more details on any of the topics discussed throughout this book, finding them may be easier than you think. You do not have to be a doctor, scientist, or medical librarian to get access to the scientific literature, nor to understand at least parts of it.

Though some papers are highly technical, a layman can comprehend a significant portion of many scientific reports. In some cases, consulting a medical dictionary a few times may be all that is needed to make sense of the findings. And while you may not understand the intricacies of the experimental design, you should have little trouble with the introduction, results, discussion, and summary—all standard parts of a research paper. Now for a plan of action.

WHAT YOU NEED TO KNOW

A few of the references cited below are books, and the information is self-explanatory. Simply locate the book title in the card (or computer) catalog, write down the call number, and proceed to the book section corresponding to the first letters of the call number. From there, use the remaining parts of the call number to find the book itself.

Because books quickly become out of date or are not thorough enough, I rely mostly on medical journals for the most complete and latest news. To find them, you simply have to know what each part of the reference (also called citation) represents.

The journal articles listed below follow the format used by the National Library of Medicine, the leader in the field of medical indexing. The first item(s) listed is the author(s). If the paper is unsigned, the word "anonymous" does not appear; the citation simply begins with the title instead.

Following the name of the author(s) is the title of the paper and the abbreviated name of the journal where it was published. From there, things get a little trickier. If available, the items after the journal name will be listed in the following order:

- The year of publication
- The month of publication
- The day of the month of publication, if more than one issue is printed per month

A slash will separate this information from the rest of the citation. Immediately after the slash is the volume number, one of the two most important pieces of information that you will need. Knowing the volume number often makes having the year of publication unnecessary, for the two generally correspond to each other. Volume 34 of the *American Journal of Clinical Nutrition*, for example, includes only papers published in 1981. Where multiple authors are cited, slashes are also used to separate names.

Nonetheless, having both the volume number and year of publication is helpful in the event of typographical errors. Also, *Lancet* and probably a few other journals number their editions in an unusual way, requiring you to have both the volume number and year.

In parentheses after the volume number is the issue number. You will rarely need it to locate a paper; in fact, the National Library of Medicine's format is one of the few that even includes issue numbers. Successive issues within the same volume take up, page-wise, where the previous issue left off. For example, if the first issue of a volume ends on page 165, the second issue will begin with page 166. As a result, the volume number and page number alone generally will lead you to the paper you want. The page number, of course, appears in the reference right after the issue number and a colon.

WHERE TO GO

Most public libraries will have few, if any, medical journals. Undergraduate libraries of universities will usually have the most common journals, but graduate school libraries will have more. The best sources, however, are medical school libraries, and, for those in the Washington-Baltimore area, the Library of Congress and the libraries at the National Institutes of Health. These include the National Library of Medicine and the Clinical Center Library, part of the NIH Hospital.

You are welcome at virtually any publicly funded library—whether at the NIH or a state-sponsored medical school. A few private schools may refuse admission to nonstudents, though many do not.

WHAT YOU WILL FIND

Most libraries have open shelves ("stacks"), where you take what you are looking for from the shelf and use it in the library. Often, the most recent journals will be on one floor, journals from the previous 10 to 20 years on another floor, and those 21 years or older still elsewhere. In other cases, all volumes of the same journal will be grouped together.

Some libraries have a limited area, often called a reading room, where current issues of the better-known journals are on open shelves. All others, however, are on closed shelves. You must request them on a "call form," and library staff will retrieve the volume for you. This saves you from trekking around the library, but often costs you more time waiting for your selections to arrive. In addition, the library may limit the number of journals that you can ask for per hour, again costing you time.

The information below gives you everything you need to fill out a call form, except for the journal's call number. The library will have printouts that list each journal it carries, along with the call number.

HELPFUL HINTS

• Take plenty of change for the copy machines.
• Don't be shy about asking questions at the reference desk; librarians, by nature, are people who like to help.
• Citations in which the name of the paper is in brackets are

written in a foreign language, but may have a short summary in English.

- Certain journals are generally more readable than others; I would say that the *Journal of the American Medical Association* (JAMA) and many state medical journals have a good percentage of papers written in clear, concise prose that is free of excessive medical jargon.

- The journal *Federation Proceedings* (abbreviated Fed Proc) contains mostly short summaries (abstracts) of work for presentation at conferences. If the citation shows the length of the item to be only one page, chances are that it is a one-paragraph summary providing few details.

- Be patient. No one feels at home in a medical library after only a few visits. With practice, you will become a pro.

GENERAL REFERENCES

Committee on Dietary Allowances. Recommended Dietary Allowances, 1980. National Academy of Sciences, Washington, D.C.

Effects of Drugs on Clinical Laboratory Tests. 1975. American Association of Clinical Chemists, Washington, D.C.

Facts and Comparisons. 1982. Facts and Comparisons, St. Louis, Missouri.

Physicians' Desk Reference. 1984. Medical Economics Company, Oradell, New Jersey.

Berkow R (ed). The Merck Manual of Diagnosis and Therapy. 1977. Merck, Sharpe, and Dohme Research Laboratories, Rahway, New Jersey.

Goodman AG / Goodman LS / Gilman A. Goodman and Gilman's The Pharmacological Basis of Therapeutics. Sixth Edition. 1980. Macmillan, New York.

McEvoy G. American Hospital Formulary Service Drug Information. 1985. American Society of Hospital Pharmacists, Bethesda, Maryland.

Pinckney C / Pinckney ER. The Patient's Guide to Medical Tests. 1982. Facts on File, New York.

Roe, DA. Handbook: Interactions of Selected Drugs and Nutrients in Patients. Third Edition. 1982. American Dietetic Association, Chicago, Illinois.

Windholz M (ed). The Merck Index: An Encyclopedia of Chemicals, Drugs, and Biologicals. Tenth Edition. 1983. Merck and Company, Rahway, New Jersey.

Vitamin A

Liver lover's headache: pseudotumor cerebri and vitamin A intoxication [letter]. JAMA 1984 Dec 28/252(24):3365.

Select Committee on GRAS Substances. Evaluation of the Health Aspects of Vitamin A, Vitamin A Acetate, and Vitamin A Palmitate as Food Ingredients. 1980. Food and Drug Administration. Washington, D.C.

Vitamin A and teratogenesis. Lancet 1985 Feb 9/1(8424):319–20.

Farris WA / Erdman JW Jr. Protracted hypervitaminosis A following long-term, low-level intake. JAMA 1982 Mar 5/247(9):1317.

Hall JG. Vitamin A: a newly recognized human teratogen. Harbinger of things to come? [editorial]. J Pediatr 1984 Oct/105(4):583–4.

Hall JG. Vitamin A teratogenicity [letter]. N Engl J Med 1984 Sep 20/ 311(12):797–8.

Herbert V. Toxicity of 25,000 IU vitamin A supplements in "health" food user. Am J Clin Nutr 1982 Jul/36(7):185–6.

Josephs HW. Hypervitaminosis A and carotenemia. Am J Dis Child 1944/ 67:33–43.

Leitner ZA / Moore T / Sharman IM. Fatal self-medication with retinol and carrot juice. Proc Nutr Soc 1975 Sep/34(2):44A–45A.

Lombaert A / Carton H. Benign intracranial hypertension due to A-hypervitaminosis in adults and adolescents. Eur Neurol 1976/ 14(5):340–50.

Marie J / See G. Acute hypervitaminosis A of the infant. Am J Dis Child 1954/87:731–6.

Mikkelsen B / Ehlers N / Thomsen HG. Vitamin A intoxication causing papilledema and simulating acute encephalitis. Acta Neurol Scand 1974/50(5):642–50.

Moore T. Hypercarotenosis and hypervitaminosis A in humans. in: Vitamin A. 1957. Elsevier, London:442–455.

Muenter MD / Perry HO / Ludwig J. Chronic vitamin A intoxication in adults. Hepatic, neurologic and dermatologic complications. Am J Med 1971 Jan/50(1):129–36.

Oliver TK. Chronic vitamin A intoxication. Am J Dis Child 1958 Jan/ 95(1):57–68.

Vollbracht R / Gilroy J. Vitamin A induced benign intracranial hypertension. Can J Neurol Sci 1976 Feb/3(1):59–61.

Carotene

Amelioration of photosensitivity by carotene. Nutr Rev 1974 Aug/ 32(8):239–40.

The use and abuse of vitamin A. Can Med Assoc J 1971 Mar 20/ 104(6):521–2.

Burry JN. Photo allergies from benzophenones and beta carotene in sunscreens. Contact Dermatitis 1980 Apr/6(3):211–2.

Cortin P / Boudreault G / Rousseau AP / Tardif Y / Malenfant M. [Retinopathy due to canthazanthine: 2. Predisposing factors.] Can J Ophthalmol 1984 Aug/19(5):215–9.

Evang K. Poisoning by carrot juice [letter]. Tidsskr Nor Laegeforen 1974 Jun 30/94(18):1214.

Gjerlow J. [Granulocytopenia as a sequel to carotenemia. A case with cutaneous xanthosis as a sequel to long-term excessive consumption of carrots.] Tidsskr Nor Laegeforen 1966 Jan 1/86(1):33–4 passim.

Hocking DR / Farrence I / Panasewycz P / Stewart M. Orange blood syndrome [letter]. Med J Aust 1981 Jan 10/1(1):44.

Komatsu S. [Teratogenic effects of vitamin A. 1. Effects of beta-carotene.] Shikwa Gakuho 1971 Oct/71(10):2067–74.

Lascari AD. Carotenemia. A review. Clin Pediatr (Phila) 1981 Jan/20(1):25–9.

Mathews-Roth MM. Neutropenia and beta-carotene [letter]. Lancet 1982 Jul 24/2(8291):222.

Page SW / Aust NZ. Golden ovaries. J Obstet Gynecol 1971 Feb/11(1):32–6.

Poh-Fitzpatrick MB / Barbera LG. Absence of crystalline retinopathy after long-term therapy with beta-carotene. J Am Acad Dermatol 1984 Jul/11(1):111–3.

Schneider W. [Dermatological side effects. Therapeutic benefits gained from their observation.] ZFA (Stuttgart) 1982 May 10/58(13):737–9.

Shoenfeld Y / Shaklai M / Ben-Baruch N / Hirschorn M / Pinkhaus J. Neutropenia induced by hypercarotenaemia [letter]. Lancet 1982 May 29/1(8283):1245.

Stampfer MJ / Willett W / Hennekens CH. Carotene, carrots, and white blood cells [letter]. Lancet 1982 Sep 11/2(8298):615.

Thiamine (Vitamin B₁)

[Demonstrated or presumed harmful or non-useful effects in therapy. Vitamin B₁.] Clin Ter 1967 Aug/42(3):267–9.

Acharya V / Store SD / Golwalla AF. Anaphylaxis following ingestion of aneurine hydrochloride. J Indian Med Assoc 1969 Jan 16/52(2):84–5.

Blum KU / Kasemir H / Scharfe W. [Pathogenesis of anaphylactic reactions following thiamine administration.] Verh Dtsch Ges Inn Med 1974/80:1369–71.

Boiko NV. [Acute allergic reaction as a result of use of vitamin B₁.] Vrach Delo 1969 May/5:116.

Boissier JR / Viars P. [On pharmacology and toxicity of thiamine.] Acta Anesthesiol (Padova) 1968/19:3–13.

Bukinich PS / Lozovoi NM. [On side effects during vitamin B₁ therapy.] Ter Arkh 1967 Jul/39(7):119–21.

Carta A / Fischer F. [The problem of intolerance to vitamin B₁.] Policlinico [Prat] 1968 Jun 24/75(26):844–7.

Causa P / Perri GC. Comparative toxicology of thiamine, its monophosphoric ester and cocarboxylase. Farmaco [Prat] 1969 Nov/24(11):712–8.

Cronin E. [Eczematous reactions following internal uptake of contact allergens.] Hautarzt 1975 Feb/26(2):68–71.

Davis RE / Icke GC / Hilton JM. High serum thiamine and the sudden infant death syndrome. Clin Chim Acta 1982 Aug 18/123(3):321–8.

Delineau MA / Bourcier J. [Circulatory arrest caused by an iodine and thiamine injection.] Cah Anesthesiol 1967 Dec/15(8):1045–52.

DiPalma JR / Ritchie DM. Vitamin toxicity. Annu Rev Pharmacol Toxicol 1977/17:133–48.

Falk RH / Protheroe DE. Ventricular fibrillation following high potency intravenous vitamin injection. Postgrad Med J 1979 Mar/55(641):201–2.

Gaudiano A / Petti G / Polizzi M / Tartarini S. [Alteration products of thiamine in injectable solutions and their acute and sub-chronic toxicity.] Ann Ist Super Sanita 1966/2(4):537–9.

Itokawa Y / Fujiwara M. Changes in tissue magnesium, calcium and phosphorus levels in magnesium-deficient rats in relation to thiamine excess or deficiency. J Nutr 1973 Mar/103(3):438–43.

Kobler E / Buhler H / Nuesch HJ / Deyhle P. [Drug-induced oesophageal ulcers (author's trans).] Dtsch Med Wochenschr 1978 Jun 23/103(25):1035–7.

Kruglikova-L'vova RP / Kozlova ED / Efimov AZ. [Study of the vitamin activity and pharmacological properties of some thiamine derivatives.] Vopr Pitan 1970 Jul-Aug/29(4):18–22.

Kushnir AS. [Study of allergic reactions in a polyclinic.] Vrach Delo 1973 Oct/10:26–8.

Lipkan GN / Pashchenko NP. [Comparative toxicity of thiamine and cocarboxylase.] Farm Zh 1973/28(1):55–8.

Markiewicz M / Uss B. [Encephalitis caused by hypersensitivity to vitamin B₁.] Pol Tyg Lek 1970 Nov 2/25(44):1661–2.

Naess K. [Allergic reactions to vitamin preparations.] Tidsskr Nor Laegeforen 1969 Jul 15/89(14):1199–200.

Nishioka K / Sarashi C / Katayama I. Chronic pigmented purpura induced by chemical substances. Clin Exp Dermatol 1980 Jun/5(2):213–8.

Ostrovski IuM / Lukashik NK / Trebukhina RV / Dosta GA / Mazhul' AG / Nepochelovich NS / Komarova BP / Karput' NS / Larin FS / Makarina-Kibak LIa. [The consequences of prolonged administration of an excess of thiamine: changes in carbohydrate, protein and lipid metabolism.] Vopr Med Khim 1970 May-June/16(3):316–22.

Ostrovski IuM / Makarina-Kibak LIa. [Pyruvate dehydrogenase activity following introduction of excessive thiamine into the body.] Biull Eksp Biol Med 1967 May/63(5):54–5.

Patlan BD / Lebedinski RI / Petukh MI. [Anaphylactic shock following administration of vitamin B₁.] Ter Arkh 1968 Sep/40(9):116–7.

Pincus JH / Cooper JR / Murphy JV / Rabe EF / Lonsdale D / Dunn HG. Thiamine derivatives in subacute necrotizing encephalo-myelopathy. A preliminary report. Pediatrics 1973 Apr/51(4): 716–21.

Wiss O / Walter P. [B and C vitamins following injuries and surgery? (letter).] Dtsch Med Wochenschr 1977 Jun 10/102(23):879–80.

Wong PW / Justice P / Smith GF / Hsia DY. A case of classical maple syrup urine disease "thiamine non-responsive." Clin Genet 1972/ 3(1):27–33.

Zheltakov MM / Skrupkin IuK / Somov BA / Butov IuS. [Allergic reactions due to group B vitamins.] Vestn Dermatol Venerol 1969 Jan/43(1):62–5.

Riboflavin (Vitamin B₂)

Alhadeff L / Gualtieri CT / Lipton M. Toxic effects of water-soluble vitamins. Nutr Rev 1984 Feb/42(2):33–40.

Brytskov VE / Avakumov VM / Kriukov VS / Egorov IA / Smirnova TN. [Biological activity of the microgranulated form of vitamin B₂.] Veterinariia 1979 May/(5):65–6.

Rivlin RS. Nutrition and cancer: state of the art relationship of several nutrients to the development of cancer. J Am Coll Nutr 1982/ 1(1):75–88.

Soloshenko EN / Brailovski AIa. [Allergic skin reactions caused by group B vitamins.] Sov Med 1975 Oct/(10):141.

Visek WJ / Clinton SK / Truex CR. Nutrition and experimental carcino-genesis. Cornell Vet 1978 Jan/68(1):3–39.

Niacin

Leads from MMWR. Niacin intoxication from pumpernickel bagels—New York. JAMA 1983 Jul 8/250(2):160.

Niacin and myocardial metabolism. Nutr Rev 1973 Mar/31(3):80–1.

Nutrition classics. Proceedings of the Society for Experimental Biology and Medicine, volume 38, 1938: Toxicity of nicotinic acid. K. K. Chen, Charles L. Rose and E. Brown Robbins. Nutr Rev 1984 Feb/ 42(2):52–4.

Select Committee on GRAS Substances. Evaluation of the Health Aspects of Niacin and Niacinamide as Food Ingredients. 1979. Food and Drug Administration. Washington, D.C.

Toxic effects of vitamin overdosage. Med Lett Drugs Ther 1984 Aug 3/ 26(667):73–4.

Bartlett PC / Morris JG Jr / Spengler J. Foodborne illness associated with niacin: report of an outbreak linked to excessive niacin in enriched cornmeal. Public Health Rep 1982 May-Jun/97(3):258–60.

Bures FA. Pruritus associated with niacinamide [letter]. J Am Acad Dermatol 1980 Nov/3(5):530–1.

Dipalma JR. Vitamin toxicity. Am Fam Physician 1978 Aug/18(2):106–9.

Einstein N / Baker A / Galper J / Wolfe H. Jaundice due to nicotinic acid therapy. Am J Dig Dis 1975 Mar/20(3):282–6.

Gass JD. Nicotinic acid maculopathy. Am J Ophthalmol 1973 Oct/ 76(4):500–10.

Harper AE / Benevenga NJ / Wohlhueter RM. Effects of ingestion of disproportionate amounts of amino acids. Physiol Rev 1970 Jul/ 50(3):428–558.

Hathcock JN. Nutrition: toxicology and pharmacology. Nutr Rev 1976 Mar/34(3):65–70.

Heninger GR / Bowers MB. Adverse effects of niacin in emergent psychosis. JAMA 1968 Jun 10/204(11):1010–1.

Herbert VD. Megavitamin therapy. J Am Pharm Assoc 1977 Dec/ 17(12):764–6.

Hoffer A. Adverse effects of niacin in emergent psychosis. JAMA 1969 Feb 17/207(7):1355.

Hotz W. Nicotinic acid and its derivatives: a short survey. Adv Lipid Res 1983/20:195–217.

Janovsky RC. Diabetogenic effects of nicotinic acid. Case reports and discussions. Ohio State Med J 1968 Oct/64(10):1139–42.

Kane JP / Malloy MJ / Tun P / Phillips NR / Freedman DD / Williams ML / Rowe JS / Havel RJ. Normalization of low-density-lipoprotein levels in heterozygous familial hypercholesterolemia with a combined drug regimen. N Engl J Med 1981 Jan 29/304(5):251–8.

Kohn RM / Montes M. Hepatic fibrosis following long acting nicotinic acid therapy: a case report. Am J Med Sci 1969 Aug/258(2):94–9.

Larson DL. On possible dangers of nicotinic acid therapy in acute burns [letter]. Plast Reconstr Surg 1977 Jan/59(1):114.

Marx R. Fibrinolytic states. Haematol Lat 1969 Jul-Dec/12(3):609–21.

Moran JR / Greene HL. The B vitamins and vitamin C in human nutrition. II. "Conditional" B vitamins and vitamin C. Am J Dis Child 1979 Mar/133(3):308–14.

Mosher LR. Nicotinic acid side effects and toxicity: a review. Am J Psychiatry 1970 Mar/126(9):1290–6.

Newbold HL / Mosher LR. Niacin and the schizophrenic patient. Am J Psychiatry 1970 Oct/127(4):535–6.

Patterson DJ / Dew EW / Gyorkey F / Graham DY. Niacin hepatitis. South Med J 1983 Feb/76(2):239–41.

Potts AM. Toxic amblyopia R.I.P. Am J Ophthalmol 1977 Feb/83(2): 278–80.

Richards AG / Brighouse R. Nicotinic acid—a cause of failed HIDA scanning [letter]. J Nucl Med 1981 Aug/22(8):746–7.

Rowe MJ / Oliver MF. Proceedings: Effect of nicotinic acid analogue on plasma free fatty acids and ventricular arrhythmias after myocardial infarction. Br Heart J 1974 Oct/36(10):1037.

Schwandt P. Drug interactions and side effects of hypolipidemic drugs. Int J Clin Pharmacol Biopharm 1979 Aug/17(8):351–6.

Sugerman AA / Clark CG. Jaundice following the administration of niacin. JAMA 1974 Apr 8/228(2):202.

Szwarcberg R / Houyet P / Dellenbach P / Gillet M. [An exceptional cause of fetal death "in utero": maternal massive digestive hemorrhage.] Bull Fed Soc Gynecol Obstet Lang Fr 1970 Apr-May/ 22(2):257–8.

Zachkeim HS / Vasily DB / Westphal ML / Hastings CW. Reactions to niacinamide [letter]. J Am Acad Dermatol 1981 Jun/4(6):736–8.

Vitamin B₆

Dangers of vitamin B₆ in nursing mothers [letter]. N Engl J Med 1979 Jan 18/ 300(3):141–2.

Pyridoxine and the anemia of cadmium toxicity. Nutr Rev 1974 Nov/ 32(11):345–6.

Select Committee on GRAS Substances. Evaluation of the Health Aspects of Pyridoxine and Pyridoxine Hydrochloride as Food Ingredients. 1977. Food and Drug Administration. Washington, D.C.

Sensory neuropathy from pyridoxine abuse [letter]. N Engl J Med 1984 Jan 19/310(3):197–8.

Vitamin B₆ in nursing mothers [letter]. N Engl J Med 1979 Jul 12/ 301(2):107.

Ananth JV / Ban TA / Lehmann HE. Potentiation of therapeutic effects of nicotinic acid by pyridoxine in chronic schizophrenics. Can Psychiatr Assoc J 1973 Oct/18(5):377–83.

Andriushchenko OM / Lamber ZP. [Case of Lyell's syndrome developing after the intramuscular administration of vitamin B₆.] Klin Med (Mosk) 1980 Nov/58(11):101–2.

Brush MG / Perry M. Pyridoxine and the premenstrual syndrome [letter]. Lancet 1985 Jun 15/1(8442):1399.

Carter AB. Pyridoxine and Parkinsonism [letter]. Br Med J 1973 Oct 27/ 4(886):236.

Carter AB. Pyridoxine contraindicated in parkinsonism [letter]. Lancet 1973 Oct 20/2(834):920.

Crawford D. Excessive use of pyridoxine [letter]. Can Med Assoc J 1984 Feb 15/130(4):343.

Dalton K. Pyridoxine overdose in premenstrual syndrome [letter]. Lancet 1985 May 18/1(8438):1168-9.

Daudon M / Reveillaud RJ / Jungers P. Piridoxilate-associated calcium oxalate urinary calculi: a new metabolic drug-induced nephrolithiasis [letter]. Lancet 1985 Jun 8/1(8441):1338.

Davidson RA. Complications of megavitamin therapy. South Med J 1984 Feb/77(2):200-3.

Ferguson RK. Where did you get those shoes? Arch Intern Med 1984 Dec/144(12):2406-7.

Fujita M / Aoki T. Allergic contact dermatitis to pyridoxine ester and hinokitiol. Contact Dermatitis 1983 Jan/9(1):61-5.

Langan RJ / Cotzias GC. Do's and don'ts for the patient on levodopa therapy. Am J Nurs 1976 Jun/76(6):917-8.

Meadow SR. Poisoning from delayed release tablets. Br Med J 1972 Feb 19/1(798):512.

Mitwalli A / Blair G / Oreopoulos DG. Safety of intermediate doses of pyridoxine [letter]. Can Med Assoc J 1984 Jul 1/131(1):14.

Mulrow JP / Mulrow CD / McKenna WJ. Pyridoxine and amiodarone-induced photosensitivity. Ann Intern Med 1985 Jul/103(1):68-9.

Petrie WM / Ban TA / Ananth JV. The use of nicotinic acid and pyridoxine in the treatment of schizophrenia. Int Pharmacopsychiatry 1981/16(4):245-50.

Podell RN. Nutritional supplementation with megadoses of vitamin B_6. Effective therapy, placebo, or potentiator of neuropathy? Postgrad Med 1985 Feb 15/77(3):113-6.

Reynolds RD. Pyridoxine dependent seizures [letter]. Arch Dis Child 1984 Sep/59(9):906-7.

Ruzicka T / Ring J / Braun-Falco O. [Allergic vasculitis caused by vitamin B_6.] Hautarzt 1984 Apr/35(4):197-9.

Vasile A / Goldberg R / Kornberg B. Pyridoxine toxicity: report of a case. J Am Osteopath Assoc 1984 Jul/83(11):790-1.

Vincent LM / McCartney WH / Mauro MA / Davidson RA. Discordant hepatic uptake between Tc-99m sulfur colloid and Tc-99m DISIDA in hypervitaminosis A. J Nucl Med 1984 Feb/25(2):207-8.

Wason S / Lacouture PG / Lovejoy FH Jr. Single high-dose pyridoxine treatment for isoniazid overdose. JAMA 1981 Sep 4/246(10):1102-4.

Yoshikawa K / Watanabe K / Mizuno N. Contact allergy to hydrocortisone 17-butyrate and pyridoxine hydrochloride. Contact Dermatitis 1985 Jan/12(1):55-6.

Folic Acid

Folic acid and the nervous system. Br Med J 1968 Dec 21/4(633):722-3.

Zinc and intestinal absoption of folates. Nutr Rev 1979 Jul/37(7):221-2.

Beal RW. Haematinics. II. Clinical pharmacological and therapeutic aspects. Drugs 1971/2(3):207–21.

Begemann H. [Does folic acid encourage tumor growth?] Munch Med Wochenschr 1969 Jan 3/111(1):62.

Blair JA. Toxicity of folic acid. Lancet 1970 Feb 14/1(642):360.

Brennan MJ / van der Westhuyzen J / Kramer S / Metz J. Neurotoxicity of folates: implications for vitamin B_{12} deficiency and Huntington's chorea. Med Hypotheses 1981 Jul/7(7):919–29.

Ch'ien LT / Krumdieck CL / Scott CW Jr / Butterworth CE Jr. Harmful effect of megadoses of vitamins: electroencephalogram abnormalities and seizures induced by intravenous folate in drug-treated epileptics. Am J Clin Nutr 1975 Jan/28(1):51–8.

Davis RE / Woodliff HJ. Toxicity of folic acid. Lancet 1970 Feb 7/1(641):308.

Emery AE. Folates and fetal central nervous system malformations [letter]. Lancet 1977 Mar 26/1(8013):703.

Gibberd FB / Nicholls A / Dunne JF / Chaput de Saintonge DM. Toxicity of folic acid. Lancet 1970 Feb 14/1(642):360–1.

Gotz VP / Lauper RD. Folic acid hypersensitivity or tartrazine allergy? [letter]. Am J Hosp Pharm 1980 Nov/37(11):1470, 1474.

Hall M / Davidson RJ. Prophylactic folic acid in women with pernicious anaemia pregnant after periods of infertility. J Clin Pathol 1968 Sep/21(5):599–602.

Hathcock JN. Nutrition: toxicology and pharmacology. Nutr Rev 1976 Mar/34(3):65–70.

Hellstrom L. Lack of toxicity of folic acid given in pharmacological doses to healthy volunteers. Lancet 1971 Jan 9/1(689):59–61.

Hollis PG. The provocation of mitosis in the mammalian kidney by folic acid. J Physiol (Lond) 1969 Jul/203(1):26P–27P.

Hunter R / Barnes J. Toxicity of folic acid. Lancet 1971 Apr 10/1(702):755.

Hunter R / Barnes J / Oakeley HF / Matthews DM. Toxicity of folic acid given in pharmacological doses to healthy volunteers. Lancet 1970 Jan 10/1(637):61–3.

Kakar F / Henderson MM. Potential toxic side effects of folic acid [letter]. JNCI 1985 Jan/74(1):263.

Katz M. Potential danger of self-medication with folic acid [letter]. N Engl J Med 1973 Nov 15/289(20):1095.

Kosik KS / Mullins TF / Bradley WG / Tempelis LD / Cretella AJ. Coma and axonal degeneration in vitamin B_{12} deficiency. Arch Neurol 1980 Sep/37(9):590–2.

MacCosbe PE / Toomey K. Interaction of phenytoin and folic acid [clinical conference]. Clin Pharm 1983 Jul-Aug/2(4):362–9.

McGeer PL / Zeldowicz L / McGeer EG. A clinical trial of folic acid in Parkinson's disease. Can Med Assoc J 1972 Jan 22/106(2):145–6 passim.

Mathur BP. Sensitivity of folic acid: a case report. Indian J Med Sci 1966 Feb/20(2):133–4.

Milne DB / Canfield WK / Mahalko JR / Sandstead H. Effect of oral folic acid supplements on zinc, copper and iron absorption and excretion. Am J Clin Nutr 1984 Apr/39(4):535–9.

Prakash R / Petrie WM. Psychiatric changes associated with an excess of folic acid. Am J Psychiatry 1982 Sep/139(9):1192–3.

Reynolds EH. Mental effects of anticonvulsants and folic acid metabolism. Brain 1968 Jun/91(2):197–214.

Richens A. Toxicity of folic acid. Lancet 1971 May 1/1(705):912.

Salter AJ. Folic acid: toxicity or placebo reactions? Lancet 1971 Jan 23/ 1(691):192.

Schubert GE / Otten G. Chronic folic acid-nephropathy. Res Exp Med (Berl) 1974/162(1):17–36.

Sesin GP / Kirschenbaum H. Folic acid hypersensitivity and fever: a case report. Am J Hosp Pharm 1979 Nov/36(11):1565–7.

Sheehy TW. Folic acid: lack of toxicity. Lancet 1973 Jan 6/1(793):37.

Stambolian D / Behrens M. Optic neuropathy associated with vitamin B_{12} deficiency. Am J Ophthalmol 1977 Apr/83(4):465–8.

Woodliff HJ / Davis RE. Allergy to folic acid. Med J Aust 1966 Feb 26/ 1(9):351–2.

Vitamin B_{12}

Select Committee on GRAS Substances. Evaluation of the Health Aspects of Vitamin B_{12} as a Food Ingredient. 1978. Food and Drug Administration. Washington, D.C.

Vitamin B_{12}. Br Med J 1968 Oct 19/4(624):167–8.

Amir J / Elian M / De Vries A. Polycythemia following folic acid and vitamin B_{12} treatment of anticonvulsant-induced megaloblastic anemia. Isr J Med Sci 1970 Jan-Feb/6(1):49–52.

Beal RW. Haematinics. II. Clinical pharmacological and therapeutic aspects. Drugs 1971/2(3):207–21.

Braun-Falco O / Lincke H. [The problem of vitamin B_6/B_{12} acne. A contribution on acne medicamentosa (author's transl).] Munch Med Wochenschr 1976 Feb 6/118(6):155–60.

Davidson NM. Withdrawal of cyanocobalamin [letter]. Br Med J 1979 Nov 10/2(6199):1219–20.

Dupre A / Albarel N / Bonafe JL / Christol B / Lassere J. Vitamin B_{12} induced acnes. Cutis 1979 Aug/24(2):210–1.

Freeman AG / Wilson J / Foulds WS / Phillips CI. Why has cyanocobalamin not been withdrawn? Lancet 1978 Apr 8/1(8067):777–8.

Hovding G. Anaphylactic reaction after injection of vitamin B_{12}. Br Med J 1968 Jul 13/3(610):102.

Ippen H. [Vitamin B_{12} acne as hypervitaminosis.] Med Klin 1977 Dec 16/ 72(50):2178.

James J / Warin RP. Sensitivity to cyanocobalamin and hydroxocobalamin. Br Med J 1971 May 1/2(756):262.

McLaren DS. The luxus vitamins—A and B_{12}. Am J Clin Nutr 1981 Aug/ 34(8):1611–6.

Malten KE. Flare reaction due to vitamin B_{12} in a patient with psoriasis and contact eczema. Contact Dermatitis 1975 Oct/1(5):325–6.

Parker AC / Bennett M. Pernicious anaemia and lymphoproliferative disease. Scand J Haematol 1976 Nov/17(5):395–7.

Pevny I / Hartmann A / Metz J. [Vitamin B_{12} (cyanocobalamin) allergy.] Hautarzt 1977 Nov/28(11):600–3.

Price ML / MacDonald DM. Cheilitis and cobalt allergy related to ingestion of vitamin B_{12}. Contact Dermatitis 1981 Nov/7(6):352.

Sawyer DR. Cyanocobalamin and cyanide toxicity [letter]. Am Fam Physician 1982 Jul/26(1):48, 50, 55.

Shinton NK / Singh AK. Vitamin B_{12} absorption by inhalation. Br J Haematol 1967 Jan/13(1):75–9.

Steiner I / Melamed E. Folic acid and the nervous system [letter]. Neurology 1983 Dec/33(12):1634.

Ugwu CN / Gibbins FJ. Anaphylactic reaction to vitamin B_{12} appearing after several years of therapy. Age Ageing 1981 Aug/10(3):196–7.

Vesey CJ / Cole PV. Cyanide antagonist [letter]. Can Anaesth Soc J 1981 May/28(3):290.

Pantothenic Acid

Haslock DI / Wright V. Pantothenic acid in the treatment of osteoarthrosis. Rheumatol Phys Med 1971 Feb/11(1):10–3.

Choline

Select Committee on GRAS Substances. Evaluation of the Health Aspects of Choline Chloride and Choline Bitartrate as Food Ingredients. 1975. Food and Drug Administration. Washington, D.C.

Austin CA / Mundy KI / Dorey S. Low dose choline chloride in cerebellar degeneration. J Neurol Neurosurg Psychiatry 1984 Sep/ 47(9):1038–40.

Davis KL / Hollister LE / Barchas JD / Berger PA. Choline in tardive dyskinesia and Huntington's disease. Life Sci 1976 Nov 15/ 19(10):1507–15.

Davis KL / Hollister LE / Berger PA. Choline chloride in schizophrenia. Am J Psychiatry 1979 Dec/136(12):1581–4.

Fischer T. Contact allergy to choline chloride. Contact Dermatitis 1984 May/10(5):316–7.

Haubrich DR / Pflueger AB. Choline administration: central effect mediated by stimulation of acetylcholine synthesis. Life Sci 1979 Mar 19/ 24(12):1083–90.

Ho IK / Loh HH / Way EL. Toxic interaction between choline and morphine. Toxicol Appl Pharmacol 1979 Nov/51(2):203–8.

Lawrence CM / Millac P / Stout GS / Ward JW. The use of choline chloride in ataxic disorders. J Neurol Neurosurg Psychiatry 1980 May/43(5):452–4.

Nasrallah HA / Dunner FJ / Smith RE / McCalley-Whitters M / Sherman AD. Variable clinical response to choline in tardive dyskinesia. Psychol Med 1984 Aug/14(3):697–700.

Tamminga C / Smith RC / Chang S / Haraszti JS / Davis JM. Depression associated with oral choline [letter]. Lancet 1976 Oct 23/ 2(7991):905.

Thal LJ / Rosen W / Sharpless NS / Crystal H. Choline chloride fails to improve cognition of Alzheimer's disease. Neurobiol Aging 1981 Fall/2(3):205–8.

Wood JL / Allison RG. Effects of consumption of choline and lecithin on neurological and cardiovascular systems. Fed Proc 1982 Dec/ 41(14):3015–21.

Vitamin C

Select Committee on GRAS Substances. Evaluation of the Health Aspects of Ascorbic Acid, Sodium Ascorbate, Calcium Ascorbate, Erythorbic Acid, Sodium Erythorbate, and Ascorbyl Palmitate as Food Ingredients. 1979. Food and Drug Administration. Washington, D.C.

Anderson TW. Large-scale trials of vitamin C. Ann NY Acad Sci 1975 Sep 30/258:498–504.

Balcke P / Schmidt P / Zazgornik J / Kopsa H / Haubenstock A. Ascorbic acid aggravates secondary hyperoxalemia in patients on chronic hemodialysis. Ann Intern Med 1984 Sep/101(3):344–5.

Basu TK. Possible toxicological aspects of megadoses of ascorbic acid. Chem Biol Interact 1977 Feb/16(2):247–50.

Bieri JG. Effect of excessive vitamins C and E on vitamin A status. Am J Clin Nutr 1973 Apr/26(4):382–3.

Clark JW. Conditioned oral scurvy due to megavitamin C withdrawal [letter]. J Periodontol 1983 Mar/54(3):182–3.

Finley EB / Cerklewski FL. Influence of ascorbic acid supplementation on copper status in young adult men. Am J Clin Nutr 1983 Apr/ 37(4):553–6.

Goldstein ML. High-dose ascorbic acid therapy. JAMA 1971 Apr 12/ 216(2):332–3.

Hoffer A. Ascorbic acid and kidney stones [letter]. Can Med Assoc J 1985 Feb 15/132(4):320.

Hoffer J. Synergistic effect of vitamin C and aspirin [letter]. Am J Clin Nutr 1979 Feb/32(2):280–1.

Holborow P. Sudden infant death syndrome [letter]. Am J Clin Nutr 1980 Apr/33(4):730–1.

Lawton JM / Conway LT / Crosson JT / Smith CL / Abraham PA. Acute oxalate nephropathy after massive ascorbic acid administration. Arch Intern Med 1985 May/145(5):950–1.

Ludvigsson J / Hansson LO / Stendahl O. The effect of large doses of vitamin C on leukocyte function and some laboratory parameters. Int J Vitam Nutr Res 1979/49(2):160–5.

McLaran CJ / Bett JH / Nye JA / Halliday JW. Congestive cardiomyopathy and haemochromatosis—rapid progression possibly accelerated by excessive ingestion of ascorbic acid. Aust NZ J Med 1982 Apr/12(2):187–8.

Mansouri A. Methemoglobinemia. Am J Med Sci 1985 May/289(5): 200–9.

Mentzer WC / Collier E. Hydrops fetalis associated with erythrocyte G-6PD deficiency and maternal ingestion of fava beans and ascorbic acid. J Pediatr 1975 Apr/86(4):565–7.

Metz J / Hundertmark U / Pevny I. Vitamin C allergy of the delayed type. Contact Dermatitis 1980 Apr/6(3):172–4.

Schrauzer GN / Ishmael D / Kiefer GW. Some aspects of current vitamin C usage: diminished high-altitude resistance following overdosage. Ann NY Acad Sci 1975 Sep 30/258:377–81.

Schrauzer GN / Rhead WJ. Ascorbic acid abuse: effects on long term ingestion of excessive amounts on blood levels and urinary excretion. Int J Vitam Nutr Res 1973/43(2):201–11.

Sharman IM. Gastrointestinal disturbances in runners. Br J Sports Med 1982 Sep/16(3):179.

Shilotri PG / Bhat KS. Effect of megadoses of vitamin C on bactericidal activity of leukocytes. Am J Clin Nutr 1977 Jul/30(7):1077–81.

Siegel C / Barker B / Kunstadter M. Conditioned oral scurvy due to megavitamin C withdrawal. J Periodontol 1982 Jul/53(7):453–5.

Stein HB / Hasan A / Fox IH. Ascorbic acid-induced uricosuria. A consequence of megavitamin therapy. Ann Intern Med 1976 Apr/84(4):385–8.

Tan SG / Cunliffe WJ. High doses of ascorbic acid [letter]. Br J Dermatol 1975 Dec/93(6):731.

Tsao CS. Ascorbic acid administration and urinary oxalate [letter]. Ann Intern Med 1984 Sep/101(3):405–6.

Van der Weyden MB. Vitamin C, desferrioxamine and iron loading anemias. Aust NZ J Med 1984 Oct/14(5):593–5.

Vickery RE. Unusual complication of excessive ingestion of vitamin C tablets. Int Surg 1973 Jun/58(6):422–3.

Wahlqvist ML / Briggs DR / Jones GP. Vitamins E, C and the B complex. Aust Fam Physician 1982 Apr/11(4):270-2, 274-8.

Walta DC / Giddens JD / Johnson LF / Kelley JL / Waugh DF. Localized proximal esophagitis secondary to ascorbic acid ingestion and esophageal motor disorder. Gastroenterology 1976 May/70(5 PT.1):766-9.

Vitamin D

New developments in pharmacology of vitamin D. Med Lett Drugs Ther 1974 Feb 1/16(3):15-6.

Renal osteodystrophy and osteosclerosis secondary to vitamin D therapy. Clin Pediatr (Phila) 1967 Dec/6(12):704-10.

Select Committee on GRAS Substances. Evaluation of the Health Aspects of Vitamin D₂ and Vitamin D₃ as Food Ingredients. 1978. Food and Drug Administration. Washington, D.C.

Anderson DC / Cooper AF / Naylor GJ. Vitamin D intoxication, with hypernatraemia, potassium and water depletion, and mental depression. Br Med J 1968 Dec 21/4(633):744-6.

Berlyne GM / Mallick NP. Arterial calcification after vitamin D. Lancet 1969 Feb 22/1(591):416.

Butler RC / Dieppe PA / Keat AC. Calcinosis of joints and periarticular tissues associated with vitamin D intoxication. Ann Rheum Dis 1985 Jul/44(7):494-8.

Dalderup LM. Ischaemic heart-disease and vitamin D. Lancet 1973 Jul 14/2(820):92.

Dalderup LM. Vitamin D, cholesterol, and calcium. Lancet 1968 Mar 23/1(543):645-6.

Duke PS. Ocular side effects of drug therapy. Med J Aust 1967 May 23/1(18):927-9.

Eskin F. Vitamin D and myocardial infarction [letter]. Br Med J 1974 Oct 26/4(5938):232.

Favus MJ. Treatment of vitamin D intoxication. N Engl J Med 1970 Dec 24/283(26):1468-9.

Fogelman I / McKillop JH / Cowden EA / Fine A / Boyce B / Boyle IT / Greig WR. Bone scan findings in hypervitaminosis D: case report. J Nucl Med 1977 Dec/18(12):1205-7.

Gabriel R / Joekes AM / Orton E. Hypervitaminosis D, anaemia and renal failure. Postgrad Med J 1970 Jul/46(537):455-7.

Goldman JM / Ahn YH / Wheeler MF. Vitamin D and hypercalcemia [letter]. JAMA 1985 Oct 4/254(13):1719.

Goodenday LS / Gordon GS. No risk from vitamin D in pregnancy. Ann Intern Med 1971 Nov/75(5):807-8.

Harris PW. An unusual case of calcinosis due to vitamin D intoxication. Guys Hosp Rep 1969/118(4):533-41.

Hirano T / Janakiraman N / Rosenthal IM. Vitamin D poisoning: from ingestion of concentrated vitamin D used to fortify milk. IMJ 1977 Jun/151(6):418–20.

Kimura K / Nozawa Y / Kitamura S / Takahashi H / Ota M. An autopsy case of hypervitaminosis D. Acta Pathol Jap 1967 Aug/17(3):377–86.

Lindahl O / Lindwall L. Vitamin D and myocardial infarction [letter]. Br Med J 1975 Jun 7/2(5970):560.

Linden V. Vitamin D and myocardial infarction. Br Med J 1974 Sep 14/3(5932):647–50.

Linden V. Vitamin D and the heart. Compr Ther 1975 Sep/1(5):34–7.

Linden V / Seelig MS. Multiple factors in the hyperlipidaemia of hypervitaminosis D [letter]. Br Med J 1975 Oct 18/4(5989):166.

Loomis WF. Vitamin D, sunlight, and natural selection. Science 1968 Feb 9/159(815):653.

Najjar SS / Yazigi A. Abuse of vitamin D: a report on 15 cases of vitamin D poisoning. J Med Liban 1972/25(1):113–22.

Omaye ST. Safety of megavitamin therapy. Adv Exp Med Biol 1984/177:169–203.

Seelig MS. Ischaemic heart disease, vitamins D and A, and magnesium [letter]. Br Med J 1975 Sep 13/3(5984):647–8.

Shetty KR / Ajlouni K / Rosenfeld PS / Hagen TC. Protracted vitamin D intoxication. Arch Intern Med 1975 Jul/135(7):986–8.

Sterling FH / Rupp JJ. An unusual case of vitamin D toxicity. Acta Endocrinol (Kbh) 1967 Feb/54(2):380–4.

Streck WF / Waterhouse C / Haddad JG. Glucocorticoid effects in vitamin D intoxication. Arch Intern Med 1979 Sep/139(9):974–7.

Taussig HB. Possible injury to the cardiovascular system from vitamin D. Ann Intern Med 1966 Dec/65(6):1195–200.

Taylor CB / Hass GM / Ho KJ / Liu LB. Risk factors in the pathogenesis of atherosclerotic heart disease and generalized atherosclerosis. Ann Clin Lab Sci 1972 May-Jun/2(3):239–43.

Taylor FE. Hypervitaminosis D.—A case report. Med Times 1966 Nov/94(11):1275–9.

Taylor WH. Renal calculi and self-medication with multivitamin preparations containing vitamin D. Clin Sci 1972 Apr/42(4):515–22.

van't Hoff W. Vitamin D poisoning [letter]. Lancet 1980 Jun 14/1(8181):1308.

Vik B / Try K / Thelle DS / Forde OH. Troms: Heart Study: vitamin D metabolism and myocardial infarction. Br Med J 1979 Jul 21/2(6183):176.

Vitamin E

Effects of vitamin E: good and bad [letter]. N Engl J Med 1973 Nov 1/289(18):979–80.

Evaluation of the Health Aspects of Calcium Pantothenate, Sodium Pantothenate, and D-Pantothenyl Alcohol as Food Ingredients. 1978. Food and Drug Administration. Washington, D.C.

Possible dangers of vitamin E [letter]. Plast Reconstr Surg 1982 Aug/70(2):274–5.

Select Committee on GRAS Substances. Evaluation of the Health Aspects of the Tocopherols and Alpha-Tocopheryl Acetate as Food Ingredients. 1975. Food and Drug Administration. Washington, D.C.

Vitamin E supplements and fatigue [letter]. N Engl J Med 1974 Mar 7/290(10):579–80.

Aeling JL / Panagotacos PJ / Andreozzi RJ. Allergic contact dermatitis to vitamin E aerosol deodorant [letter]. Arch Dermatol 1973 Oct/108(4):579–80.

Archer J. Vitamin E [letter]. JAMA 1982 Jan 1/247(1):29.

Ayres S Jr. Side effects from vitamin E [letter]. Calif Med 1973 Oct/119(4):73–4.

Ayres S Jr / Mihan R. Vitamin E as a useful therapeutic agent. J Am Acad Dermatol 1982 Oct/7(4):521–5.

Ayres S Jr / Mihan R / Scribner MD. Synergism of vitamins A and E with dermatologic applications. Cutis 1979 May/23(5):600–3, 689–90.

Cohen HM. Fatigue caused by vitamin E? Calif Med 1973 Jul/119(1):72.

Corrigan JJ Jr / Marcus FI. Coagulopathy associated with vitamin E ingestion. JAMA 1974 Dec 2/230(9):1300–1.

Farrell PM / Bieri JG. Megavitamin E supplementation in man. Am J Clin Nutr 1975 Dec/28(12):1381–6.

James P. Vitamin E and malignant hyperthermia [letter]. Br Med J 1978 May 20/1(6123):1345.

James P. Vitamin E and malignant hyperthermia [letter]. Br Med J 1979 Jan 20/1(6157):200.

Kligman AM. Vitamin E toxicity [letter]. Arch Dermatol 1982 May/118(5):289.

Lemons JA / Maisels MJ. Vitamin E—how much is too much? Pediatrics 1985 Oct/76(4):625–7 Folia Endocrinol (Roma) 1965 Jun/18(3):318–26.

Ludin EN. Vitamin E and capsular contracture [letter]. Plast Reconstr Surg 1982 Jun/69(6):1029–30.

Murphy BF. Hypervitaminosis E [letter]. JAMA 1974 Mar 25/227(12):1381.

Roberts HJ. Perspective on vitamin E as therapy. JAMA 1981 Jul 10/246(2):129–31.

Roberts HJ. Thrombophlebitis associated with vitamin E therapy. With a commentary on other medical side effects. Angiology 1979 Mar/30(3):169–77.

Roberts HJ. Vitamin E and thrombophlebitis [letter]. Lancet 1978 Jan 7/1(8054):49.

Saperstein H / Rapaport M / Rietschel RL. Topical vitamin E as a cause of erythema multiforme-like eruption. Arch Dermatol 1984 Jul/ 120(7):906–8.

Schorr WF. Allergic skin disease caused by cosmetics. Am Fam Physician 1975 Sep/12(3):90–5.

Shute EV. Vitamin E fatigue? [letter]. Calif Med 1973 Oct/119(4):73.

Sokol RJ. Vitamin E toxicity [letter]. Pediatrics 1984 Oct/74(4):564–9.

Tsai AC / Kelley JJ / Peng B / Cook N. Study on the effect of megavitamin E supplementation in man. Am J Clin Nutr 1978 May/ 31(5):831–7.

Magnesium

Advice on limiting intake of bonemeal. FDA Drug Bull 1982 Apr/ 12(1):5–6.

Magnesium—its nutritional and pharmacologic effects. Med Lett Drugs Ther 1967 Nov 17/9(23):93–4.

Multifarious magnesium—the need for a balanced outlook. Food Cosmet Toxicol 1971 Aug/9(4):571–3.

Select Committee on GRAS Substances. Evaluation of the Health Aspects of Magnesium Salts as Food Ingredients. 1976. Food and Drug Administration. Washington, D.C.

Select Committee on GRAS Substances. Evaluation of the Health Aspects of Sodium, Potassium, Magnesium and Zinc Gluconates as Food Ingredients. 1978. Food and Drug Administration. Washington, D.C.

Silicon overdosage in man. Nutr Rev 1982 Jul/40(7):208–9.

Borhani NO. Exposure to trace elements and cardiovascular disease. Circulation 1981 Jan/63(1):260A–263A.

De Silva AJ. Magnesium intoxication: an uncommon cause of prolonged curarization. Br J Anaesth 1973 Dec/45(12):1228–9.

Fassler CA / Rodriguez RM / Badesch DB / Stone WJ / Marini JJ. Magnesium toxicity as a cause of hypotension and hypoventilation. Occurrence in patients with normal renal function. Arch Intern Med 1985 Sep/145(9):1604–6.

Hendrix TR. Antacids. Am Fam Physician 1974 Mar/9(3):184–6.

Holtzman RB. Dolomite toxicity [letter]. South Med J 1983 Nov/ 76(11):1462.

Joekes AM / Rose GA / Sutor J. Multiple renal silica calculi. Br Med J 1973 Jan 20/1(846):146–7.

Karppanen H / Tanskanen A / Tuomilehto J / Puska P / Vuori J / Jantti V / Seppanen ML. Safety and effects of potassium- and magnesium-containing low sodium salt mixtures. J Cardiovasc Pharmacol 1984/ 6 Suppl 1:S236–43.

Knox EG. Anencephalus and dietary intakes. Br J Prev Soc Med 1972 Nov/26(4):219–23.

Lane MH. More on dolomite [letter]. N Engl J Med 1981 May 28/ 304(22):1367.

Levison DA / Crocker PR / Banim S / Wallace DM. Silica stones in the urinary bladder. Lancet 1982 Mar 27/1(8274):704–5.

Lotz M / Zisman E / Bartter FC. Evidence for a phosphorus-depletion syndrome in man. N Engl J Med 1968 Feb 22/278(8):409–15.

Malm OJ. Calcium and magnesium. Prog Food Nutr Sci 1975/1(3): 173–81.

Millette CH / Snodgrass GL. Acute renal failure associated with chronic antacid ingestion. Am J Hosp Pharm 1981 Sep/38(9):1352–5.

Mordes JP / Wacker WE. Excess magnesium. Pharmacol Rev 1977 Dec/ 29(4):273–300.

Ratzan RM / Chapron DJ / Mumford D / Pitegoff G. Uncovering magnesium toxicity. Geriatrics 1980 Sep/35(9):75–8, 83–4, 86.

Rude RK / Singer FR. Magnesium deficiency and excess. Annu Rev Med 1981/32:245–59.

Stowens D. Magnesium toxicity. JAMA 1973 Aug 13/225(7):751.

Calcium

Consensus Panel on Osteoporosis. Osteoporosis. 1984. National Institutes of Health, Bethesda, Maryland.

Diet and hypertension [editorial]. Lancet 1984 Sep 22/2(8404):671–3.

Select Committee on GRAS Substances. Evaluation of the Health Aspects of Calcium Salts as a Food Ingredient. 1975. Food and Drug Administration. Washington, D.C.

Select Committee on GRAS Substances. Evaluation of the Health Aspects of Carbonates and Bicarbonates as Food Ingredients. 1975. Food and Drug Administration. Washington, D.C.

Select Committee on GRAS Substances. Evaluation of the Health Aspects of Lactic Acid and Calcium Lactate as Food Ingredients. 1978. Food and Drug Administration. Washington, D.C.

The kidney and oral calcium therapy. Ann Intern Med 1967 May/ 66(5):1021–2.

Bataille P / Charransol G / Gregorie I / Daigre JL / Coevoet B / Makdassi R / Pruna A / Locquet P / Sueur JP / Fourmier A. Effect of calcium restriction on renal excretion of oxalate and the probability of stones in the various pathophysiological groups with calcium. J Urol 1983 Aug/130(2):218–23.

Carlon GC / Howland WS / Goldiner PL / Kahn RC / Bertoni G / Turnbull AD. Adverse effects of calcium administration. Report of two cases. Arch Surg 1978 Jul/113(7):882–5.

Clerkin EP / Murphy R. Hypercalcemia and the gastrointestinal tract. Med Clin North Am 1966 Mar/50(2):569–73.

Fink M / Taylor MA / Volavka J. Anxiety precipitated by lactate. N Engl J Med 1969 Dec 18/281(25):1429.

Garland C / Connor EB / Rossof AH / Shekelle RB / Criqui MH / Paul O. Dietary vitamin D and calcium and risk of colorectal cancer: a 19-year prospective study in men. Lancet 1985 Feb 9/1(8424):307–9.

Hausman P. The Calcium Bible. 1985. Rawson Associates, New York.

Heaney RP / Gallagher JC / Johnston CC / Neer R / Parfitt AM / Whedon GD. Calcium nutrition and bone health in the elderly. Am J Clin Nutr 1982 Nov/36(11):986–1013.

Henry HJ / McCarron DA / Morris DC / Parrott-Garcia M. Increasing calcium intake lowers blood pressure: the literature reviewed. J Am Ret Assoc 1985 Feb/85(2):182–5.

Ivanovich P / Fellows H / Rich C. The absorption of calcium carbonate. Ann Int Med 1967 May/66(5):917–23.

Keyler D / Peterson CD. Oral calcium supplements. How much of what, for whom, and why? Postgrad Med 1985 Oct/78(5):123–5.

Marshall RW / Cochran M / Hodgkinson A. Relationships between calcium and oxalic acid intake in the diet and their excretion in the urine of normal and renal-stone-forming subjects. Clin Sci 1972 Jul/43(1):91–9.

Nelson RW. Hypocalcemia after calcium and phosphorus supplementation [letter]. Arch Dis Child 1984 Jan/59(1):91–2.

Notelovitz M / Ware M. Stand Tall! The Informed Woman's Guide to Preventing Osteoporosis. 1982. Triad, Gainesville, Florida.

Oreopoulos DG / Velentzas C / Meema S / Meema HE / Craweller P. Dietary calcium and idiopathic hypercalciuria [letter]. Lancet 1981 Jun 6/1(8232):1269.

Pak CYC / Ohata M / Lawrence EC / Snyder W. The hypercalciurias: causes, parathyroid functions, and diagnostic criteria. J Clin Invest 1974 Aug/54(2):378–400.

Recker, RR. Calcium absorption and achlorhydira. New Eng J Med 1985 Jul 11/313(2):70–3.

Schuman CA / Jones HW 3d. The "milk-alkali" syndrome: two case reports with discussion of pathogenesis. Q J Med 1985 May/55(217):119–26.

Unfug HV. Milk-alkali syndrome reproduced by clinical trial. Rocky Mt Med J 1965 Nov/62(11):38–40.

Potassium

Enteric-coated potassium. Med Lett Drugs Ther 1974 Jan 4/16(1):2–3.

Fatal drug reactions. Lancet 1971 Jul 17/2(716):144.

Potassium in salt substitutes [letter]. N Engl J Med 1975 May 15/292(20):1082.

Select Committee on GRAS Substances. Evaluation of the Health Aspects of Carbonates and Bicarbonates as Food Ingredients. 1975. Food and Drug Administration. Washington, D.C.

Select Committee on GRAS Substances. Evaluation of the Health Aspects of Potassium Gluconate as a Food Ingredient. Supplemental Review and Evaluation. 1980. Food and Drug Administration. Washington, D.C.

Select Committee on GRAS Substances. Evaluation of the Health Aspects of Sodium, Potassium, Magnesium and Zinc Gluconates as Food Ingredients. 1978. Food and Drug Administration. Washington, D.C.

Slow-K—follow-up. Med Lett Drugs Ther 1978 Mar 24/20(6):30–1.

Who needs slow-release potassium tablets? Med Lett Drugs Ther 1975 Aug 29/17(18):73–4.

Akbarpour F / Afrasiabi A / Vaziri ND. Severe hyperkalemia caused by indomethacin and potassium supplementation. South Med J 1985 Jun/78(6):756–7.

Bacon C. Death from accidental potassium poisoning in childhood [letter]. Br Med J 1974 Mar 2/1(904):389–90.

Bhatkhande CY / Joglekar VD. Fatal poisoning by potassium in human and rabbit. Forensic Sci 1977 Jan-Feb/9(1):33–6.

Burchell HB. Dilemmas in potassium therapy. Circulation 1973 Jun/47(6):1144–5.

Burnakis TG / Mioduch HJ. Combined therapy with captopril and potassium supplementation. A potential for hyperkalemia. Arch Intern Med 1984 Dec/144(12):2371–2.

Davis RH / Fisch C. Potassium and arrhythmias. Geriatrics 1970 Nov/25(11):108–16.

Emerson DN. Potassium therapy and gastrointestinal lesions. Nebr Med J 1970 Sep/55(9):518–23.

Harrington JT / Isner JM / Kassirer JP. Our national obsession with potassium. Am J Med 1982 Aug/73(2):155–9.

Heffernan SJ / Murphy JJ. Ulceration of small intestine and slow-release potassium tablets [letter]. Br Med J 1975 Jun 28/2(5973):746.

Hultgren HN / Swenson R / Wettach G. Cardiac arrest due to oral potassium administration. Am J Med 1975 Jan/58(1):139–42.

Kallen RJ / Rieger CHL / Cohen HS. Near fatal hyperkalemia due to ingestion of salt substitute by an infant. JAMA 1976 May 10/235:2125.

Karppanen H / Tanskanen A / Tuomilehto J / Puska P / Vuori J / Jantti V / Seppanen ML. Safety and effects of potassium- and magnesium-containing low sodium salt mixtures. J Cardiovasc Pharmacol 1984/6 Suppl 1:S236–43.

Kassirer JP. Does the benefit of aggressive potassium replacement in diuretic-treated patients outweigh the risk? J Cardiovasc Pharmacol 1984/6 Suppl 3:S488–92.

Kassirer JP / Harrington JT. Fending off the potassium pushers [editorial]. N Engl J Med 1985 Mar 21/312(12):785–7.

Kolata G. Should hypertensives take potassium? [news]. Science 1982 Oct 22/218(4570):361–2.

McCall AJ. Slow-k ulceration of oesophagus with aneurysmal left atrium [letter]. Br Med J 1975 Jul 26/3(5977):230–1.

McCaughan D. Hazards of non-prescription potassium supplements [letter]. Lancet 1984 Mar 3/1(8375):513–4.

MacLeod SM. The rational use of potassium supplements. Postgrad Med 1975 Feb/57(2):123–8.

McMahon FG / Akdamar K. Gastric ulceration after "slow-K" [letter]. N Engl J Med 1976 Sep 23/295(13):733–4.

Oseas RS / Phelps DL / Kaplan SA. Near fatal hyperkalemia from a dangerous treatment for colic. Pediatrics 1982 Jan/69(1):117–8.

Palva IP / Salokannel SJ / Palva HL / Rytkonen U / Timonen T. Drug-induced malabsorption of vitamin B_{12}. VII. Malabsorption of B_{12} treatment with potassium citrate. Acta Med Scand 1974 Dec/196(6): 525–6.

Quick CA / Chole RA / Mauer M. Deafness and renal failure due to potassium bromate poisoning. Arch Otolaryngol 1975 Aug/ 101(8):494–5.

Riccardella D / Dwyer J. Salt substitutes and medicinal potassium sources: risks and benefits. J Am Diet Assoc 1985 Apr/85(4):471–4.

Scott BB. Perforation of small intestine and slow-k [letter]. Br Med J 1975 Sep 13/3(5984):649.

Treasure T. Ulceration of small intestine and slow-release potassium tablets [letter]. Br Med J 1975 Aug 2/3(5978):302.

Tyers GF / Williams EH. Potassium-induced cardioplegia [letter]. J Thorac Cardiovasc Surg 1979 Jun/77(6):929–30.

Welti CV / Davis JH. Fatal hyperkalemia from accidental overdose of potassium chloride. JAMA 1978 Sept 22/240:1339.

Wyman A / Woolley P / Nicholls AJ / Mundy K / Brown CB. Dangers of potassium in calcium supplements [letter]. Lancet 1983 Jul 23/ 2(8343):215.

Yap V / Patel A. Hyperkalemia with cardiac arrhythmia. JAMA 1976 Dec 13/236:2775–6.

Iron

Oral iron. Med Lett Drugs Ther 1978 May 19/20(10):45–7.

Reduced incidence of side effects with an iron preparation. Practitioner 1967 Jun/198(188):845–8.

Select Committee on GRAS Substances. Evaluation of the Health Aspects of Iron and Iron Salts as Food Ingredients. 1980. Food and Drug Administration. Washington, D.C.

Aronstam A / Aston DL. A comparative trial of a controlled-release iron tablet preparation ("Ferrocontin" Continus) and ferrous fumarate tablets. Pharmatherapeutica 1982/3(4):263-7.

Baker H. Erythropoietic protoporphyria provoked by iron therapy. Proc R Soc Med 1971 Jun/64(6):610-1.

Bothwell TH / Charlton RW / Seftel HC. Oral iron overload. S Afr Med J 1965 Oct 30/39(39):892-900.

Crosby WH. Bureaucratic clout, and a parable. The iron-enrichment-now brouhaha. JAMA 1974 Jun 24/228(13):1651-2.

Fischer DS / Parkman R / Finch SC. Acute iron poisoning in children. The problem of appropriate therapy. JAMA 1971 Nov 22/218(8):1179-84.

Gjone E / Stave R. Liver disease associated with a "non-constipating" iron preparation. Lancet 1973 Feb 24/1(800):421-2.

Halliday JW / Powell LW. Iron overload. Semin Hematol 1982 Jan/19(1):42-53.

Hyman S / Greengard J. Self-poisoning and accidental poisoning. Postgrad Med 1967 Jun/41(6):578-84.

Lavender S / Bell JA. Iron intoxication in an adult. Br Med J 1970 May 16/2(5706):406.

Lokken P / Birkeland JM. Dental discolorations and side effects with iron and placebo tablets. Scand J Dent Res 1979 Aug/87(4):275-8.

McEnery JT. Hospital management of acute iron ingestion. Clin Toxicol 1971 Dec/4(4):603-13.

Murray MJ / Murray AB / Murray CJ. The salutary effect of milk on amoebiasis and its reversal by iron. Br Med J 1980 Jun 7/280(6228):1351-2.

Murray MJ / Murray AB / Murray MB / Murray CJ. The adverse effect of iron repletion on the course of certain infections. Br Med J 1978 Oct 21/2(6145):1113-5.

Olsson KS / Heedman PA / Staugard F. Preclinical hemochromatosis in a population on a high-iron-fortified diet. JAMA 1978 May 12/239(19):1999-2000.

Stein M / Blayney D / Feit T / Goergen TG / Micik S / Nyhan WL. Acute iron poisoning in children [clinical conference]. West J Med 1976 Oct/125(4):289-97.

Stewart RB / Forgnone M / May FE / Forbes J / Cluff LE. Epidemiology of acute drug intoxications: patient characteristics, drugs, and medical complications. Clin Toxicol 1974/7(5):513-30.

Wallack MK / Winkelstein A. Acute iron intoxication in an adult. JAMA 1974 Sep 2/229(10):1333-4.

Whelton A / Snyder DS / Walker WG. Acute toxic drug ingestions at the Johns Hopkins Hospital. 1963 through 1970. Johns Hopkins Med J 1973 Mar/132(3):157-67.

Zinc

Select Committee on GRAS Substances. Evaluation of the Health Aspects of Sodium, Potassium, Magnesium and Zinc Gluconates as Food Ingredients. 1978. Food and Drug Administration. Washington, D.C.

Brewer GJ / Hill GM / Dick RD / Prasad AS / Cossack ZT. Interactions of trace elements: clinical significance. J Am Coll Nutr 1985/4(1):33–8.

Chandra RK. Excessive intake of zinc impairs immune responses. JAMA 1984 Sep 21/252(11):1443–6.

Cunliffe WJ. Unacceptable side-effects of oral zinc sulphate in the treatment of acne vulgaris [letter]. Br J Dermatol 1979 Sep/101(3):363.

Czerwinski AW / Clark ML / Serafetinides EA / Perrier C / Huber W. Safety and efficacy of zinc sulfate in geriatric patients. Clin Pharmacol Ther 1974 Apr/15(4):436–41.

Eby GA / Davis DR / Halcomb WW. Reduction in duration of common colds by zinc gluconate lozenges in a double-blind study. Antimicrob Agents Chemother 1984 Jan/25(1):20–4.

Feinglos MN / Jegasothy BV. Insulin: allergy due to zinc. Lancet 1979 Jan 20/1(8108):122–4.

Fischer PW / Giroux A / L'Abbe MR. Effect of zinc supplementation on copper status in adult man. Am J Clin Nutr 1984 Oct/40(4):743–6.

Fjellner B. Drug-induced lupus erythematosus aggravated by oral zinc therapy. Acta Derm Venereol (Stockh) 1979/59(4):368–70.

Gasiorek K / Bauchinger M. Chromosome changes in human lymphocytes after separate and combined treatment with divalent salts of lead, cadmium, and zinc. Environ Mutagen 1981/3(5):513–8.

Goolamali SK / Comaish JS. Zinc and the skin. Int J Dermatol 1975 Apr/14(3):182–7.

Greaves MW / Skillen AW. Effects of long-continued ingestion of zinc sulphate in patients with venous leg ulceration. Lancet 1970 Oct 31/2(679):889–91.

Herrero FA. Effect of zinc on skin and hair. Lancet 1973 Mar 17/1(803):619.

Hooper PL / Visconti L / Garry PJ / Johnson GE. Zinc lowers high-density lipoprotein-cholesterol levels. JAMA 1980 Oct 24–31/244(17):1960–1.

Lawhorn TI / Stone HH. Oral zinc therapy in thermal burns. South Med J 1971 Dec/64(12):1538–9.

Lindholmer C. Toxicity of zinc ions to human spermatozoa and the influence of albumin. Andrologia 1974/6(1):7–16.

Louria DB / Joselow MM / Browder AA. The human toxicity of certain trace elements. Ann Intern Med 1972 Feb/76(2):307–19.

Molokhia MM / Portnoy B. Bleeding gastric erosion after oral zinc sulphate [letter]. Br Med J 1978 Apr 29/1(6120):1145.

Morgan AA. Bleeding gastric erosion after oral zinc sulphate [letter]. Br Med J 1978 May 13/1(6122):1283–4.

Murphy JV. Intoxication following ingestion of elemental zinc. JAMA 1970 Jun 22/212(12):2119–20.

Muston HL / Messenger AG / Byrne JP. Contact dermatitis from zinc pyrithione, an antidandruff agent. Contact Dermatitis 1979 Jul/ 5(4):276–7.

Myers MB / Cherry G. Zinc and the healing of chronic leg ulcers. Am J Surg 1970 Jul/120(1):77–81.

Patterson WP / Winkelmann M / Perry MC. Zinc-induced copper deficiency: megamineral sideroblastic anemia. Ann Intern Med 1985 Sep/103(3):385–6.

Pories WJ / Henzel JH / Rob CG / Strain WH. Acceleration of wound healing in man with zinc sulphate given by mouth. Lancet 1967 Jan 21/1(482):121–4.

Porter KG / McMaster D / Elmes ME / Love AH. Anaemia and low serum-copper during zinc therapy [letter]. Lancet 1977 Oct 8/ 2(8041):774.

Prasad AS / Brewer GJ / Schoomaker EB / Rabbani P. Hypocupremia induced by zinc therapy in adults. JAMA 1978 Nov 10/ 240(20):2166–8.

Sandstead HH. Zinc interference with copper metabolism [editorial]. JAMA 1978 Nov 10/240(20):2188.

Shapiro S / Siskind V. Zinc and healing. Lancet 1970 Nov 28/2(683):1132.

Weimar VM / Puhl SC / Smith WH / tenBroeke JE. Zinc sulfate in acne vulgaris. Arch Dermatol 1978 Dec/114(12):1776–8.

Selenium

Amyotrophic lateral sclerosis and selenium [letter]. JAMA 1977 Nov 28/ 238(22):2365–6.

Daily selenium supplement caused toxic effects. Fam Prac News 1985 Jul 15/15(14):15.

Selenium and human health. Nutr Rev 1976 Nov/34(11):347–8.

The selenium paradox. Food Cosmet Toxicol 1972 Dec/10(6):867–73.

Buell DN. Potential hazards of selenium as a chemopreventive agent. Semin Oncol 1983 Sep/10(3):311–21.

Civil ID / McDonald MJ. Acute selenium poisoning: case report. NZ Med J 1978 May 24/87(612):354–6.

Daneshmend TK. Selenium and motor neurone disease [letter]. Br Med J 1978 Sep 16/2(6140):829–30.

Diskin CJ. Caution with selenium replacement [letter]. Lancet 1979 Dec 8/2(8154):1249.

Diskin CJ / Tomasso CL / Alper JC / Glaser ML / Fliegel SE. Long-term selenium exposure. Arch Intern Med 1979 Jul/139(7):824–6.

Ducloux JP / Ducloux B / Frantz P / Vincent V. Recording a selenium intoxication. Review of the literature. Acta Pharmacol Toxicol [Suppl] (Kbh) 1977/41(2):427.

Hadjimarkos DM. Selenium in relation to dental caries. Food Cosmet Toxicol 1973 Dec/11(6):1083–95.

Hubbard VS / Barbero G / Chase HP. Selenium and cystic fibrosis. J Pediatr 1980 Mar/96(3 Pt 1):421–2.

Jukes TH. Selenium, an "essential poison." J Appl Biochem 1983 Aug-Oct/5(4–5):233–4.

Lo MT / Sandi E. Selenium: occurrence in foods and its toxicological significance—a review. J Environ Pathol Toxicol 1980 Aug/ 4(1):193–218.

Louria DB / Joselow MM / Browder AA. The human toxicity of certain trace elements. Ann Intern Med 1972 Feb/76(2):307–19.

Robertson DS. Selenium—a possible teratogen? Lancet 1970 Mar 7/ 1(645):518–9.

Sakurai H / Tsuchya K. A tentative recommendation for the maximum daily intake of selenium. Environ Physiol Biochem 1975/5(2): 107–18.

Scott ML. The selenium dilemma. J Nutr 1973 Jun/103(6):803–10.

Snodgrass W / Rumack BH / Sullivan JB Jr / Peterson RG / Chase HP / Cotton EK / Sokol R. Selenium: childhood poisoning and cystic fibrosis. Clin Toxicol 1981 Feb/18(2):211–20.

Wilber CG. Toxicology of selenium: a review. Clin Toxicol 1980 Sep/ 17(2):171–230.

Yanagihara R. Heavy metals and essential minerals in motor neuron disease. Adv Neurol 1982/36:233–47.

Yang GQ / Wang SZ / Zhou RH / Sun SZ. Endemic selenium intoxication of humans in China. Am J Clin Nutr 1983 May/37(5):872–81.

Index

Entries referring to entire chapters appear in boldface type; entries referring to data in tables and boxes appear in italics.

509